Head Injury Rehabilitation

Dedication

To all the clients and families who have been part of the team
at the Icanho Centre, Suffolk

Head Injury Rehabilitation

A Community Team Perspective

Edited by

R GRAVELL BMED SCI, MRCSLT

AND

R JOHNSON BA, PHD, DIP CLIN PSYCH, C.PSYCHOL

both of the Icanho Centre,
Suffolk Brain Injury Rehabilitation Service, Stowmarket

W

WHURR PUBLISHERS
LONDON AND PHILADELPHIA

© 2002 Whurr Publishers

First published 2002 by
Whurr Publishers Ltd
19b Compton Terrace, London N1 2UN, England and
325 Chestnut Street, Philadelphia PA 19106, USA

British Library Cataloguing in Publication Data

A catalogue record for this book is available from the British Library.

ISBN 1 86156 274 8

Printed and bound in the UK by Athenaeum Press Limited, Gateshead, Tyne & Wear.

Contents

Acknowledgements

We would like to thank the following people:

Lesley Chapman, for assistance, advice and technological support to all contributors and for collating the final manuscript.

Daniel Sacoor for his drawings.

The Clinical Resource Centre and Library, West Suffolk Hospital, for great help in locating and providing reference material.

In addition, various people have read and made comments on the individual chapters and the authors would like to acknowledge the contributions of the following: Jenny Sheridan, Karen Davidson, Carrie Everett, Fiona Smith, Peter Coltham, Paul Herbert, Huw Williams and Anna Grief.

Contributors

Currently based at the Icanho Centre, Suffolk Brain Injury Rehabilitation Service, Stowmarket:

Kevin Baldry
Justine Fawcett BSc(Hons), DipCOT, SROT
Rosemary Gravell B Med Sci, MRCSLT
Roger Johnson BA, PhD, Dip.Clin.Psych, C.Psychol.
Tabitha Mathers BSc(Hons), MCSP, SRP
Pamela Nicholson RGN, RSCN, BSc
Julie O'Brien MSc, DipCOT, SROT
Carol Pratt CQSW

Other contributors:

Samantha Jones BA, MSc, Equalities Unit, Luton Borough Council
Kate McGlashan MBBS, MRCP, and **Kath Vick** Grad Dip Phys, MCSP, SRP, Specialist Rehabilitation Services, Colman Hospital, Norwich
David McLeod BA(Hons), DipCOT, SROT, Occupational Therapy Department, The Ipswich Hospital, Suffolk
Oliver Gravell MA, **Warren Collins** and **Susan Freeburn** BA Russell Jones and Walker, Solicitors, Swinton House, Gray's Inn Road, London

CHAPTER 1

Introduction

JULIE O'BRIEN, PAM NICHOLSON, ROGER JOHNSON,
ROSEMARY GRAVELL

It is often claimed that head injuries affect about one million people in Great Britain every year. Of these more than 150,000 are admitted to hospital. Of course, many of these people – perhaps 90% (Thornhill et al., 2000) – will have relatively mild injuries, and most will not be followed up in the community, despite some evidence of lasting effects for a few of them. Others will have moderate or severe injury and will be treated in hospital for varying lengths of time, with a variety of therapies and interventions. Nearly all will eventually be discharged into the community but they will have long-term disabilities. Frequently, such people will either be seen for short-term follow up by non-specialist services or they will fall through the net altogether. Often they and their families will be left to cope alone.

The often inadequate management of head-injured people in the community should be of concern to health-service management as well as to rehabilitation professionals. Undergraduate training courses often do not address head injury in any depth. Practitioners new to the field are often forced to learn on the job and by extrapolating from more general knowledge of neurology, despite the fact that the management of people with head injuries differs in particular ways from the management, for example, of people who have had a stroke.

This book seeks to discuss those aspects of management that are specific to working with people with head injuries and, although it is written from a community team's perspective, there will obviously be considerable overlap with rehabilitation needs at the more acute end of the spectrum. It will cover the broad range of issues that arise and outline the current approaches and work undertaken within community rehabilitation teams specializing in working with head-injured clients. The aim is to provide a text at a suitable level for students and those working for the first time in the field, which will offer practical advice and ideas to enable them to provide considered and effective services to head-injured people in the community. The intention is for it to be a practical reference, backed where possible by appropriate research, directing people to further sources when space does not allow issues to be fully discussed. It is hoped the many clinicians who are expected to work with this population as part of a general caseload, despite not being specialists in the field, will also find useful information. As far as possible, only issues specific to head injury will be covered but there is some inevitable overlap with other areas of neurological rehabilitation.

The volume will begin by addressing the service structures and the approach to rehabilitation that underlie all the subsequent chapters. It will seek throughout to move away from the strict professional lines traditionally followed by clinicians in the recognition that there is no such false distinction made within the life of the head-injured individual. Consideration will be given to physical, cognitive, behavioural, communicative, vocational and psycho-social aspects of rehabilitation. The effect of head injury on the family and friends of those affected will also be discussed.

This introductory chapter will seek to describe the way in which services for head-injured people operate and the factors that influence the current state of these services. It will also look briefly at the process or continuum of care, from acute hospitalization to community living, in order to establish the broader context in which community services operate. It will address some basic principles of rehabilitation, including the need for a team approach. In the community additional people and organizations may need to be seen as part of the rehabilitation team and the roles of some non-traditional service providers that have particular relevance to the field of head injury will be examined briefly.

Throughout the volume certain terms will be adopted for stylistic reasons. These require explanation. People who have had head injuries will be described as 'clients', which is the preferred term for many practitioners. It seeks to move away from the more medical-model term 'patient' or the emotive and negative term 'sufferer'. The pronoun 'he' will refer to those clients and the pronoun 'she' to the therapist/clinician. These pronouns do reflect the statistical probability, but the real reason is to avoid the unwieldly use of 'he or she'. The term 'head injury' seems straightforward but, for example, it covers a wide variety of severities and is not synonymous with the term 'acquired brain injury', although many policies and documents use the latter term to refer to head injury and other conditions. This would seem an appropriate point at which to define certain terms as they will be used in this volume.

What is head injury?

A head injury is defined, for the purposes of this volume, as any injury to the head causing traumatic brain injury. It refers therefore to a wide range of severity. Accurate information about the number of people sustaining head injury is difficult to obtain for a variety of administrative reasons. The annual incidence of head injury in the UK has been estimated to be 300 per 100,000 population (British Society of Rehabilitation Medicine, 1998) but with marked regional variations. Of these 300, about eight will have severe head injury, 18 will have moderate head injury and the remainder will have mild head injury. However, Thornhill et al. (2000) found a much higher incidence of disability one year after head injury than expected, citing an incidence of 100 to 150 per 100,000 population. They suggest that nearly half of all head-injured people would have severe or moderate disability, of which 90% would have initially been classified as mild injury.

The definitions of severe, moderate and mild head injury are not always based upon the same criteria, but the most common measures employed are the Glasgow Coma Scale (GCS) (Teasdale and Jennett, 1974) and the length of post-traumatic amnesia. These measures, and how they are used to define severity, are explained in detail in Chapter 2. The Thornhill et al. (2000) study above highlights dangers in classifying injuries as mild based on the GCS – such people may still have significant disabilities. Whatever the severity of the injury, there may be an enormous range of problems for any individual, and severity *per se* is not the only factor which will determine how much each individual's life is affected.

In practical terms, the injuries and their consequences discussed in this book will be the result of insults to the brain, such as concussion, shearing injuries, intra-cerebral haemorrhage and cerebral contusions. Causes vary from assaults or road traffic accidents to sports injuries and falls. Primary head injury refers to the initial insult to the brain and secondary head injury occurs following that, for example as a result of raised intracranial pressure or hypoxia. Physical aspects of these injuries will be described in Chapter 3. Subsequent chapters will discuss symptoms and consequences that follow.

It is principally the 'hidden' cognitive and behavioural disabilities, rather than the more obvious physical disabilities, which have such a devastating effect on the lives of individuals and their families. It is also worth remembering that each person is unique and no two injuries will present in the same way, so there cannot be a single recipe for rehabilitation. It must be a unique mixture of approaches and skills to meet the unique needs of each client.

Head-injury services

It is important to be aware of the context in which rehabilitation services will be provided to people who have sustained a head injury. Many factors will affect this – the historical perspective both nationally and locally, political issues and policies, legislation and funding. No service can be provided in a vacuum and, increasingly, rehabilitation staff may find themselves directly affected by these wider issues.

Chamberlain (1995) lists seven challenges faced within the field of head injury service planning. The first challenge is the frequency of injury, which increased with motorization and other social changes in the twentieth century and, secondly, the length of survival. She quotes the average length of survival for head-injured people as 50 years. Obviously this means that, each year, a significant number of severely disabled people will increase the overall numbers needing care.

Other challenges include the relatively young age of those affected, the burden of disability both on the individual and on society, the enormous variety of handicaps that may result, the family needs and, finally, the challenge of effective interagency working.

The history of head-injury services

Until the 1970s, outcome following moderate and severe head injury was often poor, with 90% of those with severe injuries dying (Social Services Inspectorate, 1996). Diagnostic techniques to determine the extent of the brain injury were less sophisticated and rehabilitation was still a relatively new speciality. There was poor information about the numbers of people with head injury and little research into the various treatment modalities used at the time. For those who did survive, there was little specialist care – people who had severe cognitive and behavioural symptoms following head injury often ended up in long-stay psychiatric institutions in the absence of more appropriate placements.

Since then, more people are surviving severe brain injury, mainly as a result of improved treatment techniques, especially in the early hours and days following the event. The emergency services provide skilled care in trying to prevent any further damage to the brain, while ensuring a rapid evacuation to hospital. Specific protocols and good teamwork in accident and emergency departments and operating theatres have improved the outcomes considerably for people with all levels of head injury, as will be seen in Chapter 2. Access to services such as occupational therapy, physiotherapy, speech and language therapy and psychology has improved and many hospitals now offer at least some rehabilitation. Nurses are also more aware of the rehabilitation needs of their clients.

There have also been social-legislative changes aiming to prevent and minimize the effects of accidents, such as the introduction of seat belt laws and increased use of cycle and riding helmets. Some of these changes have led to a fall in the number of head injuries and, overall, many more severely head-injured people are surviving and living in the community. However, services to meet their often complex needs have been slow to develop. Furthermore, even what appears to be a relatively minor injury can have long-lasting effects, and services for this group, in particular, are still poorly developed in many areas. This may be due to the small proportion of mild injuries that do develop persistent problems, but for those affected the issue is very real.

In the UK, community services have historically been defined within certain care groups, such as learning disability, mental health and so on. Services for head-injured people usually fall into the category of physical disability, despite the fact that many people are left with no residual physical problems. Because of the diversity of problems commonly seen following head injury, many individuals need a range of services, some of which may only be available to people in a particular care group. It can be difficult to overcome the invisible barriers and territoriality within the NHS to get a range of services from different departments to work together in the overall interest of the client.

An important influence in the development of services and support for people with head injury, and for their families, has been voluntary sector charitable and campaigning groups, and in particular in the UK the National Head Injuries Association ('Headway'). Headway was started in Nottingham in 1979 by a social worker and the parents of a head-injured young man. Local Headway groups, providing family support and advocacy for the needs of head-injured people, rapidly spread throughout the country. These were followed by the development of Headway Houses, which offer day services with a range of social, therapeutic and rehabilitation activities for head-injured people, as well as valuable respite for their carers.

Policies and legislation

Attitudes to disability and the responsibility of government have changed significantly during the second half of the twentieth century, with a gradual shift towards enabling people with disabilities to have choices over all aspects of their lives. The chronology of legislation, from the National Assistance Act 1948 to the Disability Discrimination Act 1995, shows a gradual focusing on individual assessment of need and the requirement to ensure equality of access to employment and services.

Various pieces of legislation affect head-injured clients, but more as a result of generally improving matters for disabled people. Legislation has not addressed the needs of head-injured people specifically. Despite this, rehabilitation staff should be aware of certain provisions. In addition to the two Acts mentioned already, relevant legislation includes The Chronically Sick and Disabled Persons Act 1970, The Disabled Persons (Services, Consultation and Representation) Act 1986, and The NHS and Community Care Act 1990. These Acts gradually strengthened the rights of disabled people to services and individual assessment of need and the 1990 Act had, at its core, the principles of choice, participation, dignity and independence.

The Disability Discrimination Act of 1995 addressed issues with regard to discrimination faced by disabled people mainly in the area of employment, in the provision of goods or services and buying or renting land or property. The Act requires schools, colleges and universities to provide information for disabled people and also allows the government to set minimum standards so that disabled people can use public transport more easily.

The Carers (Recognition and Services) Act of 1995 provided a right to carers to be assessed with regard to their ability to provide ongoing care. In 1996, the Community Care (Direct Payments) Act enabled disabled people to organize their own care by receiving payments to employ their own carers. That same year, The Housing Grant Construction and Regeneration Act included a section enabling disabled persons' homes to be adapted for use.

The 1996 Social Services Inspectorate report on head injury, *A Hidden Disability*, said that most authorities had ample information about the services needed by head-injured people but that the identified need seldom got translated into policy statements. Indeed in the past, some head-injured people, in particular those with complex needs, were offered rather piece-meal services and, on occasions, were left in the sole care of their families. This report highlighted the mismatch between disability policies that dealt principally with physical disabilities and the needs of those with cognitive problems, which are not always obvious – the 'hidden' disability.

Chamberlain (1995) states that services must be 'comprehensive, coherent, dealing with the patient from the time of accident to his final place-ment, hopefully at home'. Although the term 'final placement' may appear to suggest dependency, in fact most do return home and achieve independence. In 1988, the same author reported on behalf of a working party in West Yorkshire that suggested the framework of a four-phase service. Phase one is concerned with acute care, including primary prevention of accidents and secondary prevention of complications. Phase two focuses on inpatient rehabilitation; phase three on community-based rehabilitation. Finally, phase four is concerned with maintenance and support.

In 1992, the Department of Health, aware of the complex issues in the rehabilitation of people with acquired brain injury, invested in an initiative to develop and research different approaches to rehabilitation and to identify those approaches that successfully helped people to reintegrate into the community. The National Traumatic Brain Injury Study involved 12 pilot projects located in different parts of the country. The Centre for Health Services Studies at the University of Warwick was commissioned to coordinate and evaluate the cost-effectiveness of 10 of these different approaches by charting the progress of the patients involved.

In 1998, the research concluded 'head injury services can and have been observed to improve the likelihood of the successful reintegration into the community of persons who have suffered head injury. Such services are at present usually organized as adjuncts to acute care, but they must look outwards to the community and work jointly with the agencies, whether Health or Local Authorities or the Voluntary Sector, which operate in this arena' (Stilwell et al., 1998).

In 1999, Saving Lives: Our Healthier Nation was launched (Great Britain, 1999). It set out the government's health strategy, with the aims of improving health and addressing health inequalities. One of the areas on which it focuses is accident prevention, and in this respect, if successful, it should affect the incidence of head injury.

Within the framework of acute services there are a variety of routes for the treatment of people with head injury. The Royal College of Surgeons' report of the working party on the management of patients with head injuries (The Royal College of Surgeons, 1999) recommends that immediate care should be provided by a properly resourced and staffed Accident and Emergency Department with short-stay facilities. If further treatment is required then admission to a neurosciences unit, and not to an orthopaedic or general surgical ward, is recommended. At present it is still common in the UK, especially in rural areas, for head-injured people to be admitted to the latter wards, in the absence of more specialized units.

The same report goes on to recommend that each district should have a policy on the treatment of people with acquired brain injury, which would involve setting up protocols and guidelines. It also stresses the need for improved discharge and follow-up arrangements. Cynics may note that many reports over the past 25 years have recommended similar actions, but there remains a huge gap between recommendation and implementation.

In 2001, a report on head-injury rehabilitation by the House of Commons Health Committee was published. This highlighted many problems in current service provision and made specific recommendations, including better data collection methods, specialist inpatient and rehabilitation services, access to neuropsychiatry when appropriate, named individuals with responsibility for rehabilitation services, and the acute sector to take responsibility for establishing ongoing care plans. The committee noted the urgent need for government to formulate policy for the long-term needs of head-injured people.

Funding issues

Funding of brain-injury rehabilitation varies from country to country. In the UK there are some specialist rehabilitation services that are funded by the NHS, and are thus funded by the taxpayer, but these vary in availability and quality from area to area. However, there has been a failure within the NHS as a whole to develop a comprehensive range of appropriate services for this low-volume but high-cost client group. Health authorities have increasingly funded the use of services in the private and voluntary sector, especially where they have expertise in the field of behaviour management. This is not necessarily a cheaper option.

For some people whose complex needs cross the health and social care divide, the NHS and Social Services Departments may jointly commission care packages. In some cases, where there is a clear healthcare need, this element has been provided through NHS Trusts or is purchased separately under section 64 of the Health and Public Services Act 1968. In other instances, it has been appropriate to transfer sums to Social Services under section 28A of the NHS Act 1977. Such care packages may attract other sources of funding, such as Independent Living Fund monies, although strict criteria control access to this source of funding.

Organizational changes in the structure of the NHS, with the introduction of primary care groups and primary care trusts, have implications for the provision of specialist services for people with head injuries. There will be a need to ensure that services with a wide catchment area but with relatively few patients from each primary care group or primary care trust are not undermined. However the new regulations under the Health Act 1999 on establishing pooled budgets and lead commissioning will facilitate joint commissioning and integrated provision. Whoever funds and develops rehabilitation services has a responsibility to ensure that resources are used effectively, duplication of services is avoided and that users and carers are properly and separately involved (NHS Executive, 1997).

At the strategic and commissioning level, the funding of health services may be targeted at the acute sector so there needs to be an awareness of the long-term nature of head injury. The young man who is severely head injured in a road traffic accident is likely to have a normal lifespan yet not be able to earn his living. He may well need supported employment and ongoing health and social care support for the rest of his life. One only has to look at the settlements awarded in some compensation cases to see the huge costs of care for someone with a severe head injury. These are real costs, and when not funded from insurance monies they must be met by the taxpayer.

In some countries funding is largely from health insurers, who will require explicit treatment plans with clearly identified short- and long-term goals.

Continued funding depends on continuing to achieve the specified goals. Inequalities in terms of what services will be covered result between those who can afford private insurance and those forced to depend upon state-provided insurance. However the accountability inherent within this system has a number of advantages, in forcing professionals to look closely at what they are doing and justify their intervention programmes. The danger is in a tendency to provide prescribed programmes and a loss of flexibility to experiment with different approaches for an individual client. There may also be a tendency to oversell treatments without reliable outcome measures.

Even in a country with a funded national health service, an individual's head-injury care is frequently financed wholly or in part via compensation payments from insurance companies – for example after road traffic accidents or injuries at work. Staff working in the field will be aware of the effect this may have on the provision of care, as it may be easier for those able to claim compensation to purchase a comprehensive package of care. For example, that person may not have geographical restrictions affecting which service he can access. One problem that may occur, however, is in the length of time taken to settle compensation cases. Johnson (1998) looked at 35 successful claims and found the mean time between injury and settlement was 4.4 years, with a standard deviation of 2.8.

It is easy to say that, even without compensation monies, full assessment of needs must still be carried out and appropriate use made of local resources to achieve the best possible quality package of care. However, if no specialist service exists, there may be no possibility of an appropriate specialist assessment upon which to base decisions. In the event that needs are identified and cannot be met, local commissioners in health and social services must be made aware, to ensure that they are fully informed when planning service funding.

In addition to these main approaches to funding, there are some examples of imaginative funding through a combination of sources and a flexible approach by planners. An example of this is Icanho, the Suffolk brain injury centre that opened in 1998. Here, Suffolk health and social services jointly fund a community-based health and social care rehabilitation service provided by John Grooms, a charitable organization. Use was initially made of joint finance for the revenue funding and to make an initial contribution to the capital fund of £1.3 million, which was raised by John Grooms.

Current service provision

The lack of resources for rehabilitation following brain injury in the UK has been mentioned many times over the years (for example, London, 1967; Gloag, 1985; McLellan et al., 1988; McMillan and Greenwood, 1993). Most recently, the Royal College of Surgeons' report (1999) highlighted the inadequacy of resources, both in the acute and community setting, in many parts of the country. A majority of those with head injury are discharged from acute services to their home and into the care of their families, but appropriate community resources are limited or absent in many areas. Moreover, it has been shown that many patients have difficulty in gaining access to the rehabilitation services that do exist, or fail to do so at all (Murphy et al., 1990).

Ideally, rehabilitation should be coordinated across all services working with brain-injured people – the emergency services, casualty department, intensive care unit and acute services, as well as inpatient rehabilitation, community-based rehabilitation, and the community itself. These services should have good channels of communication between them to avoid individuals 'slipping through the net' when moving from one service to another. It is particularly important that there is good communication between inpatient and community services to avoid the individual being lost to rehabilitation services on discharge home from acute care. It is essential that other services are aware not only of the availability of community rehabilitation but also that they have realistic expectations of these services in terms of what they can provide and of their limitations.

Good channels of communication between services and the client and their family are also vital. When the patient with brain injury is being discharged from hospital into the community, or transferred between rehabilitation services, this can be a time of high anxiety and there is a need for reassurance and a good level of information and explanation to the client's family.

The approach to rehabilitation, and the kind of service required, very much depends on the stage of recovery (see McMillan and Greenwood, 1993). Individuals' rehabilitation needs will be very different in acute services compared to when they are living back in the community. In the acute stage they may have significant medical problems that must be taken into account and physical recovery may be the priority. By the time they have returned to the community the problems may be principally neuropsychological in nature. The makeup of the rehabilitation team will reflect the differing needs at each stage of rehabilitation, with more emphasis on nursing, medical input and physiotherapy in the early stages of recovery, and on occupational therapy, psychology, social work and vocational rehabilitation in the later stages. This reflects the changing needs of the individual over time (Barnes and Oliver, 1997).

The continuum of care

It is important to see rehabilitation in the community within the overall continuum of care. Figure 1.1 illustrates this continuum and some of the people and organizations involved. It highlights the need for the family to be involved from the earliest stages and for discharge planning to be taken into consideration and worked on thoroughly throughout the period of hospitalization. Like the baton in a relay race, the client must be passed from accident and emergency to the theatre, intensive care unit and ward, and thence to the community. These transitions can be turbulent times for all involved, especially families if they perceive a reduction in professional support as they go through the process. The figure also illustrates the fact that, in practice, re-entry to inpatient care may be necessary if, for example, care packages break down, clients take time to accept the need for rehabilitation, or behavioural problems develop (or are recognized) some time after the original injury.

Chapter 2 describes the process of medical care through which the more severely head-injured person may pass. Moving people through the rehabilitation process in a timely manner is important as rehabilitation is not an end in itself. It is all too easy for rehabilitation staff to become protective towards their clients, especially those who may have had major difficulties to overcome. It is especially important in what is usually the most difficult transition – that is, from hospital or rehabilitation unit to home. Much of what has been achieved through in patient rehabilitation can be lost if there is poor discharge.

Discharge planning

Discharge planning should involve hospital-based practitioners who know the client, and any relevant community colleagues, including care agency staff who may be needed for ongoing care. A detailed handover, taking community resources into account, is essential. For example, recommending daily speech and language therapy if existing services are already stretched may not be appropriate. Having said that, it is important that records are kept of ideal levels of care as ammunition in the planning and allocation of future resources. Planning must begin early with clear objectives and an agreed, realistic time frame. Four o'clock on Friday afternoon, when community services are winding down for the weekend, is not an ideal discharge time!

Accommodation and housing issues are extremely important aspects of discharge from hospital. Housing cannot be left out of the rehabilitation equation, although most people will be able to return home. Most experienced practitioners will know of people who have had to stay in hospital long after the time they should have returned home because there was no suitable accommodation. There are many different possibilities available both in terms of bricks and mortar and in support arrangements. For the small proportion of people who cannot return home, the range includes shared, supported housing or self-contained accommodation or accommodation with shared communal spaces and support from a staff team. It is also likely that these more severely head-injured people will require ongoing support in

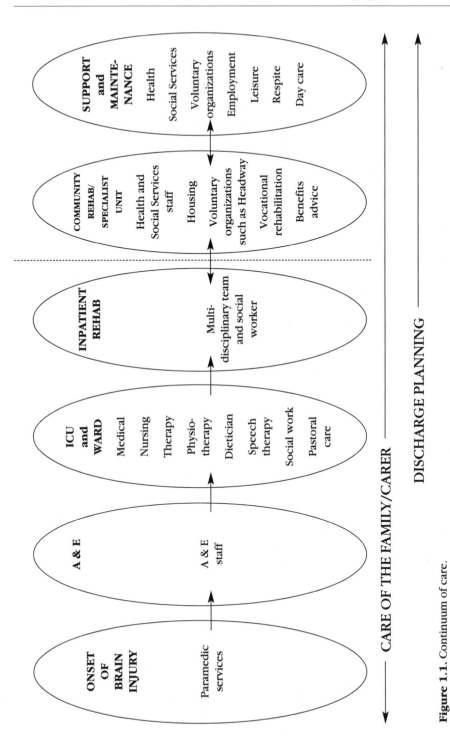

Figure 1.1. Continuum of care.

matters related to organizing their day-to-day life, their finances and their relationships with others. For a small minority of people with head injuries, residential or nursing homes may be the preferred option.

The fact that most do go home does not, of course, mean that going home is an easy process. There are almost always problems to face across a wide range of areas – functional, social, financial and so on. Many of these issues will be discussed in subsequent chapters.

If there is any question that a person may not be able to return home, assessment of housing needs must take place early in the rehabilitation process. It can take considerable time to organize, and attention must be given to the client's preferences and the amount of support necessary. It is important that there is an advocate for the client and to ensure as much choice as possible about where to live and with whom.

The incidence of head injury peaks in children, late teens and early twenties, and in old age. For the middle group, in particular, especially in severe head injury, housing can be a sensitive issue. It might seem appropriate for parents to take on a caring role, and for their children to return to the family home, but it is important to remain in touch with the parents, as years down the line they may need to relinquish this role. This can be a positive step, with the head-injured son or daughter moving to suitable supported accommodation, often with people of their own age. Living with aged parents can, in certain circumstances, be very isolating, and rehabilitation practitioners need to be aware of the options with regard to accommodation.

One of the findings of the Warwick project (Stilwell et al., 1998) was that, where there was good support from family and friends, the outcome was noticeably improved. In situations where there was severe head injury old friendships tended to fall away and considerable effort had to be made to establish a new social network.

Service inequalities and good practice

The House of Commons report into head injury rehabilitation (Great Britain, 2001) outlined barriers to successful service development. This included boundaries between acute and community services, between health and social services, and between adult and care of elderly services. Other barriers they recognized lay in a lack of understanding of the specialism among workers, limited resources, increasing demand and a lack of suitably trained rehabilitation professionals.

At all stages of the process, the current position of head-injury rehabilitation is marked by inequalities both between and within different countries. In the UK, there is a markedly uneven distribution of specialized neuroscience units and of rehabilitation consultants. Monies have tended to be targeted at acute services, perhaps because of their higher publicity and political value, rather than at community services. Often head-injured clients are not offered specialist intervention post-intensive care. Nationally, acquired brain injury rehabilitation services are often not the focus of political attention, perhaps because of the increased role of the media in publicizing more immediately emotive health issues, such as HIV or childhood meningitis.

These inequalities make it particularly useful to look at examples of good practice. It must be stressed that services should be developed to meet local need and that no one model will suit every area.

All areas need access to post-acute inpatient rehabilitation – McMillan and Greenwood (1993) suggest 20–30 such beds are needed per 2–3 million population. Rural areas will need regional units in order to offer specialized services economically. Post-acute rehabilitation is about recovery of function and independence, and may be hospital or unit based. Once back in the community, some rehabilitation aims will be similar, but the focus will shift towards integration and use of local resources.

It might be appropriate in cities to have a community rehabilitation service based in a hospital, following a traditional outpatient care model as well as staff going into people's own homes, as distances to travel will be relatively small. In contrast, the need in a rural area may be for an outreach team working alongside local community resources in developing appropriate rehabilitation services.

There are national differences that will influence good practice. Groswasser (1995), for example, describes a single-institute based service, which suits a small cohesive country such as Israel. As well as geographical factors, models of care will also be influenced by political considerations. Highly resourced countries, such as Sweden and Denmark (see, for example, Christensen and Teasdale, 1995) can focus services in a way that would be impossible, for instance, in developing countries.

In the UK, there are many examples of good practice, where services are planned to meet local needs, be they urban (see, for example, Hughes et al., 1995) or rural. Rural models vary from working through small locally based teams (for example, Evans, 1995), to developing regional centres (for example, Barnes, 1995). In practice, services vary widely in their resources and aims. In East Anglia, for example, the Icanho Centre provides day rehabilitation services for people with brain injury and covers the whole of the county of Suffolk. Staff work with clients both at the centre and within their local community. There is a full multidisciplinary team. Elsewhere in East Anglia there are some similar comprehensive services. For example, the North West Anglia Healthcare Trust operate a neurological rehabilitation team that has a catchment of both rural and urban populations. This, too, is a community-based team but it provides a coordinated pathway of care for brain-injured people that starts at the point of admission to hospital and continues through to community reintegration. Both these teams assess the needs of the head-injured client and his family. Following this an agreed goal-oriented rehabilitation programme is implemented. The teams work closely with other agencies such as education services, employment services and employers, as well as with health and social services and local voluntary organizations. One of the strengths of the teams is that they can provide a service locally to people who live in remote areas, using local facilities and resources. In contrast, there are other services in East Anglia that are much more limited and in one or two areas there is no coordinated brain injury rehabilitation at all (Seeley et al., 2001).

What is rehabilitation?

Rehabilitation is a term used to imply return of function or adaptation to changed circumstances. This extends beyond the field of medicine into many aspects of society and life in general (Ward and McIntosh, 1997). Rehabilitation was recognized as a need within healthcare during the Second World War, when many servicemen were sustaining serious and complex disabilities. This was the first time that rehabilitation was practised on a large scale and at that time it was very much based on a medical model of physical therapy following acute trauma (Ward and McIntosh, 1997). During the 1950s and 1960s there was a steep increase in road traffic accidents and in the incidence of head injury. At the same time, technical advances and new skills in the care of these patients progressed so that many more people with head injuries survived – albeit often with severe disabilities. This provided a further impetus for the development of rehabilitation as a discipline in its own right. More recently, rehabilitation has extended to include psychological, social and vocational issues. Different ways of viewing disability, with a greater involvement of the individual in the rehabilitation process, and recognition of the importance of his culture and community background, have moved rehabilitation well beyond the original medical model.

The definition of rehabilitation

The International Classification of Impairment, Disability and Handicap (ICIDH) (WHO, 1980) has been used to help understand the rehabilitation process. This introduced the terms 'pathology', 'impairment', 'disability' and 'handicap'. Wade (1992) defined these terms, beginning at the level of pathology. He describes this as 'the traditional focus of medical care. Doctors concentrate on diagnosing the disease, and then upon curing or reducing it if possible.' For example, a haematoma, which develops in the brain following a head injury, is the 'pathology'. 'Impairment' is defined as 'any loss or abnormality of psychological, or anatomical structure or function'. Thus an 'impairment' would be the loss of the use of the arm and leg on one side of the body as a result of the haematoma. 'Disability' is 'any restriction or lack of ability to perform an activity within the range considered normal for a human being', for example, the inability to walk independently because of hemiparesis. Finally, 'handicap' is described as 'a disadvantage for a given individual resulting from an impairment or disability that limits or prevents the fulfilment of a role that is normal (depending on age, sex and social and cultural factors) for that individual'. For example, this might be the individual's inability to return to his previous job because of impaired function in his arm and leg.

In 2000, the WHO revised this model in an attempt to overcome some of the shortcomings of the earlier framework, most notably in recognizing the role of the environment to a greater extent and clarifying relationships between the three dimensions. The revised model includes both positive (functioning) and negative (disability) aspects and looks at dimensions of body structures/functions (for which the negative aspect would be impairment), activity (activity limitation), and participation (participation restriction).

Activity takes into account the context of the individual's culture, and participation includes contextual factors including products and technology, physical environment, support and relationships, attitudes, values and beliefs, services, and systems and policies. Such contextual factors may be either facilitating or inhibiting. Gray and Hendershot (2000) discuss the newer model in more detail than is possible in this volume.

In the field of rehabilitation, the impairments need to be understood in terms of their functional implications for the client's life – that is, at the activity and participation level – rather than in terms of the pathology behind the signs and symptoms. When working in the area of community rehabilitation the focus is on the impact of impairments on individuals' ability to function successfully in their normal environment (Ward and McIntosh, 1997). As the revised WHO terms of activity limitation and participation restriction become more widely used it is hoped they will draw attention to the often considerable influence of environment on the rehabilitation process.

The ICIDH definition of rehabilitation states that 'rehabilitation is a problem-solving and educational process aimed at reducing the disability and handicap experienced by someone as a result of a disease, always within the limitations imposed both by available resources and by the underlying disease' (Wade, 1992). In 1997 the NHS executive published a document about rehabilitation which defines 'rehabilitation' in two ways. Firstly, it is 'a process of active change by which a person who has become disabled acquires the knowledge and skills needed for optimum physical, psychological and social function.' Secondly it is 'the application of all measures aimed at reducing the impact of disabling and handicapping conditions, and enabling disabled and handicapped people to achieve social integration.'

This highlights the complexity of the rehabilitation process. The first definition emphasizes the importance of the client's active involvement. It moves away from the model seen in a medical setting where interventions or treatments are carried out with little or no need for active participation on the part of the individual. Within the rehabilitation process it is essential that individuals are enabled to take control of their situation. The second definition highlights the importance of compensatory and adaptive processes, rather then recovery, in rehabilitation. Both these points are essential to an understanding of brain injury rehabilitation.

There are many other definitions of rehabilitation. Wade (1998) suggested that the aims of rehabilitation, acceptable to most clinicians, were:

- 'to maximize the patient's social role functioning (i.e. to minimize handicap or maximize participation)';
- 'to maximize their sense of wellbeing (i.e. to minimize somatic pain and distress)'; and
- ' to minimize the stress on and distress of the family, relatives and other emotionally involved people.'

These aims are particularly pertinent to community rehabilitation in the way they emphasize the psychological wellbeing of the client and the importance of working within the family and social structure to which the client belongs.

Aspects of rehabilitation

Rehabilitation can be considered under three headings – reducing the impairment, compensating for disability, and adjustment and adaptation to handicap.

Reducing the impairment and disability

During the first few months following head injury, reduction in impairment and disability may be achieved through efforts to facilitate the process of natural recovery and preventing secondary complications, such as contractures. This is the principal focus of acute and intermediate post-acute rehabilitation. The potential for recovery will depend on the nature and severity of the impairments. A significant head injury will result in permanent brain damage, and therefore permanent impairments. These will limit functional gains – either through the process of natural recovery or as a result of rehabilitation efforts. On entering rehabilitation clients often expect to recover fully and may require a lot of support to accept that this may not be possible.

Compensatory strategies

At least some permanent disability is to be expected following brain damage. Compensatory strategies aimed at accommodating these disabilities are the major focus of brain injury rehabilitation. This may involve learning new ways of functioning or the use of a piece of equipment to aid independence. For example, the client with a verbal memory impairment can learn to make greater use of visual aspects of memory, or simply to write things down more. The emphasis here is on maximizing the skills that an individual has whilst minimizing the difficulties that remain.

Although this is an essential part of the rehabilitation process, the first step for those with brain injury is often to improve awareness. Probably about half of all those with severe head injury show poor insight. It is often necessary to help them to gain a better understanding of the problems they have before working on compensatory strategies. When individuals are still in hospital, or have just returned home, they may not have been challenged, particularly from a cognitive point of view, and so they may be unaware of their difficulties. Sometimes it is not until they try to return to work or college that they begin to develop greater insight. It is often the neuropsychological deficits, rather than physical impairments, that are least evident to the individual and so strategies are needed to help the individual recognize these weaknesses. One method is to provide clients with the opportunity to try out their abilities in 'real' environments. For example, they may need to be encouraged to take up more demanding activities at home, or perhaps to engage in tasks that require the use of previous work skills. These activities should be introduced, in a gradual and supported way, into the community rehabilitation programme.

Thus, on the one hand there is a need to minimize the deficits while maximizing abilities, but on the other hand, the deficits need to be highlighted to clients so that they can gain insight and work on them successfully. This is a good example of the complex and at times contradictory nature of working in the field of brain injury and demonstrates the need for a flexible approach.

Adaptation to handicap

Adjustment and adaptation rehabilitation should also encompass adjustment and adaptation to permanent disabilities and handicaps that an individual may have. The adjustment process is likely to continue over a lengthy period of time and many clients never come to terms with the consequences of a brain injury. Thus the rate of adjustment, and the extent to which it is achieved, will vary between individuals. It may be difficult for the professionals involved to predict outcome accurately but it is essential that realistic goals are established from the outset. The client and his family need an honest prediction of likely outcome. Presentation of this information will need to be appropriately timed, and may need to be repeated, depending on the ability of the client and family to assimilate it.

These days, the individual does not only manage adaptation to disability but society has a greater awareness of the role it is expected to play too. Government legislation, the most recent being the Disability Discrimination Act 1995, tries to highlight the need for society to assist in the adjustment process. For example, employers are required to make reasonable adaptations to enable an individual to continue with their job (Thurgood, 1999). The Act 'imposes a new duty on employers and providers to make reasonable adjustments to their policies and physical environment to remove the barriers confronting disabled people' (Gooding, 1995).

These three areas of rehabilitation – maximizing potential, compensation, and adjustment, are not separate issues. A well-rounded rehabilitation package must be based on a combination of these. The structure will vary for each individual and according to stages of recovery in the rehabilitation process.

Rehabilitation principles

Having discussed the context in which rehabilitation services are set, the way in which those services operate will be considered. Before addressing the specific process, there are a number of generally accepted principles worth reiterating. These include adopting a multidisciplinary team approach, the need for equal access, and issues to do with the timing of intervention.

The rehabilitation team

Rehabilitation following brain injury requires multidisciplinary working. The multidisciplinary team is 'a group of people, each of whom possesses particular expertise; each of whom is responsible for making individual decisions; who together hold a common purpose; who meet together to communicate, collaborate and consolidate knowledge, from which plans are made, actions determined and future decisions influenced' (Brill, 1976). Clients and their families should always be thought of as key members of the rehabilitation team and be encouraged to play an active role in the rehabilitation process.

Wood (1997) describes the team as responsible for 'the development of a plan to which each member makes a different but complementary contribution.' Each member of a team is looking at the same problem but each will do so in a subtly different way and from different perspectives. This leads to the rich and multifaceted perspectives that can develop within a well-established team (Powell et al., 1994). A team will be working towards a common aim but its members may have different views on how this might be achieved. For example, a physiotherapist might question clients' cooperation with their rehabilitation programme because of their failure to practise mobility exercises at home. The occupational therapist might feel that the client's limited opportunities for purposeful activities at home were the basis for poor motivation. The psychologist might suspect that the client lacked confidence and was anxious about going outside his house. The social worker might focus concern on stresses within the family leading to a lack of support at home and therefore a loss of motivation.

A team approach can also enhance the understanding of the diverse and complex array of problems often experienced by people following brain injury. For example, a client may present with difficulty in carrying out a simple functional task but it is not until the occupational therapist, psychologist and speech and language therapist discuss their assessment findings that the complexity of this difficulty can be understood. Difficulty in understanding verbal information, in perceiving objects in their environment, and poor sensory feedback from their upper limbs, may all contribute to the functional difficulties experienced.

This is not to say that there is never any conflict between members of a multidisciplinary team, or between clients, their families and the rest of the team. Differences of opinion on a particular issue can often stimulate discussion, which enables the team to explore different ways of approaching a problem – ways that might otherwise have been overlooked. To illustrate this, when discussing the issue of return to work, the benefit of returning, both financially and for the emotional wellbeing of the client, may indicate an early return. On the other hand the neuropsychological difficulties that an individual has may suggest caution and a staged approach to returning to work. A compromise may have to be struck between these two considerations and the views of the client.

Differences of opinion within a team, combined with sound mechanisms for communication, will enrich the process of multidisciplinary work in the field of brain injury. It is important to note that there may be times when these discussions need to occur within the privacy of the professional team as the need for consistency when presenting information to clients and their families is essential.

An open forum between the different team members also enables each to have a greater understanding of the others' roles and allows for knowledge, ideas, skills and experience to be shared (Powell et al., 1994). This does require respect for each other's expertise, however, and a high level of trust within the team. These discussions can also play an important role in team support, as team members may be dealing with quite difficult and often stressful situations.

There may be a certain blurring of the traditional professional boundaries – this is particularly evident in community teams and is highlighted in the process of working on team rehabilitation goals. For example, the difficulty of shopping in the community may be tackled by the physiotherapist, the occupational therapist and the speech-and-language therapist, all working towards the same goal. Each professional needs to work with the client with an awareness and understanding of the skills that are being acquired in other therapy sessions. In this way they can ensure that clients are practising all aspects of their training. As Fussey and Giles (1988) state, 'those working with the brain injured need not lose their professional identity in order to belong to such a rehabilitation team; on the contrary each professional brings to the team his or her particular professional strengths.'

Team working needs to be thought of in its broadest sense. It may include people working in education, employment, housing, legal services and the voluntary sector. It must also include other specialist groups who may be working with the individual – for example, a mental health team, drug support agencies, Relate, or child care services, to name a few. An important member of the team, for clients who are able to pursue a claim for compensation, may be their solicitor. Practitioners need increasingly to understand the role of the solicitor. Although money is no substitute for recovery, compensation payments can help the client achieve the best possible quality of life in the long term. Interim payments may be negotiated to help address immediate needs. Solicitors increasingly involve themselves in the planning process for a client's rehabilitation and they will look to privately funded services where these are available. It does not always follow that this will be the best option for the client and it is important for the professional rehabilitation team to be involved in decisions of this kind. Clients need to employ a solicitor who has experience in personal injury work and of the problems that follow brain injury. An overview of legal issues, and advice on how clients can find a specialist solicitor according to their needs is given in Chapter 10.

Case management

The complexity of packages of care, perhaps involving multiple services within the community, means that there is often a need for one person to act as coordinator or case manager. The potential advantages of case management have been discussed by McMillan et al. (1988), although benefits may be small if only limited resources are available. In complex cases, or where a larger number of alternatives for rehabilitation are identified, then the need for someone to manage and coordinate a client's programme, and ensure access to facilities, will assume greater importance. Thus, case managers do not usually involve themselves in provision of services or therapy directly. Their role is to keep an eye on the whole picture, carry out reviews of the client's circumstances, and instigate change when required. 'Case managers are trained to match brain injured individuals and their families with the services that they need and to make the services accessible to them' (Winslade, 1998). The British Association of Case Managers deals with registration, competency and training in this field.

Another model of case management may be employed within this area. This is a partnership approach including representatives from the purchasers of services (health, social services, solicitors), providers of the service (care/support agencies) and specialist services (rehabilitation), in conjunction with the client and his family. This involves identified individuals from each of these areas working together as a team to manage complex cases. This model can be used where there are no compensation monies available to fund an individual as a case manager. It does, however, rely on a good understanding of individual roles and excellent communication between the different agencies.

Rehabilitation services often have a co-ordinator role built into their staff establishment. With community brain injury services, the staff group is often diverse and complex in its make up. The breadth of service that is provided is also complex and the coordination of both the staff and the service provision can be a demanding role. A coordinator can be appointed for the service as a whole but it can also be effective to allocate a member of the team to act as a coordinator or key worker for each client. This means that one person takes responsibility for overseeing an individual's rehabilitation programme and ensures that their needs are met and coordinated.

Multi-agency working

Multi-agency working and collaboration between agencies are essential both at a service-development or funding level and at the service-delivery level. This may well involve working across traditional boundaries. For instance, health and social services may need to work together to finance a rehabilitation programme for a client with brain injury and to fund jointly packages of care that will enable the individual to live in the community again. The NHS Executive report (NHS Executive, 1997) stated that: 'Organisational boundaries between agencies can often get in the way of effective, efficient and integrated ways of working at an individual and strategic level. Joint commissioning is a tool for tackling such barriers.' People with complex difficulties may need to be managed in specialist units outside the local area. For example, clients with behavioural disturbance will occasionally show extremes of aggression that may prove unmanageable in a local service. They may need funding so that they can be treated in one the few centres specializing in behavioural management.

When a client returns from a period of treatment or care outside the area, it is essential for the local services to work together in planning, implementing and monitoring the transfer back into the local community. There is likely to be a need for a complex package of care that will require joint financing and much careful planning and coordination. It is difficult on a funding level to separate the complexity of needs following brain injury into particular areas of responsibility such as those that are health issues and those that should be taken on by social services, for example. The efficient use of resources is best achieved if services can work together towards the common goal of maximizing an individual's potential and community reintegration.

The costs to the statutory agencies of care and treatment for those with very severe brain injury will often be very high, particularly if they cannot be managed within local resources. Once a client is able to return to his own community, the costs are likely to remain high and it is important that reintegration is adequately resourced. There may be a need for a community rehabilitation programme, respite care, housing and home care, day-care resources, and education or occupational opportunities. In the absence of sufficient funding, the investment in specialist treatment that has already been made may be wasted.

Clinical dilemmas

There are a number of issues that may arise after head injury that do not fall to a particular discipline, or that fall into the remit of a profession that is not represented on a particular team. Such problems may include social, emotional, financial and legal questions. It is important that this is recognized and that the team meeting is used to identify such issues and to decide the appropriate approach. This may involve either referral to a specialist outside the team, or a member of the team accepting a responsibility outside their 'normal' remit, or it may involve joint working with other agencies. It is very common to face issues that may not be entirely attributable to the head injury, although the injury may exacerbate pre-existing situations - relationship or financial difficulties for example – and it must be decided how appropriate it is for the team to become involved.

Communication

Good communication is of fundamental importance to effective work within a rehabilitation team, as well as between the team, the client and their family, and within the larger community network. The coordination of the services involved is important to make sure that everyone is working together. For example, clients might be learning strategies to assist with social communication as part of their rehabilitation programme. If they also attend a local day centre, it is important that they are able to use the same strategies, and receive support in doing so, in this environment too. Staff working in some non-specialist community services may have little or no experience in the field of brain injury. The brain injury rehabilitation team has a role to play in providing information, education and support to such services and thus enabling clients to maximize the benefit they can gain from diverse community services (Stillwell et al., 1998). For example, an individual who had a severe brain injury following a road traffic accident was in the middle of a college course at the time. The rehabilitation team worked closely with the college tutors, and at times the client's peers, to enable his smooth integration back into the college despite persisting neuropsychological disability.

This example highlights the problem of confidentiality if information about a client is to be communicated to agencies outside the rehabilitation service. Confidentiality must be maintained where the client wants this, or until he has given permission for information to be disclosed. Only the information that is relevant to a particular situation needs to be shared. Some organizations, such as Relate, normally prefer little or no information to be provided before starting to work with an individual, in case this might affect the therapeutic relationship.

It is essential that communication with the individual and his family be maintained throughout the rehabilitation process. The individual should be involved in establishing rehabilitation goals, the evaluation and review of progress made, and in planning for his discharge from the service. Communication with him needs to be clear, accurate, and well understood. Caution is needed about assuming that information has been taken in and understood properly. There is a need to check that this has been achieved. If the client has processing or memory problems, for example, then it may be important to use a written record of what is discussed and agreed, or other strategies to ensure effective communication.

The role of individuals and their families

The importance of the client at all stages of the rehabilitation process has been highlighted throughout this chapter. One of the problems that follows a traumatic injury and a long period of care in hospital and away from family members, is loss of self-confidence and the sense of self-responsibility. The client-centred approach passes some of the responsibility for their rehabilitation to individuals concerned and helps them in the process of gradually taking control of their lives again. The transfer of responsibility may take time to achieve and must be one of the implicit goals of a rehabilitation programme.

The family or network of social support around the brain-injured person plays an important part in supporting the rehabilitation process. The brain injury will have affected the family unit and the roles of each of its members. A family can have both negative and positive effects on the success of the rehabilitation programme. For example, the demands of a young family on a family member with a brain injury can exacerbate some difficulties, such as irritability. At the same time, a partner can find looking after the injured person as well as small children too great a burden, so that her capacity for support may be limited. In another instance, a partner who has a good grasp of the difficulties an individual has with memory, for example, may provide considerable emotional support, help him to learn to compensate for his impairment and minimize the level of handicap.

Other members of the family, besides the client, may have a need for support. It is important for the community rehabilitation service to be able to meet these needs, as well as those of the client. This may apply to all members of his social network, including a partner, children, parents and siblings, and sometimes friends and colleagues too. Chapter 9 addresses this in more detail.

Timeliness of intervention

At referral many clients will have a distorted perception of the likely time scale of recovery. Once fit to leave hospital and return to the community many individuals – and their families – will believe that they can get on with their lives and that things will return to normal, either immediately or very soon. In practice the reverse is often the case, with people only realizing the extent of their difficulties once they are back in a 'real' environment. Others will feel highly anxious about the loss of the support and level of care provided by an acute service or an inpatient rehabilitation facility. These factors can generate negative feelings towards community rehabilitation and it is important that such issues are discussed and negotiated at the outset. It may be that time needs to elapse before the client will accept intervention, and the service will need to ensure that the client is able to access help when he is ready.

Other clients may come to the service some time after they have returned home. It can be a matter of some months or even years after a head injury before they are referred. The study by Thornhill et al. (2000) highlights the number of clients who are not seen when they leave hospital – only 47% of those with disabilities were seen in hospital after discharge, and only 28% had any rehabilitation input during the first year.

Often clients will attach greatest importance early on to the obvious problems in a practical sense – being able to walk, to dress themselves or to talk. At a later stage, the 'hidden' disabilities become more apparent and significant to the client and the family. Returning to more demanding activities such as specific hobbies or work will highlight problems with attention, memory or executive functions. However, even at a late stage, unrealistic expectations are common. For example, a client may ask for help finding work and believe himself able to achieve this, even after years of failing to do so because of neuropsychological impairments. Clients may hold the view that they have not had the correct therapy or help. The length of time since the injury and the stage of recovery will contribute to the diversity of problems encountered in a community service. The service must be flexible and able to respond according to the very different expectations and needs at different times.

Equal access

It is obviously an accepted principle that services should be equally accessible to all, regardless of their cultural and social background or geographical location. In practice this is not as easy to ensure as it should be. To be fully accessible in a multicultural society there would need to be access to therapy services in many different languages and clinicians would need to have knowledge of cultural and social mores. This is an area of concern to which justice cannot be done in this volume, but it is important to draw attention to the issue. As has been seen already there are inequalities in the geographical provision of service.

An additional factor is that certain cohorts within the population are at greater risk of head injury and these groups may be to some extent disadvantaged premorbidly (Weller, 1985). This, in turn, will be a factor in the assessment and rehabilitation process. Previous problems with aggression, alcohol, drug use or criminal behaviour can lead to prejudice within rehabilitation services. The brain injury itself may be connected with these behaviours. For example, an individual who has an aggressive disposition may be more likely to sustain a head injury as a result of an assault. Those who take drugs or alcohol to excess are more likely to crash their cars or be involved in accidents of other kinds. Another important factor may be pre-existing mental health issues, with head injuries resulting, for example, from suicide attempts. It is essential that there are fair and equal opportunities for all in accessing rehabilitation services and this should not be prejudiced by pre-existing problems. Information about these issues is essential so that an appropriate and realistic rehabilitation programme can be planned. Where necessary, other services, such as those for substance abuse, will need to be involved. Moreover, the rehabilitation team must have a policy about clients who are attending the service, but who may take drugs or alcohol, which ensures that other clients are not put at risk in any way. With these provisos, the rehabilitation team needs to have a non-judgemental approach.

Community-based brain injury rehabilitation

As has been stated, head injury can result in a variety of neurophysical and neuropsychological symptoms. Behavioural problems are common and brain injury often has a direct effect on emotional function, motivation and insight. Pre-existing personality, abilities and experience will interact with these impairments so that each individual with head injury makes a unique presentation. Recovery is protracted and likely to be incomplete. These considerations indicate that the approach to rehabilitation for people with brain injury must be flexible. It needs to extend into the community and the context in which the disabled person must learn to function, and to involve families and others in the community. It must be able to support certain clients for a considerable length of time. Community rehabilitation programmes are particularly suited to providing the best environment for learning and training and promoting independence after brain injury (Greenwood and McMillan, 1993).

A community model of rehabilitation is appropriate once an individual has reached the point where he can live or be cared for in the community. This may be a more successful approach to rehabilitation than a residential or hospital-based programme. By working with clients in the context in which they live it is possible to offer a flexible approach and one that is highly sensitive to individual need. The structure of the service needs to allow for creativity and a problem-solving approach to accommodate the diversity of difficulties that follow brain injury. Rehabilitation may be pursued within the client's own environment. For example, rehabilitation may be based at home to increase personal independence; in the community doing the weekly shop; at their place of work, or pursuing leisure activities such as fishing at the local lake. The importance of this was emphasized by Stilwell et al. (1998): 'it is essential to see continuing problems with community re-entry in the context in which they occur and to understand the interaction between individuals and the circumstances in which they find themselves.' There is good evidence that training in new skills and compensatory strategies will be more successful for those with brain injury where it is carried out in the context in which it must be applied (*in vivo* training). Skills acquired through training within a therapy department (*in vitro* training) may not be easily transferred to the real life situation and will probably generalize less well to other similar situations (Greenwood and McMillan, 1993).

The approach of community rehabilitation is necessarily eclectic in make-up, drawing on different ways of working. For example, rehabilitation may be client centred – that is, working directly with clients on practical goals that they wish to achieve. It may be educational – helping individuals understand what has happened to them, or it may be social – working with families and social networks to support clients and promote their reintegration.

Community rehabilitation makes use of many resources, including multi-agency working, and can be enhanced by the varied views and approaches of a multidisciplinary team.

Community rehabilitation – the process

The process of rehabilitation necessarily involves four principal stages – assessment, goal planning, intervention, and evaluation (Wade, 1998). There needs to be a clear procedure by which individuals can be referred to the community rehabilitation team. Intervention will include not only direct work addressing specific problems, but also indirect input – such as education and giving information. Individual chapters in this volume will consider assessment, goal setting, intervention and evaluation from their specific perspectives, but it is worth outlining some of the common features of the process.

Access to the service

Criteria for acceptance into the service should be defined to enable appropriate individuals to be referred. Up-to-date and accurate information about clients is essential. If referrals are accepted from all sources, including self-referral, then it is essential that medical information is sought from acute and primary care sources. There should be a mechanism to screen out those referrals that are not appropriate for the service. Where needs are identified that cannot be met within the structure of the existing service – but perhaps should be – then this ought to be brought to the notice of the statutory organizations with the aim of helping to inform the process of future service development.

Assessment

Multidisciplinary team assessment will provide a baseline of the client's capabilities and identify problem areas. It is worth noting that as clients pass from team to team there is a risk of repetition of assessments and there must be procedures in place to ensure good transfer of information. The process of assessment provides the basis for planning a rehabilitation package to meet the individual's needs. It can also be used to inform the individual about his problems and the stage reached in recovery and may help to improve self-awareness. Following the assessment the team needs to work with the individual and his family to set realistic and achievable goals. Appropriate intervention can then be planned and instigated but it is essential that the goals and the rehabilitation programme are evaluated and reviewed at set intervals, and adapted according to the progress made. It is important that some longer term aims are also established as part of the planning process, and the idea of moving on beyond the rehabilitation service is introduced early. The expectation of programme completion and discharge from the service at some point in the future is an important factor in reducing individuals' reliance on the service and encourages the goal of their taking control of their lives again.

Goal setting

Goals must be tailored to match the time and stage of recovery and, as far as possible, the priorities defined by the client, so that he is motivated to achieve them (Powell et al., 1994). Therapy aims, and the timing of that input, will therefore vary. For example, early on the therapists may work with a brain-injured client to gain as much return of motor function as possible. Once it seems that no further return of movement is occurring then it may be appropriate to change the emphasis of therapy to work on compensatory and adaptive skills.

Establishing an overall or long-term aim can help to focus each individual discipline's goals. For example, if the overall aim is to gain more control in the individual's life, the rehabilitation team would need to consider what is needed to achieve this. It may mean that specific short-term goals include work on daily routine activities (for instance 'to become independent getting in and out of bed'); offering counselling to the carers to encourage them to allow the client to attempt activities without help; and the provision of a communication aid to enable a person to ask for goods in a shop.

Intervention

There are several models of treatment, which define different approaches to intervention. The medical model aims to 'reverse the pathology'. This might be relevant to recovery in the early neurosurgical management of head injury, but there are few grounds for supposing rehabilitation techniques can have direct benefits of this kind. Therapy following brain injury is usually based either on the premise that clients can be helped to re-establish functional skills as natural recovery progresses, and to use those skills and abilities they have retained more effectively, or on helping them to develop compensatory strategies and aids to circumvent their disabilities. These ideas are sometimes defined in terms of a 'problem-solving' model of rehabilitation that focuses on the practical needs and goals for each individual.

The consensus appears to be that a holistic approach of integrated therapies, tackling all aspects of the client's needs and disabilites – as pioneered by Prigatano and others (Prigatano, 1986, 1994) – shows the best outcome (Cicerone, Dahlberg and Kalmer, 2000). Malec and Basford (1996) suggested that intensive and comprehensive day treatment programmes produce the best results. The review by Cicerone, Dahlberg and Kalmer also concluded that encouraging clients to take responsibility for applying strategies for themselves may be important, together with treatments that continued over lengthy periods of time and that included long-term follow up and support to ensure that training becomes generalized and that the benefits are maintained.

Information and education

The provision of information and education to the client is of particular importance because of the 'hidden' nature of the disabilities and the difficult concepts involved in understanding the nature of some symptoms after brain injury. Information needs to be well timed, accurate and understandable. It is therefore essential that the way information is passed on is adapted to meet the needs of each client and his family. In some cases and circumstances this must be done on an individual basis but at other times there can be advantages in education through group working. Education about the brain, how it is affected by brain injury, the problems that can occur, and what can be done about these problems, is an essential part of the rehabilitation process. If individuals and their families understand their situation well then they will be able to derive greater benefit from their rehabilitation.

It is important for team members to realize the limitations to their knowledge and to be aware when it is necessary to seek information from colleagues or from elsewhere. On the same basis, a rehabilitation team should pursue an education programme that enables them to develop their skills and gain knowledge and experience from others. There is also an important role for a brain injury rehabilitation team in educating other professionals and organizations concerned with brain-injured people and for them to act as a resource centre (McMillan and Greenwood, 1993).

Review and discharge

Community rehabilitation following brain injury can vary greatly in the length of time for which therapy needs to continue. Individuals may need only infrequent input for a period of no more than two to three months in order to achieve their goals. For example, clients may have already returned to their previous activities within the community, and be functioning well, apart from some mild difficulties with memory, in the context of their employment. Advice on compensatory memory strategies and assistance in applying these in the work place may be sufficient to bring about a significant improvement.

On the other hand, other clients, who are at an early stage of recovery and have multiple disabilities, may benefit from therapy activities five days per week, involving several of the team members. This level of input is gradually reduced over time but they may continue to receive at least some therapy for a period of two years or more following referral. Clients might then progress to review or follow-up appointments that could continue, for example, over a period of a further year or more. Long-term follow-up of this kind can support clients in coping with and adjusting to the long-term consequences of their injury. Thus clients' involvement with the community rehabilitation service may last for several years.

In these circumstances, it can be appropriate for a client to have a break from therapy or contact with the rehabilitation service. This can be useful to prevent therapy from becoming tedious with a loss of motivation – sometimes for the therapist as well as the client. The opportunity to practise exercises and strategies independently at home for a while can clarify the nature of the problems for the client and enhance motivation when therapy is resumed. There is also a danger that long periods of therapy can unintentionally reinforce the expectation of an eventual full recovery – provided treatment is continued for long enough. A break in therapy encourages clients to evaluate progress and the time scale they are on, and to reconsider goals and expectations.

A follow-up or review appointment after programme completion is important in order to monitor the maintenance of the skills gained in rehabilitation and the extent to which their application has generalized into novel situations. If this vital transition does not take place then it must be questioned whether the rehabilitation programme has been of any value. Sargent and Patterson (1993) state that 'the home and the community must be used as integral parts of the rehabilitation programme'.

Follow-up also allows the individual to discuss any new difficulties that they may be experiencing. The time scale of follow-up will depend on individual circumstances. In general, once the identified goals have been achieved, it is important that individuals are helped to move on from the rehabilitation service. In order to support this transition, follow-up appointments might be set initially at three months then six-monthly intervals. Rehabilitation may therefore continue in some form over a relatively long period of time.

The importance of long-term follow-up for people with brain injury was identified by the work of the Warwick Project (Stilwell et al., 1998). It stated that 'there must be a strategy for the transition from active intervention to long-term support, and if this involves handover to other agencies, such as Social Services or General Practitioner, these agencies must be positively prepared and engaged.' This also highlights the need for the services both in rehabilitation and other areas in the community (for example, employment, education, carer support, voluntary sector and so forth) to work together to help individuals to reach their maximum potential.

Some services may choose to maintain contact with clients and their families for a period of many years (Stilwell et al., 1998). This policy needs careful consideration due to the inevitable increase in the case load for the rehabilitation team, the effect that this will have on resources for other clients, and the danger that clients and family might become overly dependent on professional support. There is a fine balance between providing support over a long period and avoiding the client coming to rely on the rehabilitation service or on particular team members. On the other hand, community rehabilitation services do need to remain responsive to future needs that may arise, perhaps several years after a head injury. Establishing a mechanism for re-referral, most probably through the general practitioner, is probably the most efficient and cost-effective strategy. This will ensure that clients are able to access rehabilitation services again should they need to do so.

The end point of any rehabilitation episode needs to be negotiated. Discharging individuals can be difficult, particularly if they feel that they have not progressed as far as they would have liked. It is unlikely that a 100% recovery can be achieved following brain injury, but some families are unable to accept this and will continue to seek further therapy in the belief that this can resolve their problems. It is therefore essential that the rehabilitation process endeavours to help the individual, their family, and often other people in their community, to adjust to the realities of the long-term disabilities that remain following brain injury.

Evaluation and outcomes

Outcomes are important both from a service planning perspective and clinically. However, trying to measure outcomes in head injury rehabilitation is, as Cope (1995) states, 'frustratingly difficult'. Measures used need to be sensitive across a range of severities and cover many dimensions – including cognition, language, physical fitness, emotional and behavioural issues, and quality of life. Measures need to be easy to administer, reliable and valid, and sensitive to what may be very small, albeit significant, changes. It is also important to consider differences between performance and capacity. It is therefore unlikely that any single measure will ever be adequate, and that a variety of evaluation materials and styles will be needed. Ideally these should include both objective and subjective measures.

Throughout the following chapters there will be reference to some of the global scales that have been employed and also some specific measures relating to certain dimensions. Methods that have been used include direct interview, rating scales, observation and psychometric assessments. As Powell (1999) points out, there are manifest differences between assessing rehabilitation outcomes in inpatient or community settings. In the latter, rehabilitation is much more participation related and should take into account beliefs, attitudes, social contacts and the environment generally. The University of Warwick study (Stilwell et al., 1998) developed a Community

Outcome Scale based on five-point scales covering engagement, social integration, occupation and mobility, and which allows for support networks to be taken into account.

One methodology that has been used increasingly is that of goal-attainment scaling (Kiresuk and Sherman, 1968). This involves selecting appropriate goals, designating time scales and an acceptable (expected) outcome level, which is rated as 0. Outcomes that would fall above or below the expected level are rated as plus or minus one or two. Goals can be weighted to reflect importance. The main drawback is that this is subjective so there are concerns about reliability and validity, but setting goals with the client can be very motivating and ensure rehabilitation focuses on areas that are of personal concern to the client (Malec, 1999).

Conclusion

This chapter has described the service context in which rehabilitation is based and offered an outline of a community-based approach to rehabilitation after head injury. Obviously there is considerable overlap with work at the inpatient stage of care – both in the principles and in specific approaches.

From a service perspective, it is apparent that there is still a shortfall between the level of service recommended in a variety of reports and policy statements, and the implementation of those recommendations. The recognition of the special needs of head-injured people is not always reflected practically in the provision of specialist services. There are historical as well as political and economic reasons for this situation, and the situation varies between countries and regions, but that does not mean the situation should be acceptable.

The aim of staff in the field must be to provide the best possible level of intervention, and this book attempts to support that aim. It would be foolish to ignore the fact that staff have to work within the constraints of their service, but to limit the practical suggestions set out in this volume to the lowest common denominator would also be foolish. The management and rehabilitation of people with head injuries needs to attract greater attention. There is still much controversy about the efficacy of rehabilitation and more research is required to establish which techniques and approaches are the most effective. However, there is evidence that rehabilitation can help head-injured people maximize their abilities and minimize their disabilities, enabling them to live as independently as possible in the community.

In relation to the effectiveness of head injury rehabilitation, Cope (1995) reviewed various studies. He posed – as many both in and outside the field have – the question of whether rehabilitation after traumatic brain injury is 'informed and well intentioned hand holding while natural recovery takes place'. In evaluating efficacy, the trend has been towards global measures of functioning in the recognition that all the components together of the rehabilitation process have a greater effect than the sum of the parts. For example, speech and language therapy may enable an individual to communicate better but that individual also needs to be able physically to get into social settings, cognitively to be aware of what is and is not safe and appropriate social behaviour, and so on. Cope concluded from available studies that, despite methodological problems, rehabilitation 'works in ways that make a worthwhile difference to traumatic brain injury victims and to society, and there is an abundance of evidence to support this assertion'.

Working with head-injured people and their families is demanding but rewarding. There is still a lot to learn about rehabilitation for this client group and many questions need to be addressed, but there are increasing numbers of examples of good practice and thoughtful work in the field. Rehabilitation specialists need to continue this work, to push the boundaries further and further and thus provide the best possible services for head-injured people and their families.

References

Barnes M (1995) A regional service: developing a head injury service. In Chamberlain MA, Neumann V, Tennant A (eds) Traumatic Brain Injury Rehabilitation. London: Chapman & Hall, pp. 37–50.

Barnes MP, Oliver M (1997) Organisation of neurological rehabilitation services. In Greenwood R, Barnes MP, McMillan TM, Ward CD (Eds) Neurological Rehabilitation. Hove: Psychology Press. 29–40.

Brill NI (1976) Teamwork: working together in the human services. Philadelphia: JB Lippincott.

British Society of Rehabilitation Medicine (1998) Rehabilitation after Traumatic Brain Injury. London: BRSM.

Chamberlain MA (1988) The Ideal Management of Head Injury. Leeds: West Yorkshire Working Party.

Chamberlain MA (1995) Head injury – the challenge: principles and practice of service organisation. In Chamberlain MA, Neumann V, Tennant A (eds) Traumatic Brain Injury Rehabilitation. London: Chapman & Hall, pp. 1–11.

Christensen A, Teasdale T (1995) A clinically and neuropsychologically led post-acute rehabilitation programme. In Chamberlain MA, Neumann V, Tennant A (eds) Traumatic Brain Injury Rehabilitation. London: Chapman & Hall, pp. 88–98.

Cicerone C, Dahlberg C, Kalmar K (2000) Evidence-based cognitive rehabiltation: recommendations for clinical practice. Archives of Physical Medicine and Rehabilitation 81: 1596-615.

Cope DN (1995) The effectiveness of traumatic brain injury rehabilitation: a review. Brain Injury 9(7): 649–70.

Evans C (1995) A rural service: developing rehabilitation in the community. In Chamberlain MA, Neumann V, Tennant A (eds) Traumatic Brain Injury Rehabilitation. London: Chapman & Hall, pp. 51–65.

Fussey I, Giles G (1988) Rehabilitation of the Severely Brain Injured Adult – A Practical Approach. London: Croom Helm.

Gloag D (1985) Rehabilitation after head injury 1. Cognitive problems. British Medical Journal 290: 834–7.

Gooding C (1995) Blackstone's Guide to the Disability Discrimination Act 1995. London: Blackstone.

Gray DB, Hendershot GE (2000) The ICIDH-2: developments for a new era of outcomes research. Arch Phys Med Rehab 81(suppl. 2): S10–S14.

Great Britain (1999) Saving Lives: Our Healthier Nation. London: HMSO.

Great Britain (2001) House of Commons Health Committee Report into Head Injury Rehabilitation. London: HMSO.

Greenwood RJ, McMillan TM (1993) Models of rehabilitation programmes for the brain injured adult: current provision, efficacy and good practice. Clinical Rehabilitation 7: 248–55.

Groswasser Z (1995) A national service: coma to community. In Chamberlain MA, Neumann V, Tennant A (eds) Traumatic Brain Injury Rehabilitation. London: Chapman & Hall, pp. 25–36.

Hughes D, Ward E, Warmock H, Hunter R, Tennant A, Chamberlain MA (1995) An urban community service for head injury: using OT to meet the challenge of community reintegration. In Chamberlain MA, Neumann V, Tennant A (eds) Traumatic Brain Injury Rehabilitation. London: Chapman & Hall, pp. 66–83.

Johnson RP (1998) How do people get back to work after severe head injury? A 10 year follow up study. Neuropsychological Rehabilitation 8: 61–79.

Kiresuk TJ, Sherman RE (1968) Goal attainment scaling: a general method for evaluating comprehensive mental health programs. Community Mental Health Journal 4: 443–53.

London PS (1967) Some observations on the course of events after severe injury of the head. Annals of the Royal College of Surgeons 41: 460–79.

Malec JF (1999) Goal attainment sealing in rehabilitation. Neuropsychological Rehabilitation 9(3/4): 253–75.

Malec JF, Basford JS (1996) Post acute brain injury rehabilitation. Archives of Physical Medicine and Rehabilitation 77: 198–207.

McLellan DL, Brooks N, Eames P, Evans C, Furth J, McClement E, Norcross K, Pentland B (1988) Report of the Working Party on the Management of Traumatic Brain Injury. London: Medical Disability Society Publications.

McMillan TM, Greenwood RJ (1993) Models of rehabilitation programmes for the brain injured adult. II: model services and suggestions for change in the UK. Clinical Rehabilitation 7: 346–55.

McMillan TM, Greenwood RJ, Morris JR, Brooks DN, Murphy L, Dunn G (1988) An introduction to the concept of head injury case management with respect to the need for service provision. Clinical Rehabilitation 2: 319–22.

Murphy LD, McMillan TM, Greenwood RJ, Brooks DN, Morris JR, Dunn G (1990) Services for severely head-injured patients in North London and environs. Brain Injury 4: 95–100.

NHS Executive (1997) Rehabilitation – A Guide. London: Department of Health.

Powell J (1999) Assessment of rehabilitation outcomes in community outreach settings. Neuropsychological Rehabilitation 9(3/4): 457–72.

Powell T, Partridge T, Nicholls T, Wright L, Mould H, Cook C, Anderson A, Blakey L, Boyer M, Davis L, Grimshaw J, Johnsen E, Lambert L, Page J, Pearce D, Smith A, Sturman S, Searle Y, Tatler, S (1994) An interdisciplinary approach to the rehabilitation of people with brain injury. British Journal of Therapy and Rehabilitation 1(1): 8-13.

Prigatano GP (1986) Neuropsychological rehabilitation after brain injury. Baltimore: Johns Hopkins University Press.

Prigatano GP (1994) Productivity after neuropsychologically oriented milieu rehabilitation. Journal of Head Trauma Rehabilitation 9: 91-102.

Royal College of Surgeons (1999) Report of the Working Party on the Management of Patients with Head Injuries. London: The Royal College of Surgeons.

Sargent M, Patterson T (1993) Postacute, home-based head injury rehabilitation: an outcome study. Rehabilitation Nursing 18(6): 380-3.

Seeley HM, Maimaris C, Carroll G, Kellerman J, Pickard JD (2001) Implementing the Galasko report on the management of head injuries: the Eastern Region approach. Emergency Medicine 18: 358-65.

Social Services Inspectorate (1996) 'A Hidden Disability' Report of the Social Services Inspectorate Traumatic Brain Injury Rehabilitation Project. Wetherby: Department of Health.

Stilwell J, Hawley C, Stilwell P, Davies C (1998) National Traumatic Brain Injury Study. Coventry: Centre for Health Services Studies, University of Warwick.

Teasdale G, Jennett B (1974) Assessment of coma and impaired consciousness. The Lancet 2: 81-4.

Thornhill S, Teasdale GM, Murray GD, McEwen J, Roy CW, Penny KI (2000) Disability in young people and adults one year after head injury: prospective cohort study. British Medical Journal 320 (17 June): 1631-5.

Thurgood J (1999) The employment implications of the Disability Discrimination Act 1995 and a suggested format for developing reasonable adjustments. British Journal of Occupational Therapy 62(7): 290-4.

Wade D (1992) Measurement in Neurological Rehabilitation. Oxford: Oxford University Press.

Wade D (1998) Editorial. Clinical Rehabilitation 12: 1-2.

Ward CD McIntosh S (1997) The Rehabilitation Process: a neurological perspective. In Greenwood R, Barnes MP, McMillan TM, Ward CD (Eds) Neurological Rehabilitation. Hove: Psychology Press. 13-28.

Weller MPI (1985) The sequelae of head injury and the post-concussion syndrome. In Granville-Grossman K (Ed) Recent Advances in Clinical Psychiatry 5. London: Churchill Livingstone.

Winslade W (1998) Confronting Traumatic Brain Injury, Hope and Healing. Newhaven: Yale University Press.

Wood RU (1997) The rehabilitation team. In Greenwood R, Barnes MP, McMillan TM, Ward CD (Eds) Neurological Rehabilitation. Hove: Psychology Press. 41-50.

World Health Organization (1980) International Classification of Impairment, Disability and Handicap. Geneva: World Health Organization.

CHAPTER 2

Setting the scene

KATE McGLASHAN

The aim of this chapter is to put the head-injured client into context. How he presents to the community rehabilitation team will be a product of what has happened to him so far in his journey through the healthcare system. The details of what occurred at the scene of the injury, the emergency treatment required, the acute-care phase ups and downs and the early rehabilitation experiences will all have had a profound influence on what sort of problems come through the door of the community rehabilitation unit. It is also important to remember that the experiences of the family, good or bad, will also come through the same door, and their pre-formed opinions and expectations may provide an added challenge.

This chapter will set out to present some of the basic background information needed to appreciate the context of the head-injured client – from a brief revision of brain anatomy and the mechanisms of head injury through to emergency treatment and the acute-care pathway. The major medical complications of head injury will then be discussed in turn.

In this chapter, the 'client' will be referred to as the 'patient' as this is appropriate for the setting being described.

Throughout this book the following definition of head injury, as put forward by the British Society of Rehabilitation Medicine (1998), will apply: 'Brain injury caused by trauma to the head, including the effects of direct complications of trauma, notably hypoxia (low oxygen concentration), hypotension (low blood pressure), intracranial haemorrhage (bleeding within the skull vault or brain substance) and raised intracranial pressure (raised pressure within the skull vault).'

Introduction

Head injuries are not a new phenomenon but the causes of head injuries have changed over the millennia. Gone are the days of the 'woolly mammoth crush injury' or the 'sabre-tooth tiger tentorial tear', these having been replaced by their modern-day equivalents resulting from road traffic accidents, injuries at work, and sporting mishaps. Sadly, assault also remains a common cause, and ballistic injuries to the head are common in times of war. Written descriptions of head injury are scarce before the twentieth century, but the Ancient Egyptians did record in some detail the sequelae of head injury such as hemiplegia, deviation of the eyes and post-traumatic epilepsy (Edwin Smith Papyrus).

The story of Phineas Gage is often quoted as the first recorded case history of a brain-injured individual demonstrating changes in personality and mental state. In his report, his physician, Dr Harlow, both elegantly and graphically describes the cognitive and behavioural manifestations of frontal-lobe damage. The year was 1848, and Mr Gage was unfortunate enough to succumb to an industrial accident, a common hazard of the times. He was a foreman, and, as he was placing dynamite down a hole with a tamping rod, the dynamite blew up and the tamping rod was fired up through his jaw and eye socket and out of the top of his head, destroying frontal lobe tissue on the way. Extraordinarily, Mr Gage not only survived the initial blast, but also the removal of the rod by the shocked Dr Harlow to whose surgery he reportedly walked. Indeed, in terms of survival he did very well, living a further 20 years after the accident, but as is often the way with stories of survival 'from the jaws of death', all was not well with Mr Gage:

General appearance good: stands quite erect, with his head inclined slightly towards the right side: his gait in walking is steady: his movements rapid, and easily executed . . . His physical health is good, and I am inclined to say that he has recovered. Has no pain in head, but says it has a queer feeling which he is not able to describe. Applied for his situation as foreman, but is undecided whether to work or travel. His contractors, who regarded him as the most efficient and capable foreman in their employ previous to his injury, considered the change in his mind so marked that they could not give him his place again. The equilibrium or balance, so to speak, between his intellectual faculties and animal propensities, seems to have been destroyed. He is fitful, irreverent, indulging at times in the grossest profanity (which was not previously his custom), manifesting but little deference for his fellows, impatient of restraint or advice when it conflicts with his desires, at times pertinaciously obstinate yet capricious and vacillating, devising many plans of future operation, which are no sooner arranged than they are abandoned in turn for others appearing more feasible. A child in his intellectual capacity and manifestations, he has the animal passions of a strongman. Previous to his injury, though untrained in the schools, he possessed a well-balanced mind, and was looked upon by those who knew him as a shrewd, smart businessman, very energetic and persistent in executing all his plans of operation. In this regard his mind was radically changed, so decidedly that his friends and acquaintances said he was 'no longer Gage'. (Harlow, 1848)

Head injury – who, why and how often?

The head injury caseload of a community rehabilitation unit will tend to reflect the national pattern for the condition. Males will outnumber females at least 2:1 and there will be an excess, of roughly 2/3 of the total, of young men in the age range 15–24 years of age. This book will only deal with the age group 16–65, but it should be remembered that children and elderly people have head injuries too, and children sustaining a significant head injury will have a lifetime of disability to contend with. Sometimes these children will be picked up by adult rehabilitation services when they are discharged from paediatric services for ongoing input and support. The older head injury cohort is largely made up of individuals aged 75 and more, often sustaining their injuries as a result of falls.

It is estimated that in the UK 200 to 300 per 100,000 of the population per year will require admission to hospital for a head injury. Of these, the majority will stay in for less than 48 hours. Five thousand of those admitted will die from their injuries, and 1,500 will be left with permanent brain damage (Jennett and MacMillan, 1981). In terms of prevalence, an average general practitioner (GP) will have two patients with persisting disability on his list at any one time. This low exposure of the GP to the head injured is important as it underlines the need for help from specialist rehabilitation services in dealing with the multiple and often complex problems that may arise as a result of the injury.

Road traffic accidents (vehicle passengers and pedestrians) are the cause of about half of the cases of head injury. The principal causes of head injury are road traffic accidents, assaults, falls, accidents at work and in the domestic setting. Sports related injuries are also relatively common, the main sporting offenders being horse-riding, rugby football and soccer. The real incidence of head injury in sport is likely to be higher than any published figures due to low reporting of injuries due to fear of a ban from the sport, even if temporary. Head injury in young men is largely caused by road traffic accidents, and the incidence of the other factors varies according to age group and geography. Alcohol plays a significant part in many cases, but on a positive note the introduction of legislation making the use of front seatbelts compulsory has resulted in a reduction in head injury statistics.

The brain: structure and function

Before detailing the mechanisms of brain injury, it is worth revisiting some of the anatomical aspects of the brain within the skull that may help explain the

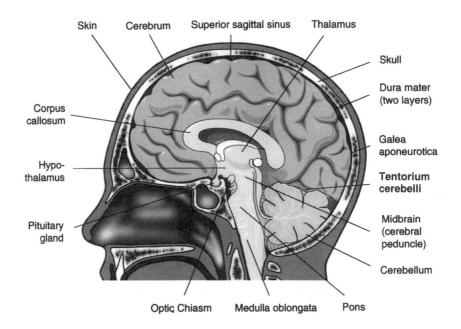

Skin   Cerebrum   Superior sagittal sinus   Thalamus

Skull

Dura mater
(two layers)

Corpus
callosum

Galea
aponeurotica

Hypo-
thalamus

**Tentorium
cerebelli**

Pituitary
gland

Midbrain
(cerebral
peduncle)

Cerebellum

Optic Chiasm   Medulla oblongata   Pons

Figure 2.1. Midline section through cranium. (Drawn by PM Ball, Senior Medical Artist, University of Cambridge.)

nature of injuries seen (see Figure 2.1). Only a limited review of basic structural and functional anatomy will be considered here. For a detailed insight into these areas of neuroanatomy the reader is referred to a neuroanatomical text.

The skull itself is a rigid, rounded box of bone that houses the brain and acts to protect it from direct damage. It can be subdivided into three main areas, or fossae (anterior, middle and posterior), which descend in a step-like manner from front to back. Prominent bony landmarks that are easy to see within the skull bound each of these fossae. Within the posterior fossa lies a central defect, the foramen magnum, through which the medulla oblongata leaves the skull. The anterior fossa, containing the frontal lobes, lies above the eye-sockets, or orbits, and has a relatively smooth floor. Its posterior limit is bounded by the sharp and prominent lesser sphenoidal wings, sweeping out to the right and left. The middle fossa, lodging the temporal lobes, lies behind and is itself bounded posteriorly by the proud petrous temporal bones, beyond which plunges the deep posterior cranial fossa containing the cerebellum, pons and medulla oblongata. It is perhaps surprising how ridged and grooved the base of the skull is, considering the delicacy of the material it is there to protect. The reader is recommended to take the opportunity to have a look inside the cranial vault of a skeleton if possible. Skeletons may often be found in physiotherapy departments, but this is not a reflection on waiting times!

A tough membrane lines the interior surface of the skull, the dura mater. This membrane is thrown into two major and fairly rigid folds: the first, the falx cerebri, lies vertically and runs front to back, lying in the groove between the two cerebral hemispheres; the second, the tentorium cerebelli, lies horizontally and separates the occipital lobes from the cerebellum. The tentorium has a gap in it anteriorly that allows the passage of the midbrain passing inferiorly. Within the margins of the falx and the tentorium lie the venous sinuses, a component of the blood drainage vessels of the brain.

The dura mater is one of three membranes, the meninges, surrounding the brain. The pia mater is a thin membrane that is closely adherent to the surface of the brain, and sandwiched between this and the dura is the arachnoid mater. The space between the pia and the arachnoid mater, the subarachnoid space, is filled with cerebrospinal fluid that bathes the central nervous system, circulating via the hollow ventricles within the brain and the central canal of the spinal cord. The subarachnoid space also contains the cerebral arteries and veins and the cranial nerves. The 'potential' space between the arachnoid and dura mater is called the subdural space, an important location for collections of blood after head trauma, which may also collect in the subarachnoid space.

The brain is supplied by two main arterial sources, the vertebral and carotid arteries. These two systems link up (anastomose) in the brain, and their smaller and smaller offshoots penetrate throughout the brain substance in the vast network of vessels that is required to deliver oxygen to the demanding tissues. This demand equates to 20% of the heart's blood output at any one time. These fragile vessels may be torn by the shearing forces common in head injury, leading to collections of free blood within the brain substance. This, in turn, may lead to the death of the brain tissue supplied by that artery, and to problems with compression of surviving brain tissue, due to the space taken up by the blood clot.

The brain itself can be divided up into the forebrain, midbrain and hindbrain. The forebrain is made up of the cerebrum and diencephalon. The cerebrum has many important functions, including those related to motor coordination and perception, and is very vulnerable to injury due to its large surface area and exposed position. The cerebrum is composed of two cerebral hemispheres, which run from the frontal to the occipital bones, and are separated by a midline cleft, the longitudinal fissure, into which projects the falx cerebri. The surface layer of the hemispheres is called the cortex, otherwise known as the 'grey matter'. This grey matter, made up of a concentration of nerve cells, is thrown into convolutions. The recesses are called sulci and the corresponding peninsulas of tissue, gyri. The surface area of the cortex is thus greatly enlarged, about two-thirds of the total surface area being hidden in the sulci. Logic dictates that direct injury to the brain will affect the 'external' gyri more than the sulci but, as will be indicated in the next section, the exposure of the brain to the bones of the skull is only one factor in producing damage to the tissues.

A number of large sulci subdivide each hemisphere into lobes that are named according to the bones of the skull under which they lie. There are thus pairs of frontal, temporal, parietal and occipital lobes (see Figure 2.2). An overview of the function of these lobes is given in Table 2.1. This is useful information when presented with acutely injured patients and their head scans, as it helps predict the functions that are likely to be compromised. However, it is worth noting that the severity of a head injury, in terms of functional outcome, cannot be directly related to the extent of damage seen on the scan, as some individuals with extensive damage can do surprisingly well, and others with fairly normal looking scans can face a lifetime of problems.

The diencephalon is embedded within the mass of the brain, and is largely made up of the thalamus and hypothalamus. The midbrain is a smaller structure, being the part that passes through the hole in the tentorium, connecting the forebrain to the hindbrain, and is therefore vulnerable to being squeezed if the pressure rises in the cranium above the tentorium, after an injury. Finally, the hindbrain is made up three regions, the pons, medulla oblongata and the cerebellum. The cerebellum is the bulbous, cauliflower-

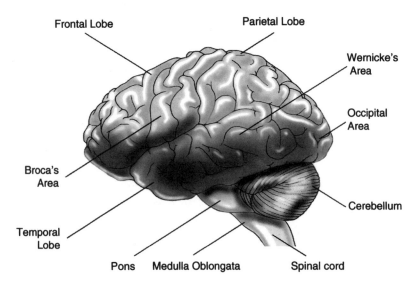

Figure 2.2. Lateral view of the brain. (Drawn by PM Ball, Senior Medical Artist, University of Cambridge.)

Table 2.1. Brief guide to functions of the cerebral hemispheres
The left hemisphere is 'dominant' in right-handed people and in up to 75% of left handed people. The non-dominant hemisphere deals with visual and spatial perception and visual (non-language dependent) memory. The dominant hemisphere deals with language and language-dependent memory.

Lobe	Function	Result of damage
Frontal	Movement of face, arm, leg, trunk Broca's area, dominant side, expressive area for speech Head and eye turning Personality, initiative Inhibition of emptying of bowel and bladder	Mono/hemiplegia Expressive dysphasia Disinhibition Poor judgement Emotional lability Apathy Indifference Poor abstract thought Unwillingness to move Incontinence Sparse verbal output
Parietal	Sensation Appreciation of posture, touch, passive movement Auditory and visual comprehension Spatial awareness (non-dominant) Calculation (dominant) Transit of visual pathways	Disturbance of posture, passive movement, localization of touch, object recognition through touch Sensory inattention Receptive dysphasia Visual field defect
Temporal	Hearing of language, music, rhythm and sounds Learning and memory Smell Behaviour Transit of visual pathways	Deafness Receptive dysphasia Difficulty hearing music Auditory hallucinations Memory/learning disturbance Aggressive or antisocial behaviour Difficulty laying down new memories
Occipital	Perception of vision	Visual field defect Blindness

shaped part sitting at the back of the brain, and is concerned with the control of muscle tone and balance. The midbrain, pons and medulla oblongata, being central structures, are relatively protected from direct and indirect injury. Damage to these areas indicates severe trauma and is often associated with a high mortality rate.

The brain substance itself can be divided in to two main tissue components, the grey and white matter. This firm grey matter is made up of a concentration of nerve cells, whereas the white matter is softer and is composed of an intercommunicating system of nerve fibres, and is supported by the scaffolding of the brain, the neuroglia. There are many different types of specialized neurone within the brain, each one consisting of a cell body, a nucleus and one or more processes (dendrites), which receive impulses, and one axon that propagates the impulse. These axons make up part of the inter-communicating fibre system of the white matter. Axons vary in both length and diameter, the longest being over one metre in length, whereas others are so short as to be microscopic. Where nerve cell bodies are clustered together, as found in the grey matter, the brain tissue is relatively solid and strong, whereas the fibre tracts of the white matter have a less robust architecture, and are thus more prone to certain types of injury.

Mode and mechanism of brain injury

Head injury may be direct or indirect. Indirect damage is caused by ischaemic insult (inadequate blood flow) or hypoxic insult (inadequate oxygenation) to the brain as a result of injury to other body parts. This may be secondary to loss of blood, causing low blood pressure, or failure of the maintenance of adequate blood oxygenation such as might occur after severe chest injury. It has been reliably demonstrated that about 90% of people that die from multiple injuries have evidence of ischaemic brain damage at post mortem, highlighting the importance of fast and effective roadside management of the emergency basics, airway, breathing and circulation.

Direct brain injury is motion related. The head may accelerate or decel-erate precipitously, such as during a sudden stop in a vehicle when the traveller is restrained by a seat-belt, or it may be propelled into a hard surface, such as the road, when a rider comes off a motorbike. Further mechanisms include being struck by a moving object such as a cosh during an assault or, more unusually, being struck at high speed by a missile such as a bullet. Associated scalp lacerations may contribute significantly to blood loss, and skull fractures may act as portals of entry for infection.

Brain injury consequent to an impact may be divided in to two distinct

Table 2.2. Primary and secondary brain damage

Primary brain damage	Cortical contusion and laceration
	Diffuse axonal injury
Secondary brain damage	Haematoma formation
	Brain swelling
	Brain shift
	Ischaemia
	Infection

etiological groups, called primary and secondary damage (see Table 2.2). Primary damage is a direct result of the impact whereas secondary damage is caused by the complications of the trauma.

Primary brain damage

Two main types of pathology are produced, which often coexist: cortical contusion (bruising) and laceration; and diffuse axonal injury.

Cortical contusion and laceration

The brain surface may be bruised or even torn by the impact. Contusions may occur either directly under the point of impact (coup), or on the opposite part of the brain (contre-coup), due to violent movement of the brain within the skull vault. Contusions are most common on the summits of the gyri, with the tips of the temporal lobes and the inferior surfaces of the frontal lobes appearing to be the most vulnerable areas (Mendelow et al., 1983). The closely adherent pia is often torn, resulting in a degree of subarachnoid haemorrhage. Contusions are often multiple, but do not in themselves contribute to loss of consciousness – this is caused by the second type of pathology to be described, diffuse axonal injury. Lacerations may occur through penetrating injury, or the sharp, bony projections of the interior of the skull vault may slice through the delicate tissues as they impinge upon them. The presence of lacerated brain tissue is a risk factor for the subsequent development of seizures.

Diffuse axonal injury

This occurs as a result of acceleration/deceleration of the brain within its rigid box. The brain may be subject to rotation that results in a swirling motion generating substantial mechanical shearing forces on the fragile axons of the white matter. Tearing of these axons occurs. The worst hit areas are often the interfaces between tissue masses of differential density and therefore strength – for example the clumps of nuclear masses will fare better than the surrounding axons they serve. It is these shearing injuries within the deep white matter that result in impairment of consciousness. Minute scattered haemorrhages may be present throughout the brain tissue indicative of patchy destruction of inter-communicating networks of neural tissue. Nerve fibres that have been shorn, now deprived of their nutrient supply, die and wither away along their entire length, and their protective myelin coats degenerate. This explains the atrophied appearance of the brain a few months down the track after severe diffuse axonal injury. This process may give the false impression of ventricular enlargement when it is actually the surrounding brain tissue that has shrunk.

It is important to stress the point that unconsciousness induced by trauma is a direct result of axonal injury and thus each 'knock-out', however short lived, is associated with neuronal damage. Neuronal regeneration is limited, hence the effects of repeated minor trauma are cumulative.

Secondary brain damage

This may start at any time after the initial injury has occurred and is a direct result of it. In contrast to primary injury, secondary damage is potentially preventable if good emergency and intensive care is available soon after the injury. The action of paramedics, accident and emergency and neurosurgical staff is therefore geared towards minimizing these complications.

The main intracranial causes of injury are the formation of a haematoma (blood clot), brain swelling, brain shift, ischaemia and infection.

Haematoma formation

Haematomas may occur either outside the dura (extradural), or inside (intradural). Extradural bleeds are due to tearing of the middle meningeal vessels in association with skull fracture. This causes release of blood into the extradural space. Intradural bleeds can involve both the intracerebral +/- subdural spaces. Subdural bleeds are sometimes the only obvious manifestation of a head injury. They may be caused by the rupture of bridging veins connecting the cortical surfaces to the venous sinuses, resulting in a subdural collection of blood.

These collections of blood may appear immediately or develop over the course of days. They cause secondary damage by either direct pressure on the brain substance or as a result of brain shift and herniation.

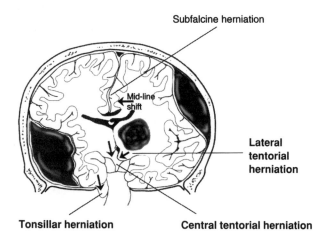

Figure 2.3. Examples of brain herniation. (Drawn by PM Ball, Senior Medical Artist, University of Cambridge.)

Brain swelling, shift and herniation (see Figure 2.3)

Brain swelling may occur either with or without intracranial haematoma formation, and is the result of a complex series of physiological responses to the trauma. These responses can set off a chain reaction that may ultimately exacerbate the situation, potentially resulting in brain shift and herniation. Herniation is a grave situation and refers to the extrusion of a portion of brain tissue down a path of least resistance, in response to a rise in pressure within an unaccommodating skull. If not reversed swiftly, death ensues.

Ischaemia

Cerebral ischaemia is a common event after brain injury and is caused by either hypoxia (low blood oxygen) or impaired cerebral perfusion. A normally functioning brain responds to a fall in blood pressure by 'auto regulating' and maintaining the head of pressure within the brain. After injury this mechanism is lost resulting in a drop in cerebral perfusion. This particularly affects the border zones of areas supplied by the major cerebral arteries.

Infection

Skull fracture with dural tear provides a portal of entry for bacteria, but this seldom happens within the first 48 hours after injury. Meningitis or cerebral abscess may ensue after months or even years.

Measuring severity and outcome after head injury

Patients with head injuries can broadly be categorized into three main groups: mild, moderate and severe. The outcome for each individual is strongly related to his initial grading, although as always there are exceptions, with patients with severe injuries recovering beyond all expectation and a minority with mild head injuries finding their lives to have been wrecked by post-concussional symptoms.

Severity and outcome of a head injury are related to both length and depth of coma and duration of post-traumatic amnesia (PTA). Patients are said to be in a coma when they do not open their eyes, obey commands or utter understandable words. Post-traumatic amnesia may be defined as 'the number of days elapsing between the injury and reinstatement of continuous day-to-day memory, as demonstrated by recall of specific items of information not of immediate relevance to the subject that had formally been presented to the subject on the previous day'. Longer periods of coma and PTA are associated with poorer outcomes. The depth of coma is graded on the commonly used Glasgow Coma Scale (GCS). This was developed by Teasdale and Jennett in 1974, and has been absorbed into everyday practice to provide a universal language for accurate description of brain injury severity. The scale has been reported as valid, sensitive and reliable, and is scored on a

Table 2.3. Glasgow Coma Scale

Score	Eye opening response
4	Spontaneous
3	To speech
2	To painful stimulus
1	None
	Best motor response in upper limbs
6	Obeys commands
5	Localizes
4	Withdraws (normal flexion)
3	Flexes abnormally (spastic flexion)
2	Extends
1	None
	Verbal response
5	Orientated
4	Confused
3	Inappropriate words
2	Incomprehensible sounds
1	None

points system. It is outlined in Table 2.3.

The scale gives valuable information with regard to both improvement and decline in the patient's condition, such as occurs with the onset of secondary complications. A state of coma is operationally defined as a GCS of eight or less for a period of six hours or longer. If the GCS remains at eight or less in the first few days after injury, this correlates with a poor outcome at six months. Prediction of outcome from the GCS alone is likely to be unreliable when applied to brief periods of coma, but is more accurate with more severe injuries. Bond (1986) defined criteria that are now widely accepted as classifying severity of trauma according to the GCS, and are set out in Table 2.4.

Duration of PTA correlates well with GCS rating. As defined above, PTA is characterized by the inability to lay down new memories from day to day. A PTA of greater than 14 days is associated with a significant likelihood of persisting deficits in cognitive and behavioural function (Brooks et al., 1987). It should be noted that both the GCS and the assessment of PTA will be influenced if the patient is sedated for any period of time, as occurs when ventilation is required. Other factors such as alcohol can also have a bearing on the assessment.

Table 2.4. Severity of head injury according to Glasgow Coma score

Mild	GCS 13 - 15, <= 20 minutes coma duration
Moderate	GCS 9 - 12, no longer than six hours coma duration
Severe	GCS <= 8, > six hours coma duration

Seeking out this information about patients, even at the stage of community rehabilitation, is useful as it is a helpful indicator of the severity of the original injury, and if gathered systematically may be used to provide a valuable insight into long-term outcomes in these individuals.

An outcome scale was developed by Jennett, and is known as the Glasgow Outcome Scale (Jennett and Bond, 1975). This scale is commonly used to describe outcome in publications, but alternative instruments such as the Disability Rating Scale (Rappaport et al., 1982) are also used. The Glasgow Outcome Scale is outlined in Table 2.5.

Table 2.5. Glasgow Outcome Scale

Score	Outcome
1	Death
2	Vegetative state
3	Severe disability, conscious but dependent
4	Moderate disability, independent but disabled
5	Good recovery

Each state in this scale covers a huge range of disabilities, a shortcoming that alternative scales attempt to address with varying degrees of success. The vegetative state will be expanded later.

From head injury to rehabilitation – the patient pathway

As already indicated, patients with head injury can present with a range of problems, but for ease of description the management of head injury will be described from the perspective of the severe case scenario. Management of mild head injuries may just involve observation in hospital overnight. The potential complications of mild head injury will be described later.

Trivial head injuries are defined by exclusion of the features set out in Table 2.6, and most accident and emergency departments and general practice surgeries would use these criteria in their assessment process.

Table 2.6. Criteria defining non-trivial head injuries

Loss of consciousness
Presence of neurological symptoms or signs
Blood or cerebrospinal fluid leakage from ear or nose
Suspicion of penetrating injury
Significant scalp bruising or swelling

If any of these features are present, then the injury is automatically not trivial and should be treated accordingly. Patients with trivial injuries can be sent home with suitable advice with regard to reporting back if anything changes, such as the development of double vision, headache, drowsiness or vomiting. If this occurs a further re-evaluation is required to exclude, in particular, the delayed development of intracranial haemorrhage.

In order to demonstrate the acute-care pathway, it is helpful to illustrate with a case scenario:

> M, a 20 year old male, was returning home at 4 AM after a night out when he lost control of his car on a shallow bend and hit a tree. M was found by the attending Ambulance crew to be in a confused and agitated state, still in the driver's seat of the car. Blood was oozing from an obvious boggy swelling on the left side of his head, and clear fluid was slowly trickling from his left nostril. M's condition rapidly deteriorated and he soon lapsed in to an unconscious state. His airway was protected and M was rapidly transferred to the local Accident and Emergency department for further management.

In this case, the worrying feature is the rapid transition from a confused, agitated patient to one that is unconscious. This obviously indicates fairly dramatic, acute compromise of brain function that could be due, for instance, to a collection of blood in the extradural space that will need prompt attention if herniation is to be prevented. The leakage of the clear fluid from the nostril indicates basal skull fracture in the region of the anterior fossa, and instantly raises the odds of infection being a secondary problem in this patient.

Accident and emergency department management

M will be transferred to the resuscitation room where immediate medical assessment will take place according to the ABCDE principles of basic life support:

- A for *airway.* The airway is checked for obstruction, foreign bodies removed and secretions sucked out.
- B for *breathing.* The adequacy of breathing is assessed clinically and by blood analysis, and the chest is checked for injuries. In M's case, a patient in an unconscious state, it is likely that he would have a tube inserted into his trachea and be ventilated immediately.
- C for *circulation.* The pulse rate, respiratory rate and other clinical indicators of the adequacy of circulation are checked. Blood pressure is a poor indicator of early blood loss, thus if the patient has a low blood pressure it is highly likely that some other injury such as a ruptured spleen has occurred. Appropriate fluid resuscitation will be instituted.

- D for *dysfunction*. An assessment using the Glasgow Coma Scale is made, and repeated every 10 to 15 minutes until the patient is deemed to be stable. Pupil size and reaction to light is measured at similar intervals, as well as pulse, respiratory rate and blood pressure. In M's case, with his rapid deterioration in condition at the scene, it is likely that his intracranial pressure is rapidly rising, and urgent management of this is required. The head is examined carefully for evidence of injury, and scalp lacerations carefully explored for evidence of a depressed fracture (a fragment of bone pushed down into the brain). The ears and nose are checked for CSF leakage – M has CSF leaking from his nose due to an anterior fossa fracture, but if the fracture had been in the petrous bone, CSF might be seen tracking from the ear. Each limb is assessed for weakness by comparing the response to a painful stimulus in the unconscious patient. The finding of limb weakness does not help in localizing the site of the trouble within the brain, as herniation may produce ipsilateral (same side) limb weakness.
- E for *exposure*. All of M's clothing would be removed and he would be checked from head to toe for associated injuries. Abdominal and bony injuries, such as fractures of the pelvis or femur, can be associated with life-threatening blood loss, so a judgement has to be made with regard to injuries and the order in which they are managed.

In the immediate post-resuscitation period, the heart rate is continuously monitored, as are the other vital signs plus the GCS. Appropriate investigations are performed, such as x-rays of the skull, cervical spine, chest and anything else indicated by the examination process. Computerized tomography scans are usually readily available for this sort of patient in most hospitals of a district general standing, and the head will be scanned as a matter of urgency.

Each region has a nominated neurosurgical unit to which referrals can be made. A patient such as M would be discussed with the on-call neurosurgical team and transferred as soon as practicable.

It is common to find that a patient such as M would start to fit in the acute stage after injury. This is usually controlled by using the drug phenytoin, which has the benefit of not depressing the breathing pattern adversely. Fits following head injury will be discussed in more detail in a later section.

Operative intervention

Most intracranial haematomas require urgent surgical evacuation in order to preserve life. The part of the brain affected is accessed via a bone flap, and the clot gently removed, along with any intracerebral blood clot and necrotic (dead) brain tissue that is present.

Some patients with very small haematomas can be managed conservatively, without resorting to operation, but they have to be observed very closely to ensure they do not deteriorate.

Management in the neuro-critical care unit (NCCU)

This sort of unit is an intensive care unit specifically for patients with neuro-surgical problems such as head injury, subarachnoid haemorrhage or tumour. Following head injury, one of the prime difficulties can be in the adequate control of the fluid pressures that exist within the body, which have a complex interrelation that can be grossly disturbed after injury. The key is to keep the head of pressure adequate to drive enough oxygenated blood through the brain to meet its needs, without allowing the pressure within the bony skull to rise so high that a vicious circle of pressure rise and resultant brain swelling is created. This is a tricky process, and requires the use of specialist monitoring equipment. The bony flap removed after craniotomy is not immediately replaced because of these very problems. Having a large hole in the head can be useful because some of the pressure can dissipate through it. Often the flap is not replaced until at least six months after the acute event, by which time everything should have settled down. In patients that require ventilation for prolonged periods it is usual practice to convert to a 'tracheostomy'. This involves having the ventilation tube passing directly through the skin in the region of the neck below the voice box, rather than down the trachea via the mouth.

Nutrition needs to be attended to carefully as patients rapidly enter a catabolic state (a state of tissue breakdown in response to stress) after severe trauma. Feeding via a nasogastric (Ng) tube is initiated early, but if it is predicted that the patient will not be capable of swallowing safely for many weeks a percutaneous gastrostomy tube is inserted. This involves passing a feeding tube directly through the abdominal wall into the stomach. In general, these 'Peg' tubes are easier to manage than 'Ng' tubes, and are certainly more comfortable for the patient.

There are many other factors that need to be considered in the immediate aftermath of a head injury. Patients confined to bed for long periods are prone to complications such as chest infections, skin breakdown, contractures of immobilized/paralysed limbs and deep vein thrombosis. The early rehabilitation of these patients is therefore directed at preventing these complications, and neurophysiotherapists and occupational therapists are involved as early as the NCCU setting. The common physical complications of head injury are dealt with in the following chapter.

Each patient's acute-care pathway will be different, with varying amounts of time being spent in the NCCU. Patients are discharged from NCCU to the neurosurgical ward and, when stable, are then sent back to the referring hospital. This is often far from ideal, as they are frequently looked after either on orthopaedic or general surgical wards, depending on the policy of the hospital. Having a confused, cognitively impaired head-injured patient sitting in the middle of a busy acute ward is not appropriate, but it still happens and will continue to do so until better facilities are provided. The best option would be for the patient to stay under the care of the neurosurgeons until a direct discharge to a suitable rehabilitation facility is possible. This approach has been recommended in a report by the Royal College of Surgeons (1999), but has significant cost and resource implications that are unlikely to be resolved quickly.

Some patients can be discharged directly home from the neurosurgical ward. This is acceptable as long as the patient's local rehabilitation service has been informed – just because patients are able to walk out of hospital this does not automatically imply that they have no problems. It is this cohort of patients – physically well, but with cognitive/emotional disturbance after a head injury, which often get 'lost' to the system, only to reappear to community services via their GP, having lost their jobs and with personal relationships in tatters. Close liaison with the regional neurosurgical unit is essential to prevent this from happening.

Management of the aftermath of traumatic head injury

The sequelae of head injury are diverse, with no two patients exhibiting exactly the same problems. As a result of this, each patient's rehabilitation programme has to be tailored to his individual needs, requiring great flexibility in the approach used. Some of the more common physical aspects of head injury that require ongoing attention in the community are dealt with in Chapter 3. A range of other medical considerations are dealt with here.

Post-concussion syndrome

This syndrome tends to follow head injuries at the milder end of the spectrum. Even a short period of unconsciousness may result in neuronal damage, and a third of patients with this type of injury will have symptoms lasting longer than six months (Bullock and Teasdale, 1990). Headache is a prominent feature, with tension headache accounting for 85% of all the headaches, with most of the remainder being associated with neck injury, occipital neuralgia (lancinating pains in the back of the head due to nerve irritation), migraine, cluster headache or injury to the tempero-mandibular joint (jaw joint) (Mandel, 1989). The features of this syndrome are listed in Table 2.7.

Table 2.7. Features of the post-concussion syndrome

Headache
Dizziness and balance problems
Impaired concentration
Impaired memory
Fatigue
Anxiety
Depression
Irritability
Indecisiveness
Impaired self-confidence
Lack of drive
Impaired libido
Alcohol intolerance

Predictive features for the development of this syndrome are: age greater than 40 years, female sex, low IQ, low socio-economic status, previous head injury, multiple trauma and history of alcohol abuse. The duration of PTA, CT scan appearances and specialized brainstem function tests are not predictive. Problems remaining at three months post injury can be predicted from a combination of emotional, organic and neuropsychological measures tested at seven to 10 days post injury (King, 1996), but the strength of prediction using these tests is diminished by six months (King et al., 1999). The Rivermead Post Concussion Symptoms Questionnaire is a useful tool for measuring the severity of the post-concussion symptoms (King et al., 1995).

Specific treatment for these symptoms is lacking, but symptomatic treatments can improve the overall picture. These include good control of pain and the restoration of a normal sleep pattern. A combination of advice and the judicious use of antidepressants can improve sleep and may also serve to help to reduce irritability and improve attention. Another key measure is support and reassurance for both the patient and his family, including advice about when and how to approach a return to work. There is no basis to the concept that these symptoms are born out of seeking compensation for the accident.

Post-traumatic stress disorder (PTSD) may be part of the clinical picture and is covered more fully in Chapter 5.

Post-traumatic epilepsy

Epilepsy after a head injury can develop as an early or late complication. Early epilepsy occurs within the first week of the trauma, and may develop in the range of 2.5% to 7% of unselected patients admitted to hospital (Annegers et al., 1980; Jennett, 1975). It is commonest in patients with a compound, depressed fracture of the skull, patients with an intracranial haematoma and those who subsequently turn out to have a prolonged PTA. Fits most commonly occur in the first 24 hours after injury. The seizures may be either focal or generalized. Status epilepticus (ongoing fitting that does not terminate naturally) may occur in up to 10% of cases. It is essential that fitting is adequately controlled as it may contribute to further brain damage due to poor brain oxygenation during the fit.

Late epilepsy occurs in approximately 5% of all patients admitted to hospital with head injury (Jennett, 1975b). It is commonest in patients with early epilepsy (25%), intracranial haematoma (35%) and compound depressed fracture (17%). Most of those destined to develop fits will do so in the first year after injury, but some may do so many years later. Generalized fits are the commonest presentation, but complex-partial seizures (local seizures, with any degree of impairment of consciousness) are also seen.

Treatment

Anticonvulsant drugs are commonly prescribed as a prophylactic measure in head-injured patients. The drug most commonly used is phenytoin, as this can be given intravenously and is an effective drug. This has been

Table 2.8. Commonly used drugs in epilepsy after head injury

Drug	Potential side effects
Phenytoin	Thickening of gums Hirsutism Acne Coarsening of facial features At toxic levels: Double vision Unsteadiness of gait Twitching eye movements (nystagmus)
Carbamazepine	Gastrointestinal upset Unsteadiness of gait Skin rash Bone-marrow suppression Antidiuretic effect
Sodium valproate	Gastrointestinal upset Low blood-platelet count (bleeding risk) Drug-induced liver inflammation Hair loss Tremor/involuntary movements

demonstrated to reduce the incidence of fits from 14 % to 5% within the first week (Schierhout and Roberts, 1998), but it has not been shown to prevent fits after one week. It should be remembered that all anticonvulsants have a side-effect profile, and the side effects of the most commonly used drugs are listed in Table 2.8. One side effect that is particularly worrying with respect to the rehabilitation of the patient is the potential for cognitive blunting by anticonvulsants. Phenytoin may be more implicated than carbamazepine in this respect, hence patients are often converted to carbamazepine from phenytoin after the acute phase.

Hydrocephalus

Dilatation of the cerebral ventricles is relatively common after severe head injury and may be due either to cerebral atrophy (loss of brain tissue mass) or true hydrocephalus. True hydrocephalus may be defined as an excessive accumulation of cerebrospinal fluid (CSF) within the head due to a disturbance of its secretion, flow or absorption. It is likely that the presence of debris such as blood or dead brain tissue, or the presence of meningitis, all of which result in an inflammatory reaction, combine to impede the free flow of CSF around the system. When CSF production exceeds resorption, hydrocephalus is the inevitable result. Hydrocephalus may be either communicating or non-communicating (obstructive) according to the site of the blockage. Communicating hydrocephalus indicates that there is flow to a level beyond the fourth ventricle, whereas non-communicating indicates that flow is obstructed at the level of the ventricular system i.e. higher up. Communicating hydrocephalus is more common after head injury.

Hydrocephalus may happen sub-acutely, in the weeks after the head injury, and can easily be demonstrated by sequential enlargement of the ventricular system on successive CT scans. Hydrocephalus occurring later becomes more difficult to assess on scan, especially in the face of brain atrophy.

The incidence of post-traumatic hydrocephalus has been reported to occur in anything from 8% to 72% of head injured patients, depending on the criteria used for its determination. Symptomatic hydrocephalus is thankfully much less common, requiring operative intervention in roughly 1% to 4% of the head-injury population (Pickard, 1997).

Clinical presentation

The classical presenting features of idiopathic hydrocephalus of dementia, gait disturbance and incontinence are not useful determinants in patients after head injury because these characteristics are frequently seen in this patient group in the absence of hydrocephalus. Relying on regression in progress to trigger investigation for hydrocephalus is also not reliable because some recovery from acute head injury can be seen even in patients with advanced hydrocephalus. Thus the only way to ensure that this treatable condition is not missed early in the rehabilitation phase is to maintain vigilance, and scan promptly if there is doubt. Patients in whom regression in status occurs are easier to spot and respond to in a timely fashion. The likelihood of reversing symptoms associated with hydrocephalus is better the shorter the duration of the hydrocephalus.

Detection of hydrocephalus

Although scanning will pick up the obvious cases, sometimes it is necessary to measure the pressures within the system directly by monitoring the intracranial pressure over 24 hours, or by doing special CSF flow studies in combination with scanning. As inserting a shunt is not a procedure to be undertaken lightly, it is important to maximize the chances of a successful response to shunting by gathering as much information as possible beforehand.

Shunting

The purpose of a shunt is to divert CSF from the ventricular system into a suitable cavity, in order for decompression to occur. The cavity most often used is the peritoneal cavity (within the abdominal cavity), hence the term ventriculo-peritoneal shunt (VP shunt). A reservoir can often be palpated on the back of the patient's head somewhere, and the tube traced down the neck before disappearing down behind the clavicle (collar bone). These tubes can occasionally cause some local discomfort, and any skin sepsis near the tube should be treated thoroughly. If a patient with a VP shunt *in situ* has peritonitis, for example from appendicitis, there is always the risk of infection ascending the tube and causing infection within the ventricles. There are a number of different types of shunt, some of the newer versions being computer programmable to allow alteration in the flow rate even after the shunt has been inserted.

Complications of shunting for hydrocephalus

The infection risk of a shunt has already been alluded to. Other complications include subdural haematoma formation, the development of a low-pressure state if the shunt is working too effectively (manifesting as headache and vomiting on attaining an upright posture) and shunt failure. Research has indicated that up to 81% of shunts will fail within 12 years (Sainte Rose, Hoffmann and Hirsch, 1989).

Cranioplasty

Patients that have required a craniotomy are usually advised that they will be left with their defect for at least six months after the original operation. This is in order to let the intracranial pressures settle down and to avoid precipitating further morbidity through premature closure. It is common for patients in the community phase of their rehabilitation process to become increasingly concerned about their residual cranial defect. The concerns are usually about either the cosmetic appearance or the vulnerability of the brain without the protective bone in place.

For patients with a large defect, or for those with mobility problems or undertaking activity that may put them at risk of injury via the defect (including vehicle travel), a protective helmet is recommended. This can often be supplied through the local surgical appliances department and is usually a fairly lightweight item, incorporating a solid plate measured to cover the defect.

Pain around the bony edge of the defect is a common complaint. This usually requires no specific treatment other than advice about analgesia, non-steroidal anti-inflammatory drugs being particularly useful. Similarly, pain can be a feature after the defect has been repaired, and this usually settles with time. The defect is usually repaired either by using the patient's original bony flap (if it is in good condition, and has been preserved), or by a synthetic plate. The operation is not without its risks, which will be explained to the patient by the neurosurgeon.

Pain management

Pain is a common complaint in the head-injured population and may arise from many sources, for example the musculoskeletal system, due to changes in demand placed upon it through muscle weakness or changes in tone. Headache is also a common complaint and, as has been stated, pain around cranioplasty sites is not unusual. As in the general population, the management of pain should follow the usual principles of pain management: a good history should be taken as to the site, nature and course of the pain, followed by a thorough examination and then institution of a management plan. Pain does not always require medication. For instance, pain arising from contracted muscles and tendons may respond to a programme of stretching, and the judicious use of orthoses may provide enough stability about a joint to relieve the pain from overstretched ligaments. Thus physical measures to relieve pain should always be considered.

Pain always has a psychological component to it and will be exacerbated if the pain is associated with fear or anxiety. It is important to ensure that the patient is not worrying that his headache is heralding further damage to his brain even if a mechanism for this seems obscure to the observer. It really is worth exploring this carefully, as simple reassurance may be enough to rid the patient of a disabling symptom.

If analgesics are required, then the 'analgesic ladder' is generally followed. This involves using the least potent painkillers first, and changing the drug to one of a greater potency in a stepwise fashion if the analgesic requirements are not met. For example, paracetamol is the drug of first choice for mild pain, but if this proves to be inadequate, a trial of a non-steroidal anti-inflammatory drug (NSAID) may be used. Drugs of increasing potency are thereafter tried, aiming for a balance between therapeutic benefit whilst keeping side effects within acceptable limits (such as constipation with codeine-based drugs). Another approach is the use of physical methods, such as the use of transcutaneous electrical nerve stimulation (TENS) machines, which pass a small electrical current through the skin to disguise pain signals to the brain.

Cranial central pain syndromes (CCPS)

Cranial central pain syndromes are defined as 'pain secondary to injury of the intracranial central nervous system' and were first described by Dejerine and Roussy on 1906 in association with thalamic stroke. More recent studies have indicated that this type of pain may be generated through lesions to parts of the brain other than the thalamus, the common feature being injury to pathways involved in pain and temperature signalling – the spinothalamic tract. The diagnosis of CCPS is made on finding clinical or radiological evidence of brain injury plus clinical evidence of decreased discrimination of pain and temperature sensation. There may well be a delay in the manifestation of this condition, which might therefore present to the community rehabilitation team.

The nature of the pain is described in different ways, the commonest description being 'burning'. Other terms used are: aching, lancinating, pricking, lacerating, pressing, shooting, squeezing, throbbing, cutting, crushing, splitting, stinging, icy, sore, stabbing, cramping, smarting and pulling (Leijon and Boivie, 1989).

Treatment of this distressing disorder is difficult and often unsatisfactory. Tricyclic drugs such as amitriptyline (in smaller doses than those required for an anti-depressant effect) are the only drugs to have been of proven worth in well-constructed trials. Anti-epileptic drugs such as gabapentin, carbamazepine, phenytoin and valproate, are also used, and may be the best choice for pain that is paroxysmal. Currently, gabapentin would be many clinicians' first-line choice. Local anaesthetics and opiates are also in the armamentarium, and specialized techniques such as electrical stimulation of the brain or spinal cord have also been used, as well as the simpler cutaneous stimulation used in

TENS. Rarely, localized neuro-surgery is performed in selected cases. Multidisciplinary input involving aerobic exercise, relaxation techniques, psychological support and physical therapies such as hot/cold treatments are all worth using. The involvement of the local pain management service in patients with recalcitrant pain problems is essential, and links should be forged with the service.

Endocrine problems after head injury

Problems resulting from pituitary gland dysfunction after head trauma usually manifest in the acute stages after head injury, and are therefore 'past history' by the time a patient reaches the community setting. However, it is worth remembering that symptoms and signs of hypopituitarism (reduced pituitary functioning) may develop very insidiously over time, taking months or years to develop, which is why it is important to bear this complication in mind in the community rehabilitation setting. The most likely manifestation of this would be a condition called hypogonadotrophic hypogonadism. This is a defect in the production of sex hormones by the anterior part of the pituitary gland. A steady failure of hormone production may eventually manifest as impotence in the male, with infertility, loss of libido and genital atrophy in both sexes, associated with scanty periods in the female. If the diagnosis is confirmed, treatment with suitable hormone replacement can be initiated. The help of an endocrinologist is strongly recommended.

It should be noted that the initial absence of periods (amenorrhoea) in females after head injury is a relatively common feature in the absence of damage to the pituitary gland, and is likely to be a response to the stress of the trauma. The majority will resume normal cycles with time. Despite this, amenorrhoea with the associated low oestrogen levels is an important finding, as it has implications for loss of maintenance of bone mass in these individuals, mimicking the menopause in terms of the deleterious effect on the bones. If the same individual has motor impairment resulting in poor mobility, or is liable to fall over, it should be remembered that the threshold for bone fracture will be lower. It should also be remembered that amenorrhoea is not a guarantee of infertility, and that appropriate contraceptive measures should be used even if amenorrhoeic!

Pressure sores

Pressure sores are a product of immobility, a factor common in patients recovering from brain injury. Pressure sores not only retard the rehabilitation process, but also have the potential to kill through overwhelming sepsis or the development of secondary complications of long-term inflammation, an outcome all too frequently not appreciated. Prevention of pressure sores is far easier than healing them once they have occurred, and every effort should be made to stop them developing in the first place. Pressure sores are often referred to as 'bedsores'. This is an inappropriate term as they can develop from sitting in a wheelchair just as easily as from lying in bed. 'Pressure sores' also infers that they can occur at any time in the rehabilitation process, and are not just an acute hospital phenomenon.

Pressure sores are formed when the forces of pressure, shear and friction on the skin over a bony prominence cause failure of blood supply to the skin resulting in local tissue damage and death. Exposure of the skin to urine and faeces is an exacerbating factor, as well as intrinsic factors such as acute illness, poor nutrition, dehydration, fever, low blood pressure and advancing age (Warren and Bennett, 1998). In bed-bound patients, sores are commonest on the sacral area, heels and sometimes the back of the head from pillow pressure. Seated patients tend to develop sores on the sacral area and the lateral aspects of the thighs where they rest against the sides of the wheelchair. In the normal situation, local skin pressures are not allowed to stay high for long, as a shift in body position occurs automatically, thus releasing the pressure. In unconscious or otherwise immobile patients, such as those with paralysis after brain injury, the individual is unable to automatically shift position in response to discomfort and therefore has to rely on vigilance, as well as specific management tools, to prevent pressure sores. Handling techniques are important, to prevent shear injuries from, for example, pulling the patient up the bed or further back into the seat of the wheelchair.

The key to preventing pressure sores is remembering the risk of their development in the first place. Various scoring systems have been developed to predict the risk involved, such as the Norton score, or the Waterlow (Bridel, 1993). Patients are then stratified according to risk and appropriate preventative measures are put into operation. The preventative measures used are as appropriate in the community as in the hospital setting and are outlined in Table 2.9. As an easy means of description, pressure sores may be graded as indicated in Table 2.10.

Treatment of pressure sores

The detailed treatment of sores is beyond the scope of this book but the main principle is one of pressure avoidance whilst the healing process is allowed to occur. Pressure sores soon become infected, which retards healing and brings with it the risk of septicaemia. Long-standing pressure sores can be associated with a condition known as amyloidosis that can affect the kidneys causing renal failure and subsequent death. Pressure sores are not to be taken lightly.

The development of a pressure sore is a disaster for the patient. Often patients are reluctant to adhere to advice regarding bedrest, especially if the rehabilitation programme is suspended in the meantime. However, all temptation to be lenient should be resisted – sores will not heal if subjected to ongoing pressure. A short period of bedrest in the initial stages of a sore (with appropriate positioning in relation to the sore), may well prevent months of misery and all the risks that infection in the sore brings.

Table 2.9. Basic measures for the prevention of pressure sores

Regular skin inspection
Regular position shift
Control of continence to ensure skin kept dry
Use of appropriate pressure care products such as mattresses/cushions
Use of appropriate patient handling techniques, such as glide sheets
Ensuring adequate nutrition

Table 2.10. Grading of pressure sores

Grade 1	Non-blanching erythema, skin intact.
Grade 2	Superficial skin break, involving epidermis or dermis.
Grade 3	Full thickness skin loss involving subcutaneous tissues.
Grade 4	Full thickness skin loss involving muscle, bone or tendon.

Bowel problems

General enquiry about habitual and current bowel habit in the head-injured patient is essential, as upset is a common result of the disruption to routine that occurs after head injury. It is surprising how often the patient's bowels are forgotten in the melee of an acute care/early rehabilitation programme, but most previously constipated patients will say it was the single most distressing symptom of the lot for them. Constipation makes patients feel bad and in no mood for rehabilitation! Loss of control of faecal continence is also highly distressing, demeaning and humiliating, and for the large part can be brought under fairly rapid control with a little common-sense management. Once a patient is back in the community, hopefully being nourished by a well-balanced diet with appropriate fibre content, his bowel habit can usually be 'normalized' once again without the need for intervention. A review of the drug list is essential, and liaison with the district nurse in difficult cases will usually result in success. For those patients unable to swallow, and therefore fed through a gastrostomy tube, some feeds used are well known to cause diarrhoea, so liaison with the dietician may be helpful.

Bladder problems

As with patients after stroke, voiding dysfunction is a frequent problem in the early stages after injury, but may continue and become a long-term issue. Impaired control of bladder function can have two major manifestations, either frequency or incontinence through the failure of the bladder to retain an adequate volume of urine or the failure of the bladder to empty properly resulting in urinary retention. Gelber et al. (1993) summarized the major mechanisms for post-stroke incontinence as being disruption of the neuromicturition pathway resulting in bladder hyperreflexia and urge incontinence; incontinence associated with cognitive and language deficits, with normal bladder function; and bladder hyporeflexia and overflow incontinence associated with concurrent neuropathy or medication. This summary is pertinent to post-head-injury patients also, and provides a useful way of thinking about the presenting problem.

Urethral catheterization is common in the early stages after head injury. It is necessary for monitoring of the output of urine and is also a necessity in an unconscious or sedated patient. The effect of the head injury on bladder control is therefore not known until the catheter is removed, and may be influenced by the presence of infection that is common in the catheterized patient. It is quite common for patients to require a prolonged period of bladder retraining before continence is once again established. In some instances, despite the above regime and exclusion of infection, the patient remains incontinent. In these individuals, it is worth performing an ultrasound of the renal tract to exclude overt pathology, and also to measure the volume of urine in the bladder after voiding. In normal individuals the bladder should empty completely, but retained volumes of greater than 100 ml require attention, as they predispose to infection and the formation of bladder stones. 'Urodynamics' – tests designed to examine the response of the bladder to filling with fluid via a catheter tube – are also useful. The most likely finding in head-injured patients will be a bladder that gets 'twitchy' at relatively low urine volumes, resulting in the desire to pass urine frequently. This twitchiness can be reduced by using drugs such as oxybutinin that help the bladder to retain more urine before signalling the need to empty.

Some patients will have ongoing bladder problems, not so much as a direct result of the head injury, but because they either had bladder problems previous to the injury or because of the treatment in the acute phase. An example of the former is the older male with benign prostatic hypertophy (enlarged prostate) causing outflow obstruction, or the female with long-term stress incontinence following childbirth. Establishing the previous history is therefore critical. Some men will be unfortunate enough to develop a stricture (tightening) in the urethra after catheterization, which can also impede bladder emptying. Using ultrasound to check on residual volumes in the bladder after micturition (urination) is thus a very useful approach.

Some patients will have sufficiently difficult problems with their bladder control that they require long-term catheterization. Excluding those with treatable outflow obstruction, this is most often seen in patients with significant cognitive impairment who are unable to comply with a bladder-training regime – frequently in those with frontal lobe damage. It is also necessary for those that have a level of disability that makes frequent transfer on to the bedpan or toilet impractical. Long-term catheterization is therefore seen in individuals at the more severe end of the head injury spectrum. It can create problems, and should only be resorted to when all other reasonable measures have failed. Infections, bladder stones and bypassing (leakage of urine around catheter) are all complications that may occur, with considerable associated morbidity. Sometimes, a suprapubic catheter is inserted, where the catheter tube is passed directly through the lower abdominal wall instead of the urethra. This has the advantage of being easier to keep clean, and easier to change. It is also more comfortable for the patient and avoids irritation of the urethra.

Bladder problems often take a long time to sort out, so they are often a feature of the patient in the community rehabilitation phase. As with bowel problems, bladder dysfunction is a cause of a lot of misery for patients, so every effort must be paid to achieving the best possible management plan.

Outcome after head injury

Head injury carries with it a significant mortality and morbidity rating, often affecting young men at the start of their lives. Of patients comatose for a period of greater than six hours, 40% will be dead within six months (Lindsay and Bone, 1997). Although the majority of recovery can be expected to be seen in the first six months after injury, further changes will be seen in the following months. A means of grading outcome is through using the Glasgow Outcome Scale, which has already been outlined. In general, about 40% of patients with severe injury will regain an independent existence, but this does not imply all will return to their previous social and occupational status. Less than 2% will be left in a vegetative state. Jennett et al. (1979) produced the following figures in Table 2.11.

There are a number of specific outcome issues that prove to be of great concern to some patients once they return to the community. One such issue is the return to driving. There are many obvious reasons why, following brain injury, a patient might be suspended from driving. These include cognitive impairment, physical impairment, visual disturbance, a tendency to experience seizures, and intracranial bleeding with or without operative intervention. When this issue arises, unless the answer is very clear cut with respect to the regulations governing return to driving, it is sensible to refer patients to one of the national driving assessment centres for expert assessment of their driving capabilities. Although the final decision about an individual still rests with the DVLA, their decision-making process is helped by the detailed assessment provided at these centres. It should be made clear that the legal responsibility lies with patients to inform the DVLA of their incapacity and often occupational therapy colleagues will take up this issue with patients and guide them through the administrative process required.

It is common for patients to express anger and discontent at a driving ban, in view of the social/occupational impact this may have on their lives. It is useful to remind them that the decision of the DVLA is based on the law, and that persuasive letters from either the doctor or the patient cannot sway the outcome.

As this issue is one that arises very often in community rehabilitation, it is considered in greater detail in Chapter 10, where more specific guidance on how rehabilitation staff should deal with clients who wish to return to driving is offered.

Another issue about which advice is often sought is when to return to sport after head injury. Aerobic exercise is beneficial in reversing the physical deconditioning that inevitably occurs after head injury due to disruption of normal patterns of physical activity. Return to non-contact sports is therefore a reasonable aim once a basic level of fitness has been acquired.

Contact sports are a different matter. Repeated head trauma is cumulative, hence sports that are liable to result in head trauma, such as boxing, rugby, jockeying and possibly even heading the ball in football, cannot be advised. If an individual decides to return to the sport against this advice, it is essential that the club or other appropriate officials be made aware of the individual's past history. However, this remains the responsibility of the patient.

Sexual problems after head injury are common and again it is an issue that causes great anxiety. This subject is a very important aspect in the rehabilitation of an individual, and is dealt with in the chapter on psychosocial issues.

Table 2.11. Outcome after head injury

	Poor outcome (GOS 1-3) (%)	Favourable outcome (GOS 4-5) (%)
Patients in coma >6 hrs	61	39
Best GCS >11	18	82
Best GCS 8-10	32	68
Best GCS <8	73	27
Pupillary response - reacting	50	50
Pupillary response - non-reacting	96	4
Age < 20 years	41	59
Age > 60 years	94	6

The vegetative state

Depending on the remit of the community team, it is quite possible that individuals diagnosed as being in a permanent vegetative state may be seen in either community hospitals or nursing homes by team members. The vegetative state is defined as 'a clinical condition of unawareness of self and environment in which the patient breathes spontaneously, has a stable circulation, and shows cycles of eye closure and opening which may simulate sleep and waking'. It has a wide range of causes, but head injury is probably the commonest. The condition came to the fore in the case of Tony Bland in 1993, when the High Court ruled that once a diagnosis of a permanent vegetative state had been made it was lawful to withhold active medical treatment.

It is usual to consider a person to be in a permanent vegetative state (PVS) if a period of 12 months has elapsed with no behavioural evidence of awareness of self or the environment. It is also vital to be certain that the situation of the patient will not change and cannot be altered. The drug list must be scrutinized and the patient re-examined after drug withdrawals as appropriate. Hydrocephalus is occasionally overlooked and should be excluded. The exact process of examination to establish unawareness is beyond the scope of this book, but involves testing all sensory modalities for meaningful response – hearing, vision, somatic awareness and motor response (Wade and Johnston, 1999).

The 'rehabilitation' of these patients is a rather depressing process as there is usually no prospect of recovery. With good nursing care, patients may remain alive for many years after the diagnosis has been made. The primary management aims in dealing with a patient in a low level state include establishing the diagnosis, careful attention to nursing and physical needs and, very importantly, supporting the family of the individual. In order to establish a diagnosis, an appropriate environment in which organized episodes of sensory stimulation are given to the patient should be provided. The stimulation should embrace all sensory modalities, and is used as a vehicle to establish if there is any meaningful response from the patient. Physical care needs are addressed by careful nursing with the aim of maintenance of an intact skin and control of contractures. Involvement of the physiotherapy and occupational therapy teams is therefore also required. Often these patients are fed by gastrostomy, and have a tracheostomy for tracheal toilet. Placement of the patient is variable, some residing in community hospital settings, and others in nursing homes. All should be under the care of a consultant.

Family support is a major management focus both before and after a diagnosis of PVS is made. Families and friends, quite naturally, hope against hope that their loved ones will improve and recover from their injuries, and a year is a long time to wait for a diagnosis, even if the diagnosis seems inevitable. Distress is ongoing throughout, and may often be accompanied by episodes of despair and anger. Anger may well be directed towards the health professionals involved in the care of the patient, and is understandable considering the context. The relatives should be offered plenty of opportunity to talk through their feelings, and should be given as much information about the management plan as is appropriate to the circumstances. It is also likely, in this day and age, that the relatives will seek information on PVS from the Internet. This may be either constructive or destructive, depending on the quality of the information and its relevance to their relative's situation. It is worth being prepared for this eventuality by having a look at the information available oneself. If available, the offer of counselling may be well received, and family members should be advised to let their GP know of their circumstances so that support is maintained through this route also. These individuals remain under great strain throughout the remaining life of the patient, and are often unable to finish the grieving process until death has occurred, which may be many years away. Support should therefore be maintained for the duration.

It is also important to remember that healthcare professionals may find the situation difficult too. Looking after a patient who one is told is in PVS, but who has sleep/wake cycles and whose eyes move around the room, albeit not fixating, can be disconcerting and takes time to get used to. This should not be forgotten and the staff should have the opportunity to express their feelings too.

Conclusion

The medical sequelae of head injury are many and varied. Some, such as transient hormonal imbalances, will only influence the patient's course during the acute phase, but others, such as the development of a central pain syndrome, may have a long-term negative impact on the patient's wellbeing. Having an understanding of what has happened to patients in the acute phase of their injury and rehabilitation sets the scene for their future rehabilitation in the community. Obtaining this information is another matter, but efforts should be made to encourage the communication of details about the patient. Part of providing a seamless service for patients is the communication of relevant information about the patient, but all who are familiar with working in the community will recognize the paucity of detail available to them by the community stage. This is an area we all need to work on, and could be helped by adopting a system of 'patient-held notes'.

The key role of the doctor in this rehabilitation setting is not only to manage ongoing medical problems, but also to seek out and tidy up any 'loose ends' that may be outstanding from the acute system – the nocturnal incontinence, the problem with pain, the worsening muscle tone. Defining the residual problems and using the resources of the multidisciplinary team to solve them is the best therapeutic approach to the head-injured patients at this stage of their recovery.

References

Annegers JF, Grabow JD, Groover RV, Laws ER Jnr., Elveback LR, Kurland LT (1980) Seizures after head trauma: a population study. Neurology 30: 683-9.
Bond MR (1986) Neurobehavioural sequelae of closed head injury. In Grant I, Adams KM (Eds) Neuropsychological Assessment of Neuropsychiatric Disorders. New York: Oxford University Press, 347-73.
Bridel J (1993) Assessing risk of pressure sores. Nursing Standard London 7(25): 32-5.
British Society of Rehabilitation Medicine (1998) Rehabilitation after Traumatic Brain Injury. London: BSRM.
Brooks N, McKinley W, Symington C, Beattie A, Campsie L (1987) Return to work within the first seven years of severe head injury. Brain Injury 1: 5-19.
Bullock R, Teasdale G (1990) Head injuries II. BMJ 300: 1576-9.
Dejerine J, Roussy G (1906) Le syndrome thalamique. Review Neurology (Paris) 14: 521-32.
Gelber DA, Good DC, Laven LJ, Verhuist SJ (1993) Causes of urinary incontinence after stroke. Stroke 24: 378-82.
Harlow JM (1848) Passage of an iron rod through the head. Boston Medicine and Surgery Journal 39: 389-93. Cited in O'Driscoll L, Leach JP (1998) 'No longer Gage': an iron bar through the head. British Medical Journal 317: 1673-4.
Jennett B (1975) Epilepsy after non-missile head injuries. Second edition Chicago Year Book.
Jennett B, Bond M (1975) Assessment of outcome after severe head injuries Lancet 1: 480-5.
Jennett B, MacMillan R (1981) Epidemiology of head injury. British Medical Journal (Clinical Research Edition) 282(6258): 101-4.
Jennett B, Teasdale G, Braakman R, Minderhoud J, Heiden J, Kurze T (1979) Neurosurgery 4: 283-9.
King NS (1996) Emotional, neuropsychological, and organic factors: their use in the prediction of persisting postconcussion symptoms after moderate and mild head injuries. Journal of Neurology Neurosurgery and Psychiatry Jul 61(1): 75-81.
King NS, Crawford S, Wenden FJ, Moss NE, Wade DT (1995) The Rivermead Post Concussion Symptoms Questionnaire: a measure of symptoms commonly experienced after head injury and its reliability. Journal of Neurology 242(9): 587-92.
King NS, Crawford S, Wenden FJ, Caldwell FE, Wade DT (1999) Early prediction of persisting post-concussion symptoms following mild and moderate head injuries. British Journal of Clinical Psychology 38(1): 15-25
Leijon G, Boivie J (1989) Central post-stroke pain – a controlled trial of amitriptyline and carbamazepine. Pain 36: 27-36.
Lindsay KW, Bone I (1997) Localised neurological disease and its management. A. Intracranial. In Lindsay KW and Bone I (1997) Neurology and Neurosurgery Illustrated. London: Churchill Livingstone, p. 232.

Mandel S (1989) Minor head injury may not be 'minor'. Postgraduate 85: 213-25.

Mendelow AD, Teasdale G, Jennett B, Bryden J, Hessett C, Murray G (1983) Risks of intracranial haematoma in head injured adults. British Medical Journal (Clinical Research Edition) 287(6400): 1173-6.

Pickard JD (1997) Post traumatic hydrocephalus. In MacFarlane R, Hardy DG (eds) Outcome after Head, Neck and Spinal Cord Injury: A Medicolegal Guide. Oxford: Butterworth-Heinemann, pp. 130-3.

Rappaport M, Hall KM, Hopkins K, Belleza T, Cope DN (1982) Disability rating scale for severe head trauma: coma to community. Archives of Physical Medicine and Rehabilitation 63: 118-23.

Royal College of Surgeons of England (1999) Report of the working party on the management of patients with head injuries. London: RCS.

Sainte-Rose C, Hoffmann HJ, Hirsch JF (1989) Shunt failure. Concepts in Pediatric Neurosurgery 9: 7-20.

Schierhout G, Roberts I (1998) Prophylactic antiepileptic agents after head injury: a systematic review. Journal of Neurology, Neurosurgery and Psychiatry 64: 108-12.

Teasdale G, Jennett B (1974) Assessment of coma and impaired consciousness: a practical scale. Lancet 2(7872): 81-4.

Wade DT, Johnston C (1999) The permanent vegetative state: practical guidance on diagnosis and management. British Medical Journal 319: 841-4.

Warren K, Bennett G (1998) Wound care. Prescriber's Journal 38: 115-22.

CHAPTER 3

Physical issues following head injury

TABITHA MATHERS, KATE MCGLASHAN, KATH VICK, ROSEMARY
GRAVELL

Introduction

Many severely head-injured people will have physical impairments, such as
movement disorders and contractures, somatosensory disturbances,
vision/hearing problems and swallowing problems. Some will experience
difficulties in a number of these areas; others may have isolated, specific
problems. The impairments *per se* are not specific to traumatic brain injury
but may occur as a result of a variety of neurological pathologies.
Impairment-based treatments will often therefore be generally applicable.
Working with this client group's physical problems differs in the way in
which cognitive and behavioural factors influence therapeutic decisions.
Healthcare professionals still have a tendency to focus disproportionately on
the impairment, forgetting the life of the individual at the heart of their intervention. It is important to remember, particularly in the community setting,
that 'the aim of rehab is to return people to an active lifestyle, not merely an
existence' (Tyson, 1995). Many individuals in this group may find themselves
and their families having to adopt a completely new lifestyle and therapists
have a critical role to play in helping them come to terms with this, and not
fuelling unrealistic expectations of recovery. In addition, the high proportion
of young adults affected by head injury is reflected in the functional issues
that will need to be considered.

This chapter will consider the main physical issues that may be faced by
people after head injury – movement disorders, tone disorders, joint
problems, somatosensory issues, cardiovascular fitness, vision and hearing,
and swallowing. Beginning with a background explanation of normal
movement and its components, each topic and specific management strategies will then be considered individually. Physiotherapeutic intervention,

approaches to treatment, assessment, measurement and mechanisms of recovery will be addressed later, ending with carer involvement.

Normal motor control

In order to identify the movement deficits that a client may face there needs to be an understanding of how the client's movement patterns and postures differ from normal. It is important, therefore, to consider what is 'normal'.

Normal movement can be described as the achievement of a motor goal (implying voluntary motion or action) consisting of patterns made up of selective movements (or desired active movement), which are based upon neuromuscular innervation, which is influenced by afferent input (incoming information from the environment).

Normal movement has several vital components, namely normal postural tone, reciprocal innervation, sensory-motor feedback, balance and normal muscle biomechanics. Normal postural tone is the 'state of readiness of the body musculature in preparation for the maintenance of a posture or the performance of a movement' (Bernstein, 1967). Reciprocal innervation is the 'graded and synchronous interaction of agonists, antagonists and synergists throughout the body' (Bobath, 1990). This allows harmonious interplay of muscle activity to give selective posture and movement. It is facilitated through postural fixation of proximal (central) parts of the body with regulation of smooth interaction of the muscles of the moving parts (Davies, 1990). An agonist is a muscle whose active contraction causes movement of a body part. The opposite antagonist muscle has to relax to allow the movement to take place. A synergist acts together with an agonist to produce a movement. Sensory-motor feedback occurs with the sensitivity of the central nervous system (CNS) to both intrinsic and extrinsic sensory information, which is assimilated to produce effective activity (Edwards 1996). Balance includes righting and equilibrium reactions. These are the postural adjustments and adaptations, which occur constantly to maintain alignment of body posture within the base of support (Edwards, 1996). Equilibrium reactions are automatic adaptations of postural tone in response to gravity and displacement. Righting reactions allow maintenance of and movement around the midline through sequences of selective movement in patterns in response to displacement. Normal muscle biomechanics relate to 'normal' proportions of the various different properties of muscle and the way that they can alter their characteristics depending upon their usage (Dietz, 1992).

Disorders of movement after head injury

A wide range of disturbances of motor function may be seen after head injury, some of which may be easily explained by the known pathology seen on scans and other investigations. Sometimes impairments that are present cannot readily be attributed to known lesions within the brain, leading clinicians to surmise that unidentified microdamage has occurred. In the rehabilitation context, the cause of the impairment becomes less important in the face of the disability that arises from it.

For ease of description it is convenient to try to categorize the motor sequelae of head injury into three main clinical groups – paralysis, post-traumatic Parkinsonism, and post-traumatic ataxia, with or without tremor. Physiotherapy of the head-injured patient however is not prescriptive and adopts a problem-solving approach whereby functional deficits and the underlying cause are identified and treated.

Paralysis

Paralysis is said to have occurred when motor function is either impaired or lost. There are various ways to describe the degree of paralysis affecting the body as outlined in Table 3.1.

The weakness seen is often associated with either an increase or a decrease in the tone of the muscle (the resistance of the muscle to passive stretch). The tone of a paralysed limb can have a great influence on the rehabilitation outcome of a client, and will be discussed further later in this chapter. Paralysis after brain injury occurs following damage to the descending nerve pathways involved in control of the motor function resulting in the inability of the CNS to recruit appropriate activity. The severity and longevity of the paralysis is dependent on the nature of the damage. Destruction of nerve tissue, for example from a missile, will produce irreversible damage. In contrast, some of the immediate weakness seen after contusion (bruising) will improve as the effects of the local swelling diminish.

The human nervous system is set up in such a way that if there is muscle weakness following brain injury, the weight bearing muscles are affected more than their antagonists (the anti-gravity muscles). Thus the extensor muscles of the arms, which straighten the joints. are affected more than the flexors, causing the joints to bend; and the flexor muscles of the legs are often weakened more than the extensors, causing the joints to straighten.

Table 3.1. Paralysis: descriptive terms

Monoplegia: paralysis affecting one limb only.
Paraplegia: paralysis affecting legs.
Hemiplegia: paralysis affecting one side of the body, including the arm and leg.
Quadriplegia: paralysis affecting all four limbs.

Interestingly, the sloth, which spends its life hanging upside-down from trees, is affected in the converse way. The relative preservation of strength in the 'anti-gravity' muscles is fortuitous, and is an essential underlying component of the rehabilitation of standing and walking after head injury.

Over the course of time, as well as weakness of central derivation from the brain injury, the disused muscle itself becomes weak from withering of the muscle fibres. This may make an important contribution to the level of disability, and is important to consider when devising a programme of rehabilitation. While the damaged nerve tissue itself may not recover, other pathways may be uncovered with time. These theories of recovery are dealt with later in the chapter as are the various therapeutic approaches used to maximize the return of 'normal' selective movement and thereby optimize function.

It is often the later secondary changes that significantly hinder the return of selective or volitional movement. These include, firstly, loss of cortical representation of the affected part, where the area of representation in the brain of a particular area of the body reduces in size. Secondly, muscles and joints may become malaligned in positions of which the CNS has no memory. Lastly, disruption of the 'normal' properties of the soft-tissues involved occurs with resultant loss of range of movement and muscle strength (Carr and Shepherd, 1998). Cognitive issues such as reduced motivation and insight, and a general inability on the part of the client to participate fully in the rehabilitation process, may compound these problems. Involvement of other team members and carers and a flexible, positive approach is invaluable for the therapist working with this client group.

Post-traumatic Parkinsonism

The development of Parkinsonian features in an individual after head trauma is well described (Ward et al., 1983), although there may be a delay between the trauma and the development of symptoms. Idiopathic Parkinson's disease itself may also present after trauma. The key differences between these two conditions are that idiopathic Parkinson's is a progressive disorder, whereas post-traumatic Parkinsonism is not, and that idiopathic Parkinson's responds well to pharmacological treatment, unlike post-traumatic Parkinsonism which is generally resistant to treatment. There is debate over the exact mechanism of the pathological process underlying post-traumatic Parkinsonism, but it probably involves either direct disruption of the substantia nigra or its vascular supply by the trauma. (The substantia nigra is the part of the brain that degenerates in idiopathic Parkinson's, producing the well-known triad of symptoms of tremor, rigidity and slow movement.) Other suggestions are that brain injury just accelerates the general degenerative mechanisms of the brain, especially prominent in the 'punch-drunk' syndrome seen in boxers. In this condition there is a syndrome of deterioration in personality, memory impairment, dysarthria, tremor and ataxia, associated with Parkinsonian features (Lancet, 1973).

Treatment

As already mentioned, drug therapy is often disappointing in post-traumatic Parkinsonism, but may be worth a trial. The aims of physiotherapy in this condition are modelled on those approaches used in idiopathic Parkinson's disease, and include aiming to maximize function by maintaining joint range of movement, mobility and fitness (Banks, 1991). This could be done through the introduction of a fitness and exercise regime, which the client may be able to carry out independently or with the assistance of a carer. In the community it may be beneficial to carry out this type of rehabilitation in a group setting as a means of improving motivation and morale (Sanford, 1989).

Post-traumatic ataxia and tremor

The three main types of ataxia are cerebellar, sensory and vestibular ataxia. The individual with traumatic brain injury may present with one type, or a combination depending on the sites of impairment.

Cerebellar ataxia involves damage within the cerebellum itself and/or its connections. The signs and symptoms exhibited will depend upon the areas affected. Lesions involving the midline structures and flocculonodular lobe produce problems with equilibrium, with stance and gait, with occular movements and with titubation (tremor of the head and upper trunk). Lesions affecting the lateral and intermediate zones produce ipsilateral, abnormal limb movements (Thompson and Day, 1993). Clinical signs of cerebellar ataxia include dysmetria, tremor, dysdiadochokinesia, dysynergia postural sway and occulomotor incoordination. Dysmetria refers to inaccurate movement of a limb and is highlighted by finger-nose or heel-shin tests. The person may overshoot (hypermetria) or undershoot (hypometria) the target. There may also be slurred, slow speech. Tremor can involve kinetic tremor (oscillations during limb movement), intention tremor (present at the end of a movement), postural tremor (oscillations of the limbs when held outstretched), titubation, postural truncal tremor (of the lower trunk and legs) and rubral tremor (involving a combination of rest tremor, severe intention tremor and postural tremor) (Thompson and Day, 1993). Dysdiadochokinesia is seen where the individual is unable to perform rapidly alternating movements – for example rotating the palm up and down quickly. Dysynergia is a decomposition of movement. The individual shows difficulty in compensating for movements that occur with multi-joint movements. Postural sway is where the individual overshoots in their postural response. Occulomotor incoordination can lead functionally to reduced hand-eye coordination. Other signs include involuntary, rapid movements of the eyeball (nystagmus) and dysmetric saccades where the eyes may simultaneously over or undershoot when changing the point of fixation on an object. The muscle tone in these clients is usually low, but clients may develop spasticity in some muscle groups in order to provide themselves with some postural stability.

Sensory ataxia involves impairments in the sensory cortex or its afferent connections from proprioceptive receptors. The individual will demonstrate a positive Romberg's test. This is where, when standing with heels together, clients show a marked increase in sway on closing their eyes. Walking involves a wide-based gait with an emphasis on visual feedback at all times. There is increased latency of postural adjustments with inappropriately scaled postural responses. The balance strategies at the ankle will be reduced with the individual relying on the hip muscles to compensate.

Vestibular ataxia involves peripheral or central vestibular lesions. The individual's gait may be affected with reduced righting reactions; gait may be wide based, there may be a tendency to lean back (in bilateral labyrinthine dysfunction) or towards the side of the unilateral lesion, reduced head, trunk and arm movement, worsening of symptoms in the dark or on uneven surfaces, reduced balance strategies at the hip, and reduced head and trunk stabilization control (Borello-France, Whitney and Herdman, 1994). The individual may suffer recurrent episodes of vertigo secondary to decompensation following labyrinthine concussion, associated with head trauma, and may complain of symptoms of dysequilibrium (Luxon and Davies, 1997). There may also be occulomotor signs if the vestibular occular reflex is reduced (oscillopsia) or reduced head-eye coordination. Vertigo and nausea are often associated with vestibular dysfunction.

Treatment

Tremor disorders and ataxia can be very disabling and are often difficult to treat. The management may be the same for either condition but it is important to assess and analyse the cause of the problem. For instance, is it a muscle imbalance problem and does this originate centrally or from the periphery? How are posture, movement and function affected? Do stress or fatigue increase the symptoms? The treatment approaches can be divided into three groups – exercise, compensation (including use of equipment), and medical management.

For an individual with cerebellar ataxia, treatment is often aimed at trying to help the client achieve proximal (central) stability through exercise. The therapist should encourage performance of smooth movement, sustained force generation and activities requiring an initial burst of agonist activity. For uncompensated peripheral vestibular damage the individual may respond well to an aggressive vestibular rehabilitation programme. This may include Cawthorne-Cooksey exercises (Cawthorne, 1945; Cooksey, 1945), individualized exercises relating to specific symptoms, gait and balance training and specific manoeuvres. The reader is referred to Luxon and Davies (1997) for details of techniques. Central vestibular disorders are more difficult to treat but may respond to re-education of gait and postural control.

Compensatory techniques may be appropriate for many clients with the aim of stabilizing the affected limbs and reducing the tremor. Approaches may include anchoring the elbow into the side of the body or placing the elbows on a table and stabilizing the wrist with the non-dominant hand. The client may require assessment for supportive, specialized seating. For some clients, the provision of weighted walking aids or weighted wristbands that act as damping devices could facilitate the functional ability of the client (Thornton and Kilbride, 1998), although removal of the weight may show a return of the tremor in greater measure than before. The client should be encouraged to keep activities close to the body, to slide objects up the body or over surfaces and to move the object rather than reaching. Specialized tools used for eating, such as the 'neater-eater', can help maintain independence in feeding by using a dampening mechanism to control the movement of, for instance, a spoon towards the mouth. The use of 'lycra suits' is receiving some attention. To date these have primarily been used in the treatment of children with spasticity, but some evidence does exist to suggest that they may be helpful in the treatment of ataxia. The exact mechanism for their success is unclear but it is possible that they provide a dampening effect, which reduces the tremor (Edmondson, Fisher and Hanson, 1999). These effects appear to be associated with normalization of posture, tone, increased stability and improved muscle balance as well as promoting sensory feedback to the brain.

Drug management is largely ineffective. There are suggestions that treatment with clonazepam, baclofen, cinnarizine or carbamazepine may be effective in symptom treatment (Luxon and Davies, 1997). Very occasionally patients are put forward for specialized surgery to the brain, again with variable results.

Disorders of tone after head injury

Muscle tone can be defined as the amount of resistance offered by a muscle when a joint of a relaxed client is moved passively (Britton, 1998).

Assessment of tone

Quantifying tone has been difficult within the clinical setting. Measurement of tone has been based on scales that rely heavily on observational judgement. The most commonly used scale appears to be the Ashworth scale, which records qualitative data (Bohannon and Smith, 1987). Other measurements used in clinical trials have recorded aspects of the upper motor neurone features of spasticity (Katz and Rymer, 1989). These have been criticized in light of the more recent evidence suggesting that spasticity may also be the result of mechanical changes within the tissue itself (Carr, Shepherd and Ada, 1995). Standardization of the measurement of tone also provides some difficulty as it can vary with factors such as stress, heat and pain (Thornton and Kilbride, 1998). Carr, Shepherd and Ada (1995) state that as the aim of treatment is to enable the client to regain or maintain motor function through the management of tone, clinical testing should involve the use of functional scales such as the Motor Assessment Scale (Carr et al., 1985) or the FIM and FAM (Hall et al., 1993).

Spasticity

There is still not complete agreement over the exact mechanism of spasticity and a whole book could be devoted to this discussion. For the purposes of this chapter, two theories, which are widely believed to be the predominant causes of pathologically increased muscle tone, will be considered.

Lance (1990) defined spasticity as 'a motor disorder characterised by a velocity-dependent increase in tonic stretch reflexes with exaggerated tendon jerks resulting from hyperexcitability of the stretch reflex as one component of the upper motor neurone syndrome'. This reflects the view that spasticity is the result of abnormal upper motor neurone features, upper motor neurone features being any neural component within the brain or spinal cord. Clinically this is characterized by tendon jerk hyperreflexia that becomes more obvious when the velocity of the stretch applied to the muscle to elicit the reflex is increased.

The second theory suggests that soft tissue changes within the muscle itself also contribute to the resistance that is felt when moving a spastic limb (Thilmann, Fellows and Garms, 1991). Immobility of a limb as a result of paralysis following a head injury may mean that a muscle is held in a short-ened position relative to its normal physiological length. This can lead to adaptive biomechanical changes occurring within the muscle (Goldspink, 1976). Immobilization of a muscle in a shortened position results in a decrease in the number of sarcomeres, the contractile unit of a muscle. The muscle therefore becomes contracted. The loss of sarcomeres and subse-quent reduction in muscle length leads to a proportional increase in collagen relative to muscle fibre tissue. This means that the muscle will feel stiffer to move (Goldspink and Williams, 1990).

The presence of spasticity results in abnormal posture and mass movement patterns. There is inappropriate co-contraction of muscles and an inability or difficulty in moving one joint independently of another in the same limb. The site of the injury influences the initial severity and distribution of spasticity. External factors such as stress, illness and temperature of the surrounding environment also have an effect on the level of spasticity experienced. These triggers cause associated reactions of abnormal motor behaviour that are beyond the individual's level of inhibitory or modulatory control. They may range from a barely noticeable alteration in muscle tone to an extensive change in position of a whole limb or side of a body. They are capable of change. The presence of spasticity affects the ability of the client to move normally and subsequently affects his ability to function. Movement requires greater effort, which in itself can exacerbate spasticity, further frustrating the client's ability to achieve a physical task (Barnes, McLellan and Sutton, 1993).

A client presenting with spasticity may well have learnt ways of coping through abnormal mass movement patterns; for example, clients with lower limb extensor spasticity may use this as a brace to enable them to walk (Ko Ko and Ward, 1997). In the long term this can sometimes be self-defeating as abnormal movement can lead to excessive wear and tear on joints and result in painful musculoskeletal problems that could prevent movement later on in life. It would be unreasonable, however, to expect the client to discontinue walking. The team must therefore work in close partnership with clients to provide strategies that may help prevent the side effects of their poor movement control, such as contractures, whilst still enabling them to achieve their maximum motor function.

Drug treatment

Treatment of spasticity may include the use of drugs or traditional physiotherapy techniques. The drugs most commonly used in the treatment of spasticity are baclofen, dantrolene, and tizanidine, and increasingly botulinum toxin as a local muscle injection.

Baclofen is a derivative of gamma-aminobutyric acid (GABA), an 'inhibitory neurotransmitter' found in the central nervous system. Neurotransmitters are the chemical messengers that transmit signals between nerve cells. Baclofen is thought to reduce the release of excitatory neurotransmitters in the system and hence reduce both spinal and cerebrally induced spasticity. Side effects include drowsiness, nausea and light-headedness, but these can be minimized by starting with a low dose and increasing gradually. Muscle weakness can also be induced, and there has to be a trade-off between the positive and negative effects of the drug.

Another mode of delivery of baclofen is the direct infusion of the drug into the intrathecal space via a small catheter. This involves delivery of the drug into the space containing the cerebrospinal fluid, with the catheter often being inserted in the lumbar region. A computer programmable pump that is implanted underneath the skin, usually in the anterior abdominal wall controls the drug delivery. This mode of treatment can be very helpful in refractory cases of severe spasticity, but should not be undertaken lightly as the maintenance programme for the pump is demanding, requiring two or three monthly top-ups, usually at a specialist centre.

Dantrolene sodium has a peripheral action on spasticity, in contrast to baclofen and the other agents listed, which all act centrally. This means it can be used in conjunction with centrally acting drugs. Dantrolene depresses the release of calcium within muscle cells, hence inhibiting the strength of contraction of the muscle. Nausea, vomiting and diarrhoea are included within the side-effect profile of this drug, but the most serious side effect is liver damage, which, rarely, can be fatal. Hence, liver function tests should be monitored throughout therapy and the drug withdrawn if no benefit is evident after six weeks.

Tizanidine is a relatively new drug on the market in the UK. It acts centrally to inhibit transmission of certain nerve pathways within the spinal cord and is marketed as producing less muscle weakness than baclofen and diazepam. Other side effects include drowsiness and a dry mouth, and a dose-dependent slowing of the heart rate and lowered blood pressure. Again, these can be minimized by a gradual increase in the dosage of the drug.

Botulinum toxin is a neurotoxin produced commercially from the bacterium clostridium botulinum. It has been used in the treatment of dystonias such as torticollis for a number of years, but has more recently been applied to the treatment of spastic muscles. Botulinum toxin is given in the form of an injection directly into the affected muscle and produces temporary weakness by inhibiting presynaptic release of acetylcholine (a neurotransmitter) at the junction between the nerve and muscle. The effects are not seen for seven to 10 days and often longer. The presynaptic block leads to muscular atrophy and paralysis with rapid nerve regrowth occurring in response over a period of six weeks or so. Effective neuromuscular reconnections are not made for several more weeks when neuromuscular transmission is once more possible and the effect wears off (Richardson and Thompson, 1999). It is important that botulinum toxin is used in conjunction with a planned physiotherapy programme for the affected limb, to make the most of the opportunity that its use affords.

Richardson and Thompson (1999) provide a comprehensive literature review of studies looking at the use of botulinum toxin in spasticity, and draw the conclusion that, although there is evidence to support the use of botox in the treatment of spasticity, further trials need to carried out. Until these trials are carried out, however, they suggest guidelines for the use of botox in the treatment of spasticity, including EMG studies to determine the degree and extent of the neural component of spasticity within the identified muscle group(s), identification of desired functional outcome, and follow-up management of the client once the injection has been given, including splinting, stretching and activities.

Physical treatment

Treatment techniques are listed in Table 3.2.

Stretch

Applying a long slow stretch to the affected muscle is believed to inhibit the hyperexcitable stretch reflex, one component of the upper motor neurone feature of spasticity (Od'een and Knutsson, 1981). Stretching has also been shown to prevent the adaptive changes that occur within a muscle held in a shortened position (Goldspink and Williams, 1990). The duration of the stretch required to inhibit the upper motor neurone features and prevent length-associated changes seems to remain unclear. Tardieu et al. (1988) determined that a stretch had to be applied to the soleus muscle for six hours a day to prevent contractures in children with cerebral palsy. In normal immobilized muscle 30 minutes of stretching a day was found to be sufficient to prevent the soft tissue changes from occurring (Williams, 1990). Stretch has also been found to be important in disused muscles to prevent atrophy or wasting. Protein turnover in the soleus muscle in the calf was found to increase after immobilization in a lengthened position. The length of time to gain the maximal effect from stretching in this case though also remains poorly defined (Goldspink and Williams, 1990). A therapist can instigate a passive stretching regime for the client. If the client or carer is able to participate then this can be achieved actively and more frequently in the home situation.

Weight bearing

Weight bearing is considered to be one way of applying a stretch so standing or weight bearing through the affected arm often forms an integral part of

Table 3.2. Physical techniques used with spasticity

- Stretch
- Weightbearing
- Splinting
- Positioning and seating
- Facilitation of movement
- Ice and heat
- Functional electrical stimulation (FES)

therapy (Thornton and Kilbride, 1998). Weight bearing is also believed to provide valuable sensory input to the joints. In the severely physically disabled client standing may be achieved using pieces of equipment such as a tilt table or an Oswestry standing frame. In the community this strategy may be used in conjunction with another technique, as it will not always be possible for clients to have these pieces of equipment at home. The only time they may be able to use them is when they visit the rehabilitation unit. If the client is able to achieve standing independently or with minimal assistance then an active weight-bearing regime can be implemented at home.

Splinting

Splinting is often used as a means of providing a long slow stretch. This can be in the form of plaster casts or back slabs made specifically for the patient. These can be applied at night or when the patient is resting; careful monitoring of the skin condition is however essential to prevent the formation of pressure sores (Edwards and Charlton, 1996). Splinting can also be used correctively to restore range of movement in a contracted joint; this will be discussed later during the treatment of contractures.

Positioning and seating

Good positioning and seating are considered essential in order to maintain soft tissue length and provide enough stability to enable clients to move successfully so that they do not increase their spasticity by using compensatory movements. This will also be discussed under the treatment of contractures.

Facilitation

Facilitation of movement via key points is also believed to influence tone. Bobath (1990) suggests that movement of the head, trunk, pelvis and shoulder girdles are influential in altering spasticity. The positioning of each of these parts of the body relative to one another is believed to be able to alter muscle tone throughout the body. This theory is based on the belief that the upper motor neurone features of spasticity may occur as a result of the plastic adaptation of the central nervous system following the brain injury (Musa, 1986). Therefore if the therapist can provide normal peripheral sensory or afferent input by facilitating movement of key areas in the body she may be able to change the upper motor neurone features of spasticity by plastically reorganising the central nervous system.

Ice and heat

Ice and heat have also been used in the treatment of spasticity. After applying cold bags to spastic muscles for 15 to 20 minutes Knutsson (1970) found an average increase in range of movement of 35 degrees in most people. This treatment does not have a long-lasting effect but it can prove a useful adjunct to other treatment.

Heat has also been shown to relax spastic muscle temporarily and may prove more comfortable for the client (Lehman and Delateur, 1982).

Functional electrical stimulation (FES)

FES has been used most notably in the rehabilitation of clients with paraplegia following a spinal cord injury. Electrodes are placed over selected leg muscles to stimulate a muscle contraction and enable the client to stand independently without the use of callipers. Development of this standing system has led to the use of FES in the treatment of clients following a stroke. Several studies have found that by electrically stimulating the 'paralysed' anterior calf muscles of stroke patients sufficient to dorsiflex the foot, reciprocal inhibition of spasticity in the posterior calf muscles has occurred (Merletti, Andina and Galante, 1979; Carnstam, Larsson and Prevec, 1979).

To date there do not seem to be any studies supporting the use of FES to reduce spasticity in clients following a head injury. Despite this lack of specific evidence, it is still possible to apply what has been learnt through its use in the rehabilitation of stroke clients and consider it as a potentially useful adjunct to the treatment of spasticity and movement disorders in clients following a head injury.

Hypotonia

Low muscle tone or hypotonia can also present following a head injury. This can be detected clinically when moving the affected limb, as there will be very little resistance to the movement. Clients often present with a mixture of both hypertonia and hypotonia. Where hypotonia is detected it is very important that joint protection strategies, such as client and carer instruction and the provision of orthoses, are used to avoid damage to the soft tissue structures. As there is little or no resistance to movement at the end of range it is very easy for a joint to become over stretched and painful (Thornton and Kilbride, 1998).

The shoulder joint is particularly vulnerable in a client with hypotonia as it relies on the musculature surrounding it for its stability. If the muscles are effectively paralysed as a result of a head injury the shoulder relies on the joint capsule and ligaments for its stability. These structures are normally quite loose to enable the shoulder to be able to move through large ranges of movement so, without the support of the rotator cuff and other shoulder muscles, the shoulder joint can become subluxed or partially dislocated (Griffin, 1986; Culham, Noce and Bagg, 1995).

Treatment

Treatment strategies are usually aimed at increasing the muscle tone, stimulating the muscle directly through the application of ice or quick stretching
or by stimulating the receptor in the joint through weight bearing. Emphasis
again is on providing normal sensory and motor input to try to influence the
central nervous system (Musa, 1986). Splints or orthoses may be provided
such as a 'foot drop splint' so that the client can walk without having to use
compensatory strategies to bring his affected leg through (Edwards and
Charlton, 1996), and these will be discussed in more detail later in the
chapter.

   In order to ensure that damage does not occur to the shoulder joint, a
physiotherapist will often supply a shoulder support (Edwards and Charlton,
1996). It is important, however, that the client and carer are educated in
positioning and looking after the arm in order to prevent damage to the
shoulder and maintain the range of movement. Shoulder malalignment has
also been found in the presence of spasticity, when management is aimed at
preventing soft tissue damage and correcting alignment (Culham, Noce and
Bagg, 1995).

Problems with joints after head injury

Contractures

Contractures are tackled separately within this chapter because of the huge
impact that they can have on the physical management of a head-injured
client. Contractures can affect up to 80% of severe traumatic brain-injured
clients (Watson, 1997). In the initial stages of recovery from head injury
when the client may be unconscious, contractures can simply result from
being kept in one position for too long – for example toes pointed down due
to the weight of the bed clothes can lead to shortened calf muscles. In this
case adaptive changes occur within the muscle as previously described and
the muscle shortens. In order to prevent these changes occurring the physiotherapist may initiate a preventative stretching and splinting programme. If
clients make a good physical recovery with no abnormal muscle tone
changes and begin to bear weight, any adaptive soft tissue changes may
reverse without direct intervention. If they do not get better straight away
the physiotherapist can advise on a stretching programme to facilitate the
lengthening.

   Within the community setting contractures will have probably developed
as a result of postural incompetence. Postural incompetence develops
because the client, in trying to achieve maximum functional ability, develops
extraordinary postures to overcome movement disorders, such as spasticity

or tremor, which have resulted from the head injury. If these postural adaptations are continually reinforced then contractures will develop, as soft tissue structures will adapt to this new positioning. Thus the development of contractures is a strategy for establishing a fixed and stable posture. The presence of contractures will inevitably adversely affect the client by, for example, causing pain, an increase in spasticity or pressure sores (Pope, 1996).

The following two examples illustrate how a client may develop contractures and what might happen as a result. Two years ago, following a blow on the head, X was left with spasticity in the extensor muscles of his right leg. In order to walk he used this spasticity to keep his right leg straight as a prop to enable him to step his left leg through. The recurrent use of this extensor spasticity caused his right foot to point downwards and turn in, so that he walked on the outside of his right ankle. He was referred to the community rehabilitation team because he was suffering from pain in his right ankle and back, and could not walk as fast as previously.

Mrs Y was in a car accident 10 years ago. She was referred to the community rehabilitation service because her swallowing problems had worsened and she was continually suffering from chest infections as a result of aspiration. On examination the team assessed that Mrs Y's wheelchair was not providing enough postural support. This meant that she had adopted a fixed slumped posture, which was gradually worsening. This posture resulted in poor head and trunk alignment and meant that she was unable to achieve a successful swallow. The slumped posture also made it impossible for her to achieve good chest expansion during breathing, making it more difficult for her to recover from her chest infections.

Assessment

Assessment of the client with contractures is very important. If a contracture has developed in order to provide the client with stability then reduction of the contracture without providing the client with other means of obtaining stability could adversely affect their motor function. The range of movement of the affected joint will be limited with a solid end feel. The angle should be noted, perhaps using a goniometer. The functional effect on the client with regard to activities of daily living should be investigated and a record of this made.

Treatment

If as a result of the head injury the unconscious client suffers from muscle tone changes such as spasticity, the physiotherapist may choose to apply splints to inhibit spasticity and prevent contractures occurring. As the client regains consciousness other methods of stretching, such as weight bearing or an active assisted stretching regime may be adopted. Therapy techniques useful for the treatment and prevention of contractures include positioning and provision of orthotics (specialized splinting). Positioning and seating are important, as the case of Mrs Y illustrated so clearly. These are dealt with comprehensively by Pope (1996) and will only be addressed briefly here. In the more severely motor-impaired client some contractures may be prevented if appropriate advice and management has been given with regard to specialized seating, at an earlier stage in their rehabilitation. An appropriate seating system should provide the client with a stable base of support so that the client does not have to use abnormal motor control to stabilize himself. If clients have already developed established contractures and correction is not possible, moulded seating may be required to obtain the best alignment possible for them and prevent further deterioration in their physical condition. Positioning and seating should be reviewed regularly throughout the rest of their life as age and other factors such as systemic illness can alter their postural requirements.

Splints or orthotics can be used to prevent loss of range of movement, to increase range of movement, or to stabilize a body segment (Edwards and Charlton, 1996). As previously mentioned, they are also used in the treatment of spasticity. Any splint that applies stretch or is used to provide normal body segment alignment is believed to have an inhibitory effect on the neural component of spasticity. This function of splinting has already been discussed.

Preventative splinting may be used in the presence of spasticity or because the patient has no active muscle activity, but in both cases the aim would be to prevent soft tissue shortening and subsequent contracture (Edwards and Charlton, 1996). In the lower limb these splints tend to be made out of some form of plaster and can be worn at night so that a long stretch can be applied without the plaster boots becoming a nuisance to the client who would then be less likely to wear them. Splints may also be used to maintain a good position in the hand and wrist and a variety of hand splints can be found, depending on which group of muscles is being stretched.

Splinting to regain muscle length may take the form of serial casting or drop-out splints. Serial casting is a means of applying a progressive long-term stretch. A cast is applied to hold the muscle group in a stretched position and left in place for a period of seven to 10 days (Watkins, 1999). After this time the splint is removed. A small gain in range of movement should have been achieved by the addition of sarcomeres in the muscle. The cast can then be reapplied holding the muscles on a stretch in their new position. In this way a gradual increase in the range of movement at a joint can be achieved. A regimen of casting and prolonged stretching has been shown to increase range of movement in the calf muscles of a group of head-injured adults (Moseley, 1997).

Drop-out splints allow active movements of the antagonistic group of muscles – that is, the muscles that normally oppose the action of the contracted muscles – to occur whilst stretching the shortened muscles. If spasticity is present this may enable the client to use the opposing muscle group to the ones that are spastic to try and inhibit the spasticity. In PNF much emphasis is placed on the theory of reciprocal inhibition whereby one muscle group is used to relax and inhibit the action of the opposing group (Kabat and Knott, 1954). This theory, however, needs to be further explored and researched.

Splinting to correct movement deficits and control body segment align-ment, particularly in the lower limb, can involve strapping and the provision of ankle-foot orthoses (AFOs). Strapping is a widely used form of splinting in the treatment of sports injuries. It is applied to protect the joint from further injury by preventing strain on injured soft tissue structures and to limit unwanted joint movement. It can also be applied as a means of improving proprioception in a joint after an injury (Macdonald, 1996). Strapping can therefore be used to achieve joint alignment in some cases following a head injury.

The AFO is used to enable correct foot and ankle alignment. If the client is predominantly hypotonic or low tone he may not be able to lift the foot up against gravity. This makes walking difficult as the client has to pick his affected leg up very high in order to swing it through. The provision of an AFO preventing the foot from dropping can therefore make walking easier. It will also help to maintain range of movement of the posterior group of ankle muscles. Spasticity in the legs seems predominantly to affect the extensor group of muscles. This means that the foot will point down and turn in. If patients are unable to control this then it can also mean that they will have difficulty walking. The provision of an AFO could lead to an improvement in their gait pattern if it can control the effects of the spasticity (Edwards and Charlton, 1996). A variety of AFOs can be obtained depending on the goal, and the provision of any orthotics should be planned with podiatrists, who have knowledge of what is available or could be custom made.

The use of splinting and casting to improve the range of joint movement as one part of the physical management of head-injured clients seems to be the one area that has been researched most thoroughly. Evidence does suggest that these methods can be successful as one part of the physical management but further research is needed to see if this can be related to any improvement in function (Tolfts and Stiller, 1997).

Heterotopic ossification

This strange condition sometimes occurs after head injury and can be quite devastating. It involves the laying down of new bony material around joints. The mechanism for this is unknown, and the treatment unsatisfactory. It tends to happen in the early stages of rehabilitation and can cause considerable problems with pain and restriction of movement of the involved joint. Non-steroidal anti-inflammatory drugs sometimes help, and occasionally the ectopic ossification is surgically excised, but this is usually delayed for 18 months to two years to reduce the risk of recurrence. It is therefore worth considering x-raying a joint that is restricted if soft tissue contraction is not felt to be the culprit.

Cardiovascular fitness

In a study comparing the physical work capacity of head-injured clients to a matched control group, Becker et al. (1978) found that the head-injured group exhibited lowered physical work capacity and a decreased resistance to physiological fatigue. Scherzer (1986) and Jankowski and Sullivan (1990) have also supported these findings more recently. This loss of physical conditioning occurs because of the clients' initial inability to participate in any activity as a direct result of their head injury. The client may then be further prevented from participating in any exercise programmes by subsequent physical disability and/or cognitive problems such as reduced motivation, poor attention span and memory problems. Once lost, this lack of physical conditioning and this fatiguability can become self-defeating (Sullivan, Richer and Laurent, 1990).

Physical conditioning programmes are recommended as part of the rehabilitation process for clients with a head injury for several reasons. Firstly, it improves their cardiovascular function and subsequently increases their resistance to fatigue (Sullivan, Richer and Laurent, 1990). This has the longer term effect of enabling the client to be able to handle the physical demands of returning home and possibly returning to work (Novak, Roth and Boll, 1988). Secondly it can improve self-confidence and satisfaction by achieving targets (Eames and Wood, 1985). Thirdly it encourages participation in general healthy behaviour (Sullivan, Richer and Laurent, 1990). Fourthly increasing activity is a method of combating depression, emotional lability and regression (Moran, 1976). Finally, there has been some evidence recently to suggest that aerobic exercise can have a positive effect on cognitive function (Rosenfeld, 1998).

In the community setting a physiotherapist may be called upon to advise regarding levels and types of activity or identify this as a specific problem as part of her assessment. If she feels that an exercise programme is necessary then she must choose the best way for this to be prescribed. For some clients it may be sufficient to provide them with a written programme and review them regularly. If they require the involvement of their carer for assistance in some of the activities then time must be spent with the carer or assistant to make sure that they are confident in assisting with these activities. The client may have previously been a member of a gymnasium and may wish to start attending there again but may lack the initial motivation and self-confidence to start going by himself. In this case some liaison between the therapist, client and the staff at the gym may be appropriate. It is usually possible for the therapist to attend the initial session so that the client can be confident that he will not be doing anything that would adversely affect his rehabilitation.

The therapist may feel that the client will be unable to carry out this programme on his own because of cognitive problems such as poor motivation or memory. She may therefore choose to see the client individually at the rehabilitation centre or invite him to attend a group session. The physiotherapist will need to work closely with other members of the team in order to establish an independent exercise programme for that client.

Mr Z was referred to the community rehabilitation team following a head injury as a result of a car accident a year previously. On assessment Mr Z was complaining of stiffness in his left ankle, which had been broken at the time of the accident. As a result of private funding Mr Z's family had been able to employ a full-time rehabilitation assistant to work with Mr Z, as he required 24-hour input due to reduced mobility and a very poor memory. Mr Z was mildly ataxic and could walk with the use of a walking frame but had to have supervision at all times because of his lack of confidence; this resulted in his using the wheelchair whenever he was outdoors and sometimes refusing to walk at home with his family. He was grossly unfit and could only manage 5 minutes of the exercise bicycle at its lowest resistance, he exhibited muscle wastage and reduced range of movement predominantly in his hips and ankles.

Following a brief period of physiotherapy in the rehabilitation gym, which was quite a distance from Mr Z's home, Mr Z agreed to go to his local gymnasium. The physiotherapist, sports instructor, rehabilitation assistant and Mr Z attended the first session. A programme was planned and because of his continuing cognitive problems Mr Z would continue to rely on the rehabilitation assistant to help him carry out this programme. It was decided that the sports instructor would progress the programme as necessary. When followed up by the physiotherapist several weeks later Mr Z could sustain 15 minutes cycling at resistance 6, and both muscle bulk and joint range of movement had increased. He was also more willing to walk at home and outdoors with his family and complained less of pain in his ankle.

Somato-sensory disturbance after head injury

Tactile and proprioceptive deficits

There are no accurate data on the incidence of somato-sensory disturbance after head injury but, as in the stroke population, it is common. Feigenson et al. (1977) reported that up to 60% of people following stroke have impairment of tactile and proprioceptive sensation. These impairments may result in a significant amount of functional disability because, even if motor recovery is good, having poor sensory feedback regarding a task, such as holding a cup, may result in the cup being dropped despite adequate strength being present.

The location and extent of sensory disturbance depends on the site of the underlying lesion. Resulting deficits may manifest in either the complete absence or reduced intensity of sensation (hemianaesthesia or hemianalgesia) either on the same or opposite side to the lesion. There is no effective, well-defined approach to treating these sensory impairments, and there is no firm evidence to indicate either way if changes in sensory recovery can occur after the early stages.

Proprioceptive deficits are, similarly, very disabling. Again, even in the face of good strength, if an individual is unaware of where his limb is in space, then function will inevitably be impaired. Tactile impairments such as astereognosis (an inability to identify, through tactile information, common objects) and decreased two-point discrimination (an impairment of the ability to recognize as separate two simultaneous points of contact on the skin) may also be present.

Assessment

Tactile sensation may be assessed by touching the skin of the affected part, starting peripherally and asking the client to indicate when and where he feels the sensation, whether the sensation received through one side masks the other and whether he can distinguish between light and deep touch and identify two-point discrimination.

Proprioception may be assessed by working from the periphery on one limb, moving each joint and noting whether the client can sense any movement, the direction of movement and the final position. This is best done using the unaffected part to mirror the movement but it can be verbalized if necessary.

Communication and cognitive difficulties limit this type of formal testing. A fairly accurate idea of clients' sensation levels can be gained simply by observing their reaction to handling and to movement. It is useful to be aware of the spectrum of sensory tests that exist, although in practice only one or two tests will be appropriate for each client (Carr and Shepherd, 1998).

Management

The aim of intervention for sensory impairments is twofold. Firstly, the therapist aims to promote plastic recovery and to prevent further loss of cortical representation of the affected limb within the sensory cortex. This involves the therapist teaching the client and carer methods of sensory stimulation, through massage and use of differing stimuli, in order to keep the part 'interesting' to the CNS. The second aim is to teach the individual care of the affected part in order to avoid physical damage. For example, an affected arm should be placed in front of the client and the affected foot safely positioned on its foot plate to avoid entanglement with the working parts of a wheel chair or to avoid contact with, for example, sharp or hot surfaces. Visual compensation is crucial. Client-carer participation and collective cognitive ability are key to the successful management of sensory impairment.

Unilateral neglect

A further deficit that may be encountered is unilateral neglect, which is also termed sensory hemi-inattention. This is a condition in which there is a failure to respond to stimuli presented to the opposite side to that of the brain injury. This is discussed further in Chapter 4, but is worth outlining briefly at this point. The stimuli can involve space, the body or the visual field on that side, and even though the stimuli are sensed – that is, heard, seen or felt – they are not interpreted correctly as being of consequence to the client. For example, an affected individual may only eat food from one half of the plate, or may only shave one side of his face or attend to only one half of a doorway when passing through in a wheelchair (as evidenced by the defects seen in the paintwork in the doorways of all rehab units). This impairment is often accompanied by denial that there is a problem – a condition termed anosognosia. Unilateral neglect is a very disabling condition, disrupting everyday activities and causing difficulty with cognitive skills such as reading, writing and calculation, and stopping the client from driving. Physical injury frequently follows – for example, with the ignored arm being allowed to get trapped in the spokes of the wheelchair.

Unilateral neglect is more commonly seen in clients with right-sided brain damage, with the lesion likely to lie in the parietal lobe. It is often associated with a worse rehabilitation outcome than, for example, motor impairment on its own. It is important to realize that a visual inattention may co-exist with a homonymous hemianopia on the same side, and it can be difficult to sort out which is which.

The commonest tasks given to demonstrate visual hemi-inattention are the line-bisection test or the star cancellation test. The former requires the client to draw either a line through the centre of a series of scattered lines on a piece of paper, the latter to score through small stars distributed randomly over a page of larger stars. Management is considered in Chapter 4.

In terms of prognosis, one longitudinal study of 20 clients found that the majority of symptoms of gross neglect improved within one month and resolved completely within one year, but that 25% of the clients showed little or no improvement after the first year (Colombo, De Renzi and Gentilini, 1982). Residual deficits are, in general, very resistant to therapy. In the earlier stages however, rehabilitation using compensatory strategies has been shown to improve outcome in structured tasks (Diller and Weinberg, 1977; Diller and Gordon, 1981).

In summary, unilateral neglect is associated with considerable disability and a very poor prognosis if recovery has not occurred within the first year after injury. Indeed, the issue of this neglect may well be the most challenging aspect of a client's rehabilitation in the community setting.

Vision, hearing and balance disorders

Visual disturbance

Visual disturbance may result from direct trauma to the eye itself, to the optic nerve, to the nerves controlling eye movement, to the occipital cortex where the information is processed or to the fibre tracts within the brain transferring visual information. Estimates of the frequency of optic nerve damage with head trauma vary according to the data collected, but Roberts (1979) reported a figure of 2.7%. Retinal or optic nerve damage may produce one of three patterns of visual field loss: peripheral field loss, arcuate field loss or a central field loss. There is no regeneration of nerve fibres within the optic nerve so any damage is permanent. The damage may be sustained either directly or indirectly, and secondary damage can be done to the optic nerves as well as to the rest of the brain, as already described. Damage to the parietal cortex will produce a relatively congruous homonymous hemianopia, denser below than above, often characterized by a lack of awareness of the field defect. Occipital lobe damage may produce bilateral homonymous hemianopias of varying degrees, depending on the exact site of the trauma.

It is beyond the scope of this book to go into the assessment and management of each of these possibilities in detail, but thorough clinical examination and knowledge of the history and the pathology of the injury should help to locate the source of the visual impairment. Referral to an ophthalmologist is often required, for guidance with regard to exact diagnosis, prognosis and for inclusion on the blind register when necessary. There are no specific treatments available for injury to the visual pathways posterior to the optic nerves. Surgical decompression +/- high dose steroid treatment is used on occasion for optic nerve lesions, but the jury is still out on the merits of this (Sarkies, 1997).

Eye movement

Damage to the cranial nerves associated with the control of eye movement (the oculomotor, trochlear and abducens nerves) after head injury is the second commonest cause of acquired palsy to these nerves (Keane and Baloh, 1992). The oculomotor nerve (III nerve) is particularly vulnerable to injury through contusion or stretching, due to its firm attachment to the dura within the skull. The pupil served by the affected nerve dilates and becomes unresponsive to light, the eyelid may droop (ptosis) and the eye is pulled into a 'down and out' position. Some spontaneous recovery may occur over time (roughly a 12-month period), and squint surgery/surgery for the ptosis may be required. Green et al. (1964) reported that, in a group of 130 people with traumatic oculomotor palsy, 36% showed incomplete recovery with the remaining 64% unchanged.

Trochlear palsies (IV nerve) are evidenced by failure of downgaze and problems with reading, and the patient tends to adopt an automatic head tilt to accommodate the diplopia produced. Closed head trauma is thought to cause avulsion of the rootlets of the nerves as they emerge from the brainstem, hence both nerves may be affected. More minor trauma may result in a unilateral problem only, as may direct ocular trauma. Approximately 40% to 50% of unilateral palsies will recover spontaneously (Rush and Younge, 1981; Sydnor, Seaber and Buckley, 1982), often within eight months, but only 25% of bilateral palsies will resolve (Sydnor, Seaber and Buckley, 1982). As it may take up to 12 months for spontaneous recovery to occur, any operative correction will be deferred until after this time has elapsed.

The abducens (VI nerve) may similarly be stretched with trauma to the head, resulting in either unilateral or bilateral palsies (manifesting as failure of sideways movement of the eye). Rush and Younge reported that approximately 40% of traumatic VIth nerve palsies improve within six to 12 months so, again, surgical correction will usually be deferred until after a 12 month period has elapsed. Eye patching may usefully be employed to relieve the diplopia, and prism lenses may also be used as an interim measure to help relieve symptoms.

Injuries resulting in hearing disturbance

Individuals who have sustained significant trauma to the temporal region are at risk of hearing loss. Injuries can either affect the conductive hearing apparatus or the sensorineural hearing apparatus. Conductive apparatus damage may involve injuries to the external auditory canal from bony fracture, the tympanic membrane may be torn or there may be disruption of the chain of ossicles (the tiny chain of bones that transmit sounds). Ossicular damage requires operative exploration and repair. In the absence of temporal bone fracture, inner ear injury may be due to 'labyrinthine concussion' – damage to the highly sensitive tissues within the inner ear. Aural rehabilitation may involve fitting a hearing aid.

Vertigo after head injury

Injuries to the temporal bone after head injury may result in an array of damage to the vestibular system (the balance organ) involving some or all of its parts, from the inner ear to the collections of nerve cells that make up the 'vestibular nucleus' in the brain. Manifestation of the injury may be delayed, and may be compounded by concomitant injury to other elements of the nervous system involved in balance and eye movement coordination such as the cerebellum and higher cortical centres.

Benign paroxysmal positional vertigo is seen relatively frequently after head injury. Bergman and Fredrickson (1978) report an incidence of 34% of clients with minor head injury, and 50% after major head injury. It is associated with considerable morbidity. It is thought to be due to the dislodgement of particles within the vestibule that become free floating and cause havoc by randomly stimulating the inner ear as they float around in response to changes in the patient's position. Clinical examination may reveal an associated nystagmus (twitching of the eyes). The body has a tendency to try and compensate for this disturbance by resetting central controls, but this compensation may be delayed by the presence of other deficits such as visual/proprioceptive impairments. A form of physiotherapy known as vestibular physiotherapy can be used in this difficult client group, and has been shown to enhance central compensation and reduce the incidence of balance disorders after head injury (Luxon and Davies, 1997).

Occasionally, patients may present with fluctuating vestibular symptoms due to a leakage of fluid from the inner ear. Episodic vertigo, hearing loss and tinnitus are the hallmarks of this condition, which can be ameliorated by operative repair of the leak. Referral to the ear, nose and throat specialists is essential for help with the diagnosis and appropriate treatment of these disabling conditions.

Physiotherapeutic intervention

The role of the physiotherapist with the community-based brain-injured individual begins with observation and identification of the primary sensori-motor impairments, any associated physical injuries that remain active and the secondary problems in the musculoskeletal and cardiovascular systems. Added to this, she requires an understanding of the cognitive, communicative and socio-economic factors impacting on the individual. This information assists in the discussions with clients to establish their concerns and aims and to plan realistic, meaningful goals for intervention.

Approaches to treatment

Neurophysiology is continually evolving and it is important that therapists remain up to date with theoretical models underlying therapy techniques. Many therapists will adopt an approach that combines elements of several models and techniques. Indeed, therapists that restrict themselves to one particular approach limit the outcome for patients (Punt, 2000). It is important, however, that within the boundaries of current knowledge the therapist is able to justify treatment and show that a change has been made because of it. Specific treatment techniques for potential motor impairments are discussed throughout this chapter; however, over the years, a number of physiotherapeutic treatment approaches for managing neurologically impaired clients have evolved. The evolution of these approaches is closely linked to the advances that have been made in the understanding of neurophysiology and recovery following brain injury. Each treatment approach requires specialized training to acquire the skills required to implement it. The approaches include the Rood approach (Goff, 1969; Edwards, 1996); conductive education (Robinson, McCarthy and Little, 1989); Proprioceptive Neuromuscular Facilitation (Kabat and Knott, 1954); the Johnstone technique (Johnstone 1983); Bobath (Edwards, 1996; Davies, 1990) and the Motor Relearning Programme (Carr and Shepherd, 1998).

To date there is little evidence to suggest that any of these approaches are the 'gold standard' in treatment of the brain-injured client (Edwards, 1996).

In an extensive literature search, Tolfts and Stiller (1997) discovered that whilst a multidisciplinary approach to the treatment of brain injury had a positive effect on recovery, there is no substantial scientific evidence to suggest that any of the previous physiotherapy approaches are effective in the treatment of brain injury.

This lack of scientific data belies positive clinical experience that has found physiotherapy to be a major factor in influencing recovery after brain injury but, clearly, effective, well designed studies that allow for the heterogeneity of this population need to be conducted to support this.

Physiotherapy assessment

The motor impairment that a client can present with following a brain injury will depend on the severity and site of the brain injury (Hewer, 1993). The degree and type of disability experienced by the client in the community is a combination of the initial impairment and any secondary complications that have arisen over time as a result of this, together with any social or physical limitations set by the individual's environment. For the rehabilitation team this means that each client needs to be individually assessed because no two brain injured clients are going to present in exactly the same way.

In the community setting a client may be referred to the physiotherapist for follow-up following an inpatient period of rehabilitation to assist integration of that client into the community. They may also receive referrals for clients who have been living in the community for some time, if it is perceived that the clients are deteriorating in their ability to achieve activities of daily living. If it is felt that the client has recently improved and would benefit from a period of therapy to maximize this achievement then he may also be referred for therapy.

Often a client remains on review for several months, if not years, so that any deterioration or improvement can be monitored by the specialist team. Physiotherapy assessment of the client within the community is usually functionally based and is influenced by determining what the client perceives to be the problem. It is important to balance function, client goals and risk assessment in order to arrive at realistic goals.

The client may present in the community without any medical notes so a thorough assessment by the team is necessary to establish what difficulties the client has that might affect his therapy. This assessment should involve the whole team so that each member has an holistic knowledge of the client. It has already been mentioned that the cognitive and behavioural difficulties that may be the result of a head injury could influence a client's physical rehabilitation; therefore it is important that the physiotherapist is cognizant of these problems as highlighted in the MDT assessments.

There is no definitive physiotherapy assessment procedure and the order and content will vary depending on the therapist and the presentation of the individual. A sample format is set out as an appendix to this chapter. It is one used at the Icanho Centre in Suffolk, UK, and is constantly evolving.

There are various important pieces of information to include. The history of present condition (HPC) should include all appropriate details relating to the incident, any neurosurgery, musculoskeletal injuries and so forth, where they were treated, any ongoing secondary-based care and future clinic appointments, and any previous or ongoing physiotherapy intervention. The past medical history (PMH) should include any previous and ongoing conditions unrelated to the incident that may affect rehabilitation. The social and family history (SFH) should include carer details, such as their health and their potential to be involved with rehabilitation, the type of accommodation and access and details of previous sporting and leisure interests. The aim is to obtain an idea of the clients' pre-morbid level of physical activity at work and home. The drug history (DH) should include details of any anti-inflammatory, analgesic and anti-spasticity medication, noting when they were prescribed and why, and the current dose.

At the end of the subjective examination, it is important to note the clients' perception of their physical difficulties and what they hope to achieve with rehabilitation. Questioning can provide an indication of what specific functional activities they are still unable to do at home and what they hope to achieve. Discussion should give the therapist valuable insight into the clients' level of expectation and motivation, as well as providing some early pointers for specific goal setting. It should be discussed at this point that, as part of intervention, the client might be required to remove items of clothing as necessary and to be physically handled by the therapist. Consent, if given, should be noted.

The objective examination will include factors such as the client's dominant hand, pain, neglect, sensation, vision, hearing and cognition. When investigating pain it is important to include location, any aggravating/easing factors, severity, incidence and nature. This information may be difficult to establish where the client has limited communication. For tactile sensation, assessment is done by touching the skin of the affected part, working from the periphery, and asking clients to indicate when they feel the sensation. Kinaesthetic awareness testing would start distally on the affected limb, each joint being moved and a note made as to whether the client can sense any movement, the direction of movement and the final position. As discussed earlier in the chapter, this is best done using the unaffected part to mirror the movement, but it can be verbalized if necessary. Communication and cognitive difficulties do limit this type of formal testing. A fairly accurate idea of the clients' sensation level can be gained simply by observing their reaction to your handling and to movement. When assessing vision and visual field deficits pre-existing impairments and any aids should be noted. Equipment should be noted, such as any aids to mobility currently in use and any problems with these, and the need for wheelchair/seating assessment checked. Information on cognition should relate particularly to motivation, insight and the clients' ability to participate in therapy. Other multidisciplinary team assessments can be invaluable, including those of neuropsychology and occupational therapy, to highlight cognitive issues and also to indicate spatial and perceptual problems.

When assessing the upper limbs, lower limbs and trunk, the therapist should note the range of movement (ROM), the selective movement, muscle strength, muscle tone (and associated reactions), posture, joint alignment and symmetry relating to these areas. Balance findings should include observations on righting and equilibrium reactions in sitting, standing and walking and should cover both static and dynamic activities. The use of Romberg's test, previously described, should also be noted. Observations concerning coordination should include such tests as heel-shin, finger-nose, and heel-toe, depending on the level of ability of the client. The presence of ataxia, and type if possible, should be evaluated. A general opinion regarding the level of cardiovascular fitness is useful, considering whether it affects functional activity. A fitness test can be included if appropriate.

When assessing functional activity, each manoeuvre is checked and for each one the level of assistance needed to perform the activity safely is noted – that is, the number of people and the level of skill required, whether verbal, standby or physical assistance is needed and what type of equipment. One aim of the assessment if appropriate is to gain enough information for a risk assessment relating to physiotherapy and non-physiotherapy trained staff. For every movement that the client does a note should be made of how they do it and any deviations from 'normal' in the way that the movement is carried out. Actions such as sitting, transferring, walking and so on all require skilful coordination of movement and are considered to be important elements in the functional skills of daily life (Van Sant, 1999). The summary should include an analysis of the particular deficits that may be inhibiting the client from achieving successful functional independence in his chosen task.

Formal assessment

In order to assist with the decision-making and goal-setting processes, various measurement and outcome tools have been developed. The aim of physiotherapy in the physical rehabilitation of the head-injured client is to 'enable patients to attain their optimum level of function with regard to effectiveness and economy of movement' (Edwards, 1996). In order to evaluate this there are a variety of motor assessment tools that have been tested with head-injured clients and these are listed in Watson (1995).

Within a multidisciplinary community setting it is often useful to review client progress with global measures such as the Functional Assessment Measure (FIM + FAM). This measure has been specifically validated for use with the brain-injured population and enables multidisciplinary input so that all aspects of the client's rehabilitation can be considered (Hall, 1992). A common measurement of motor function needs to be identified so that management of this client group can be optimized (Watson, 1995; BSRM, 1998).

Physiotherapists often find gross motor function scales such as the Functional Assessment Measure to be too insensitive and therefore not useful for measurement on a treatment to treatment basis and not always directly relevant to the client. For example, Mrs D was able to walk 17 m independently and therefore attained the highest measurement on that section of the

Functional Assessment Measure. Her walking pattern, however, was very laborious and she could only walk a maximum of 25 m before she became so tired that she had to sit down. Mrs D found this very disabling as her local shops were twice that distance and she was therefore unable to go to buy herself a pint of milk without having to ask for help. Prior to therapy the physiotherapist chose to time how long it took for Mrs D to walk a distance of 10 m and also used the Physiological Cost Index (PCI). It is assumed that as quality of gait improves, the time taken to walk 10 m is reduced and the effort that is required to make that walk will be less (Ladouceur and Barbeau, 2000). These measurements are easily reproduced in the therapy situation and motivated Mrs D to continue coming to the rehabilitation unit, as she was able to see an improvement each time.

Many additional tools are also cited in Wade (1998). The choice of each specific tool will depend on the problems highlighted by the assessment. The Rivermead motor assessment and Motor assessment scale (Wade, 1998) both give an overview of function as well as quality of specific limb movements. The disadvantage of these and others is that they are designed for a client with defined hemiplegia and make no allowance for the diverse disabilities that accompany traumatic brain injury. The motor assessment scale is timed in parts and therefore lends itself to clients with a higher level of recovery. It is less sensitive with clients who may have recovered functional ability but lack speed and therefore can fail to measure independence. The Rivermead has sections devoted to gross function and to upper limb both of which are hierarchical, and sections for lower limb and trunk which are not (Adams et al., 1997). Balance can be assessed by the Berg balance scale for clients with the relevant problems.

Simple goniometric measurements may be relevant for noting limitations in range of movement due for example to malalignment or contractures resulting from tonal changes, trauma or abnormal posture (American Academy of Orthopaedic Surgeons, 1986).

Goal setting

To ensure an individual approach for each client, a list of his or her specific physical and functional issues should be compiled, drawing from the assessment findings. From this list and on further discussion with the client, specific, short-term goals can be set. These are timed and measurable and should be reviewed on a six-to-eight week basis to check progress and the appropriateness of that goal. Joint goal setting that involves the physiotherapist, the client and other members of the team is to be encouraged as this provides goals that are usually functionally relevant and more meaningful to the client. Clients' motivation is likely to be higher if working on tasks that are important to them (Campbell, 2000).

Physical recovery following head injury

There are two main mechanisms underlying physical recovery, namely neuroplasticity and compensatory strategies.

Neuroplasticity

Recovery within the brain following a head injury relies on plastic adaptation and reorganization. Studies have shown that there can be multiple pathways to one area of the brain but only one dominant pathway will show any functional activity. If that pathway is damaged as a result of brain injury then the secondary pathways can immediately show functional connections and start to take over that role. This plastic adaptation is continually occurring within the brain influenced by peripheral inputs (Kidd, Lawes and Musa, 1992).

In order to demonstrate this phenomenon, experiments were carried out using monkeys. On the cortex of the brain, areas have been accurately mapped that respond to sensory information from all parts of the body. In one such experiment the median nerve (which innervates the cutaneous regions of the hand) was severed. One would then expect this area on the cortex to become non-functioning; however, surgery showed that neighbouring areas expanded and took over the role of the denervated area. This adaptation continued to occur over the following weeks (Merzenich et al., 1983).

Clinically, this could lead to the conclusion that some recovery will occur immediately following brain injury as a result of immediate adaptation and that further longer term changes can also follow. Traditionally literature has suggested that maximum motor recovery occurs within the first six months to a year following traumatic brain injury (Bond, 1975). Watson (1997) conducted a review of appropriate literature and found that significant motor recovery in a client with severe traumatic brain injury extended beyond six months and potentially up to 10 years. This review did suggest, however, that most recovery occurred earlier rather than later. It should be noted that this study was based on only a small number of papers, indicating a need for further research. This evidence of late stage motor recovery may be particularly positive for therapists treating head-injured clients within the community as some referrals for rehabilitation can be received a number of months or even years after the original injury.

When discussing the time scales for motor recovery following a brain injury it is important to take into consideration that some clients may not be able to participate actively in physical rehabilitation for some time after the incident. This may be as a result of severe cognitive and behavioural difficulties which can limit physical recovery (Jackson, 1986) or severe fractures sustained during the time of the head injury.

Compensatory strategies

Physical recovery and improvements in functional ability also occur through the development of compensatory strategies. It is vital for the client that the therapist recognizes when these strategies should be adopted. This is often when the client has either stopped responding or, for cognitive reasons, is unable to participate in treatment approaches that focus on quality and neuroplasticity.

These strategies may occur internally, for instance in the development of an 'abnormal' gait pattern to enable walking using the high tone in the affected leg to give stability in stance. The potential disadvantage with this is the risk of the unnatural, new joint alignment and adaptation of soft tissue structures resulting in, for example, accelerated joint degeneration or chronic pain. There are also external strategies through appropriate, timely adaptations to the environment, such as provision of assistive devices or provision of appropriate rails to assist with transfers. Here again the advantages and disadvantages should be weighed up, as overuse of the unaffected side (in, for example, repeated pulling up from sitting to standing using a rail) is likely to promote increased tone and learned non-use in the affected side. Regular review and updating clients and carers on techniques can minimize these potential hazards.

It is also important to consider the acceptability of such 'external' strategies. A 22-year-old head-injured woman had great difficulty accepting a stick as an aid to walking, partly because she felt it drew attention to the nature of her disability and partly because she saw sticks as something suitable for old people. However, she did accept a crutch because she felt this would suggest to other people that she had had a sports injury – in her view a more 'normal' injury for someone of her age.

Despite evidence for later stage motor recovery there do seem to be times when the client's ability to benefit from therapy plateaus. Cessation of treatment can be difficult if the client has had unrealistically high expectations of the outcome. In order to avoid this conflict, clear treatment goals and time scales should be set prior to starting treatment (Rosenthal and O'Leary, 1995).

Physical treatment

In principle physical rehabilitation of the head-injured client should aim to improve function and prevent secondary complications that may arise as a result of the impairments that can occur following a head injury (Barnes, McLellan and Sutton, 1993).

A physiotherapist may use any of the physiotherapeutic approaches mentioned previously but as clients who present with physical disabilities following a brain injury can exhibit a variety of problems it is important not to become prescriptive.

Physical rehabilitation of the head-injured client should be carried out within an interdisciplinary environment. Shumway-Cook and Woollacott (1995) believe that motor control evolves from the 'dynamic interplay between perceptual, cognitive and action systems'. The term 'action systems' includes both the neuromuscular properties and the physical properties of the musculoskeletal system. The physiotherapist must therefore learn how to influence cognitive and perceptual problems as part of the physical rehabilitation process of the head-injured client. A close working relationship between all members of the therapy team and the client needs to exist, if rehabilitation goals are to be met.

The following case study illustrates the importance of considering cognitive factors in planning how to approach a specific physical impairment. C was referred as an outpatient to the community rehabilitation team, one year after a road traffic accident in which he had sustained a head injury. He presented with severe memory and associated behavioural problems. At the time of the assessment he was able to transfer with the assistance of one person. The behavioural problems manifested themselves in a refusal to come to therapy. If his family did manage to get C to therapy he would refuse to carry out his programme and become verbally aggressive. The multidisciplinary team believed that a new environment, and the fear of trying to overcome his physical problems in this new environment, made him very anxious, especially as he was unable to remember what he had achieved in previous sessions and what he was doing at home.

The team felt that if strategies could be used to enable him to remember what he had achieved in each session then this might help decrease his anxiety. Video recordings of C's therapy sessions and a diary for the therapist to document progress in were started. These were then used at home to reinforce how much he was able to achieve and that this had been achieved in the rehabilitation gym. Continuity was also very important, so C always saw the same therapist and within the limitations of the service always came at the same time and on the same day. Gradually over a number of months, despite little improvement in his memory, C's compliance improved and he began to make progress in his physical abilities, to the point where he is now attending gym sessions at his local sports centre with the help of a facilitator.

Swallowing and eating

Swallowing is a complex process that safely conveys food and drink from the oral cavity to the stomach, via oral, pharyngeal and oesophageal stages. The entire act of eating would also encompass getting the food to the mouth. Swallowing and eating problems often result from head injury.

Once a client has emerged from coma and is alert enough for evaluation, swallowing and oral intake must be considered. Adequate nutrition is vital and brain-injured clients have a significant increase in resting metabolic expenditure, which puts them at risk of excessive weight loss (see, for example, Pepe, Morgan and Mackay, 1997). Mackay, Morgan and Bernstein (1999) looked at risk factors for swallowing problems (dysphagia) and found lower admitting GCS score, severe cognitive dysfunction, longer ventilation time and having a tracheostomy were all related, although not necessarily directly.

At the stage of acute rehabilitation, the incidence of dysphagia after head injury has been variably cited, for example as 27% (Weinstein, 1983) and 41.6% (Cherney and Halper, 1996). This difference may be explained by methodological differences, as may Yorkston et al.'s (1989) figure of 77.5% of acute patients. However, they compared acute and outpatient treatment settings, and found a marked decrease to only 13% of outpatients. When they considered only those who were so severe they could not meet their nutritional needs orally, the decrease was from 45% to 2%. It is likely in a community setting that many clients will refer to swallowing problems that have resolved, with only a few experiencing persistent severe problems.

Problems may be physiological or cognitive-behavioural. After head injury, physiological deficits may affect swallowing at the oropharyngeal level, with delayed or absent swallow reflex, reduced tongue control and reduced pharyngeal contraction. A smaller proportion have laryngeal and cricopharyngeal problems. Aspiration was found in between a third and a half of subjects studied by Lazarus and Logeman (1987) and Field and Weiss (1989). Cognitive-behavioural factors may also cause or accentuate eating and swallowing difficulties. Yorkston et al.'s (1989) data suggested that the frequency of dysphagia decreases as clients improve cognitively and behaviourally.

To illustrate the possible impact of cognitive-behavioural factors, at an extreme level of severity, attention deficit may mean clients do not attempt to manipulate food even when it is placed in the mouth. This degree of dysfunction is unlikely in a community setting, but attention disorder can still create problems. For example, a client is more likely to aspirate if unable to maintain attention, is more likely to have difficulty using compensatory strategies and is more likely to take a long time over meals. Impulsive behaviour can result in clients rushing their food and increases the risk of aspiration. Memory deficits will affect the ability to retain instructions and make use of adaptive strategies and techniques.

Apathy may lead to reduced initiation of eating and lack of interest. Appetite may be affected centrally or because of decreased sensory reception or perception. The use of strategies will also potentially be affected by executive dysfunction and problem-solving/sequencing problems. Language disorder may make following instructions about modifying swallowing difficult. Cognitive abilities may also affect the selection of and preparation of food, which for the community-based client may be a crucial area to consider.

Assessment

Dysphagia needs a systematic and careful assessment. At the physiological level, once beyond the acute stage, what to assess is the same as in other groups of clients, but how to adapt to the cognitive changes will affect the approach to assessment. Mackay, Morgan and Bernstein (1999) offer a useful summary of procedure, including the use of videofluroscopic studies. Cherney, Cantieri and Pannell (1986) suggest seven functional severity levels for oral intake, from severe to normal. They incorporate considerations such as oral versus non-oral intake, need for supervision, use of new techniques, prescribed diet and safety.

Assessment should, within a case history, include medication, as some drugs may affect respiration (and thus pose aspiration risks), swallowing, or appetite.

Management

Management of eating and swallowing disorders after head injury will need to encompass both physiologic and cognitive-behavioural aspects. Treatment will differ in acute and community settings as the needs of clients differ, but care at the acute stage is outside the scope of this chapter. At any stage oral hygiene needs to be encouraged, and cognitive issues may affect individual's ability and motivation to maintain this aspect of personal care.

In general, intervention can be described as oropharyngeal, postural, dietary, behavioural, and environmental. Orophayngeal work addresses the physiological issues, and may be direct, via eating and drinking, or indirect, via oral muscle strength and range exercises. At times it may help to teach physical manoeuvres, such as an adapted swallow pattern. Such issues are the same for other groups of clients, and are covered in most general dysphagia texts.

Postural changes may be to do with seating and whole body posture or more specifically positioning of the head/neck – for example, head flexion may be a useful technique to protect the airway. Dietary modifications may include advice on consistency, texture and type of foods or liquids. Again, these issues are covered in general texts.

Behavioural management encompasses such advice as having short, frequent meal times, if attention is a problem for instance. Similarly, using prompts (visual and/or verbal) may be helpful with people who have attention, memory or executive problems – for example, to slow down, to take small bites/sips, or to swallow twice after each mouthful. Written advice is important and can be presented pictorially if reading comprehension is an issue.

Environmental manipulation may mean adapting the physical environment or the social environment. The former would, for example, include suggesting the person with an attention deficit eat in a quiet, distraction-free room or the restriction of utensils to one at a time. Social manipulation involves using people in the environment to provide necessary prompts and assistance to the dysphagic person, or ensuring the number of people present at mealtimes is kept to a minimum.

Education of the client, family and other members of staff can be critical to a programme. Hutchins (1989) offers an outline of a teaching session for families and advice on setting up such a programme. It is useful to describe the normal swallow, before explaining what has changed in the individual client. Then videotapes and assessment results can illustrate information to do with dietary and other advice.

The few clients who arrive in a community setting unable to eat orally may well need help to adjust to long-term, or even lifelong, non-oral feeding – usually via a PEG. Eating is very often part of social events and it is very hard for people who can no longer join in family meals or social outings. However, the huge majority will, by the time they are in the community, be able to eat orally. Some might need long-term support to continue with the strategies and techniques that have been used successfully, but most will have no persistent difficulty.

Outcome

Dysphagia therapies are effective in restoring oral intake – Schurr et al. (1999) found 83% of their head-injured sample responded to dietary, postural and behavioural modifications. There appears to have been no attempt to study dysphagia after head injury in a community-based population, but at the Icanho Centre in Suffolk, UK, only two clients with non-oral feeding were seen over a three-year period, one of whom then did establish oral feeding successfully.

Carer involvement

The involvement of carers within the whole rehabilitation process will be discussed in Chapter 9; however it is important that the carer is involved in the physical management of the brain-injured client. This may be by supporting the client in general or, if the carer feels able and is physically able, encouraging them to take part in specific programmes. Some of the specific physiotherapeutic treatments will require carer assistance, such as certain stretching and positioning techniques. It is necessary for the therapist in this case to ensure that she has spent sufficient time with both the client and carer to make sure that they are both confident and comfortable with what is being asked of them. Lack of such support to carry out programmes outside the formal rehabilitation setting could directly affect what is planned.

An example of a situation when the carer has a crucial physical role is in transfers and mobility. Severely affected brain-injured clients may not have the ability to move themselves either in bed or between bed and chair independently and so will require assistance to do so. Techniques for assisting the client to move and transfer should be carefully taught so that injury to either client or carer can be avoided. The provision of a hoist may be recommended if the therapist assesses that the risks to the client and/or carer are too great to use manual transfer procedures. There are a variety of hoists that can provide more or less assistance dependent on how much the client can do. The Royal College of Nursing has published a guide to the handling of patients and this contains precise guidelines about what to do and what not to do when moving and handling clients.

Another example may be seen in people who have dysphagia and depend on a carer to provide an appropriate diet, and to offer consistent reminders about how to position, eat and swallow. In a more general way, clients with visual problems will often no longer be able to drive and will become dependent upon a carer for transport, particularly in rural communities, where public transport is poor. This can be upsetting for the client, who feels a loss of independence, and it places a considerable burden on the carer.

Conclusion

'The goal of successful community reintegration should guide all rehabilitation intervention' (Carr and Shepherd, 1998). As the individual progresses through his 'formal' rehabilitation, therapists can assist him to adapt to his physical disabilities and help him to move on from being a passive recipient of treatment to an active institutor of his own long-term rehabilitation using services in the community. Formal therapy will not continue ad infinitum; however therapists should not simply withdraw at the end of the formal treatment stage leaving the client high and dry. The role of the therapist gradually becomes that of advisor and trouble-shooter, a state which may justifiably exist for years, as many of the individuals concerned are young adults with many years and life changes ahead of them.

Appendix

ICANHO PHYSIOTHERAPY ASSESSMENT
(source: whether GP letter, medical assessment and/or client)

CLIENT NAME: CLIENT NUMBER:
DATE OF BIRTH: DATE OF ASSESSMENT:

HISTORY OF PRESENT CONDITION:
PAST MEDICAL HISTORY:
SOCIAL AND FAMILY HISTORY:
DRUG HISTORY:
    Client's perception of rehabilitation
    Consent to treatment

ON EXAMINATION

Dominant hand (pre-morbidly):
Pain
Neglect
Tactile sensation
Proprioception/kinaesthetic sensation
Visual field
Hearing
Equipment
Cognition

PHYSICAL ACTIVITY:
    Upper limbs
    Lower limbs
    Trunk
    Balance
    Coordination
    Exercise tolerance

FUNCTIONAL ACTIVITY:
    Bed mobility
    Lying to sitting to lying
    Sitting
    Sit to stand to sit
    Transfers (involving wheel chair, bed, toilet and car as appropriate)
    Standing
    Walking
    Stairs

SUMMARY OF FINDINGS

References

Adams SA, Ashburn A, Pickering RM, Taylor D (1997) The scalability of the Rivermead Motor Assessment in acute stroke patients. Clinical Rehabilitation 11: 42–51.

American Academy of Orthopaedic Surgeons (1986) Joint Motion. Method of measuring and Recording. Edinburgh: Churchill Livingstone.

Banks MA (1991) Physiotherapy in Rehabilitation of Parkinson's Disease. London: Chapman & Hall.

Barnes M, McLellan L, Sutton R (1993) Spasticity in Neurological Rehabilitation. Edinburgh: Churchill Livingstone.

Becker E, Bar-Or L, Mendelson L, Najenson T (1978) Pulmonary responses to exercise of patients following cranio-cerebral injury. Scandinavian Journal of Rehabilitation Medicine 10: 47–50.

Bergman JM, Fredrickson JM (1978) Vertigo after head injury: five year follow up. Journal of Otolaryngology 7: 237.

Bernstein N (1967) The co-ordination and regulation of movements. Oxford: Pergamon.

Bobath B (1990) Adult Hemiplegia: Evaluation and Treatment. 3 edn. Oxford: Butterworth-Heinemann.

Bohannon RW, Smith MB (1987) Interrater reliability of a modified Ashworth scale of muscle spasticity. Physical Therapy 67: 206–7.

Bond MR (1975) Assessment of the psychosocial outcome after severe head injury. CIBA Foundation Symposium 43: 141–51.

Borello-France DF, Whitney SL, Herdman SJ (1994) Assesment of vestibular ypofunction. In Herdman SJ (ed.) Vestibular Rehabilitation. Philadelphia PA: FA Davis.

Britton TC (1998) Abnormalities of muscle tone and movement. In Edwards S (1998) Neurological Physiotherapy. St Louis and London: Mosby.

BSRM (1998) A Working Party Report of the British Society of Rehabilitation Medicine. London: British Society of Rehabilitation Medicine.

Campbell M (2000) Rehabilitation for Traumatic Brain Injury: Physical Therapy Practice in Context. Edinburgh: Churchill Livingstone.

Carnstam B, Larsson LE, Prevec TS (1979) Improvement of gait following functional electrical stimulation. Investigations on changes in voluntary strength and proprioceptive reflexes. Scandinavian Journal of Rehabilitation Medicine 9(1): 7–13.

Carr JH, Shepherd RB (1998) Neurological Rehabilitation: Optimizing Motor Performance. Oxford: Butterworth-Heinemann.

Carr JH, Shepherd RB, Ada L (1995) Spasticity. Research Findings and Implications for Intervention in Physiotherapy 81(8): 421–9.

Carr JH, Shepherd RB, Nordholm L, Lynne D (1985) Investigation of a new motor assessment scale for stroke patients. Physical Therapy 65: 175–80.

Cawthorne TE (1945) Vestibular injuries. Proceedings of the Royal Society of Medicine 39: 270–3.

Cherney LR, Halper AS (1996) Swallowing problems in adults with traumatic brain injury. Seminars in Neurology 16(4): 349–53.

Cherney LR , Cantieri CA, Pannell JJ (1986) Clinical Evaluation of Dysphagia. Rockville MD: Aspen.

Colombo A, De Renzi E, Gentilini M (1982) The time course of visual inattention. Arch Psychiatry Neuro Science 231: 539–46.

Cooksey FS (1945) Rehabilitation of vestibular injuries. Proceedings of the Royal Society of Medicine 39: 273–8.

Culham EG, Noce RR, Bagg SD (1995) Shoulder complex position and glenohumeral sub-luxation in hemiplegia. Archives of Physical Medicine and Rehabilitation 76(9): 857–64.

Davies PM (1990) Right in the Middle. Berlin: Springer-Verlag.

Dietz V (1992) Human neuronal control of automatic functional movements: interaction between central programs and afferent input. Physiological Reviews 72(1): 33–69.

Diller L, Gordon WA (1981). Rehabilitation and clinical neuropsychology. In Filskov S, Bell T (eds) Handbook of Clinical Neuropsychology. New York: Wiley.

Diller L, Weinberg J (1977) Hemi-inattention in rehabilitation: the evolution of a rational remediation programme. Advanced Neurology 18: 521–32.

Eames P, Wood RW (1985) Rehabilitation after severe brain injury: a follow-up study of a behaviour modification approach. Journal of Neurology, Neurosurgery and psychiatry 48: 613–19.

Edmondson J, Fisher K, Hanson C (1999) How effective are lycra suits in the management of children with cerebral palsy? APCP Journal (March): 49–57.

Edwards S (1996) Neurological Physiotherapy: A Problem-solving Approach. Edinburgh: Churchill Livingstone.

Edwards S, Charlton P (1996) Splinting and the use of orthoses in the management of patients with neurological disorders. In Edwards S (1996) Neurological Physiotherapy: A Problem-solving Approach. Edinburgh: Churchill Livingstone.

Feigenson JS, McCarthy ML, Greenberg SD, Feigenson WD (1977) Factors influencing out-come and length of stay in a stroke rehabilitation unit. Part 2. Comparison of 318 screened and 248 unscreened patients. Stroke 8: 657–62.

Field LH and Weiss CJ (1989) Dysphagia with head injury. Brain Injury 3: 9–26.

Goff B (1969) Appropriate afferent stimulation. Physiotherapy 51: 9–17.

Goldspink DF (1976) Changes in size and protein turnover of skeletal muscle after immo-bilization at different lengths. Proceedings of the Physiological Society: 263(2): 269–70.

Goldspink G, Williams P (1990) Muscle Fibre and Connective Tissue Changes Associated with Use and Disuse. In Canning AL (ed.) Key Issues in Neurological Physiotherapy. Oxford: Butterworth-Heinemann.

Green WR, Hackett ER, Schelzinger NF (1964) Neuro-opthalmologic evaluation of occulo-motor nerve paralysis. Archives of Opthalmology 72: 152–67.

Griffin JW (1986) Hemiplegic shoulder pain. Physical Therapy 66(12): 1884–93.

Hall KM (1992) Overview of functional assessment scales in brain injury rehabilitation. Neurorehabilitation 2: 98–113.

Hall KM, Hamilton BB, Gordon WA, Zasler ND (1993) Characteristics and comparisons of functional assessment indices: Disability Rating Scale, Functional Independence Measure and Functional Assessment Measure. Journal of Head Trauma Rehabilitation (June): 60–74.

Hewer RL (1993) The epidemiology of disabling neurological disorders. In Greenwood R, Barnes MP, McMillan TM, Ward CD. Neurological Rehabilitation. Edinburgh: Churchill Livingstone.

Hutchins BF (1989) Establishing a dysphagia family intervention program for head injured patients. Journal of Head Trauma Rehabilitation 4(4): 64–72.

Jackson H (1986) Psychological aspects of physical rehabilitation after severe head injury: a case study. Physiotherapy Practice 2: 47-51.

Jankowski LW, Sullivan SJ (1990) Aerobic and neuromuscular training: effect on the capacity, efficiency, and fatigability of patients with traumatic brain injuries. Archives of Physical Medicine and Rehabilitation 71: 500-4.

Johnstone M (1983) Restoration of Motor Function in the Stroke Patient: a Physiotherapist's Approach. Edinburgh: Churchill Livingstone.

Kabat H, Knott M (1954) Proprioceptive facilitation therapy for paralysis. Physiotherapy 40: 171-6.

Katz RT, Rymer WZ (1989) Spastic hypertonia: mechanisms and measurement. Archives of Physical Medicine and Rehabilitation 70: 144-55.

Keane JR, Baloh RW (1992) Post traumatic cranial neuropathies. Neurology Clinician, Nov 10, 4: 849-67.

Kidd G, Lawes N, Musa I (1992) Understanding Neuromuscular Plasticity: a Basis for Clinical Rehabilitation. London: Edward Arnold.

Knutsson E (1970) Topical cryotherapy and spasticity. Scandinavian Journal of Rehabilitation and Medicine 2: 159-63.

Ko Ko C, Ward A (1997) Management of spasticity. British Journal of Hospital Medicine 58(8): 400-5.

Ladouceur M, Barbeau H (2000) Functional electrical stimulation-assisted walking for persons with incomplete spinal injuries: changes in the kinematics and physiological cost of overground walking. Scandinavian Journal of Rehabilitation Medicine 32(2): 72-9.

Lance JW (1990) What is spasticity? Lancet 335: 606.

Lancet (1973) Boxing brains. Lancet 2: 605.

Lazarus C, Logeman JA (1987) Swallowing disorders in closed head trauma patients. Archives of Physical Medical Rehabilitation 68: 17-84.

Lehman JF, Delateur BJ (1982) Therapeutic heat. In Lehman JF (Ed) Therapeutic Heat and Cold. 3 edn. Baltimore: Williams & Wilkins.

Luxon LM, Davies RA (1997) Handbook of Vestibular Rehabilitation. London: Whurr.

MacDonald R (1996) Taping Techniques: Principles and Practice. Oxford: Butterworth Heinemann.

Mackay LE, Morgan AS, Bernstein BA (1999) Swallowing disorders in severe brain injury: risk factors affecting return to oral intake. Archives of Physical Medical Rehabilitation 80: 365-71.

Merletti R, Andina A, Galante M (1979) Clinical experience of electronic peroneal stimulators in 50 hemiparetic patients. Scandinavian Journal of Rehabilitation Medicine 11: 111-21.

Merzenich MM, Kaas JH, Wall JT, Sur M, Nelson RJ, Felleman DJ (1983) Progression of change following median nerve resection of the hand in the cortical representation of the hand in areas 3b and 1 in adult owl and squirrel monkeys. Neuroscience 10: 639-65.

Moran AJ (1976) Six case studies of severe head injury treated by exercise in addition to other therapies. Medical Journal of Australia (20 March): 396-7.

Moseley AM (1997) The effect of casting combined with stretching on passive ankle dorsiflexion in adults with traumatic brain injuries. Physical Therapy 77: 240-7.

Musa IM (1986) The role of afferent input in the reduction of spasticity: an hypothesis. Physiotherapy 72(4): 179-92.

Novak TA, Roth DL, Boll TJ (1988) Treatment alternatives following mild head injury. Rehabilitation Council Bulletin 31: 313-24.

Od'een I, Knutsson E (1981) Evaluation of the effects of muscle stretch and weight load in patients with spastic paraplegia. Scandinavian Journal of Rehabilitation Medicine 13(4): 117-21.

Pepe J, Morgan AS, Mackay LE (1997) The metabolic response to acute tbi and associated complications. In MacKayl E, Chapman PE, Morgan A (1997) Maximising brain injury recovery: integrating critical care and early rehabilitation. Gaitnersburg MD: Aspen, pp. 396-443.

Pope PM (1996) Postural management and special seating. In Edwards S (1996) Neurological Physiotherapy: A Problem-solving Approach. Edinburgh: Churchill Livingstone.

Punt TD (2000) No success like failure: walking late after stroke. Physiotherapy 86(11): 563-6.

Richardson D, Thompson AJ (1999) Botulinum toxin: its use in the treatment of acquired spasticity in adults. Physiotherapy 85(10): 541-51.

Roberts AH (1979) Severe Accidental Head Injury. London: Macmillan.

Robinson RO, McCarthy GT, Little TM (1989) Conductive education at the Peto Institute, Budapest. British Medical Journal 299: 1145-9.

Rosenfeld J (1998) Psychological/Cognitive Benefits of Aerobic Training. London: University of East London.

Rosenthal M, O'Leary JF (1995) Strategies for Community Integration: Physical Therapy for Traumatic Brain Injury. Edinburgh: Churchill Livingstone.

Rush JA, Younge BR (1981) Paralysis of cranial nerves III, IV, and VI: cause and prognosis in 1000 cases. Archives of Ophthalmology 53: 82-97.

Sanford B (1989) Group Exercise. In Hollis M, Fletcher-Cook P (eds) Practical Exercise Therapy. Oxford: Blackwell Scientific Publications.

Sarkies NJC (1997) Neuro-ophthalmological aspects of head injury. In MacFarlane R, Hardy DG (eds) Outcome after Head, Neck and Spinal Trama. A Medico-legal Guide. Oxford: Butterworth Heinemann, pp. 163-75.

Scherzer BP (1986) Rehabilitation following severe head trauma: results of a three year programme. Archives of Physical Medicine and Rehabilitation 67: 366-74.

Schurr MJ, Ebner KA, Maser AL, Sperling KB, Helgerson RB, Harris B (1999) Formal swallowing evaluation and therapy after TBI improves dysphagia outcomes. Journal of Trauma Injury Infection and Critical Care 46(5): 817-23.

Shumway-Cook A, Woollacott M (1995) Motor Control. Theory and Applications. Baltimore: Williams & Wilkins.

Sullivan SJ, Richer E, Laurent F (1990) The role of and possibilities for physical conditioning programmes in the rehabilitation of traumatically brain-injured persons. Brain Injury 4(4): 407-14.

Sydnor CF, Seaber JH, Buckley EG (1982) Traumatic superior oblique palsies. Ophthalmology 89: 134-8.

Tardieu C, Lespargol A, Tabary C, Bret MD (1988) For how long must the soleus muscle be stretched each day to prevent contracture? Dev Med Child Neurol 30: 3-10.

Thilmann AF, Fellows SJ, Garms E (1991) The mechanism of spastic muscle hypertonus. Brain 114: 233-44.

Thompson PD, Day BL (1993) The anatomy and physiology of cerebellar disease. Advances in Neurology 61: 15-31.

Thornton H, Kilbride C (1998) Physical management of abnormal tone and movement. In Stokes M. Neurological Physiotherapy. St Louis, London: Mosby.

Tolfts A and Stiller K. (1997) Do patients with traumatic brain injury benefit from physiotherapy? A review of the evidence. Physiotherapy Theory and Practice 13: 197-206.

Tyson SF (1995) Stroke rehabilitation: what is the point? Physiotherapy 81(8): 430-2.

Van Sant AF (1999) Rolling over and rising from supine. In Durward BR, Baer GD, Rowe PJ (eds) Functional Human Movement: Measurement and Analysis. Oxford: Butterworth-Heinemann.

Wade DT (1998) Measurement in Neurological Rehabilitation. Oxford: Oxford University Press.

Ward CD, Duvoisin RC, Ince SE, Nutt JD, Eldridge R, Calne DB (1983) Parkinson's disease in 65 pairs of twins and in a set of quadruplets. Neurology 33: 815-24.

Watkins CA (1999) Mechanical and neurophysiological changes in spastic muscles. Serial casting in spastic equinovarus following traumatic brain injury. Physiotherapy 85: 603-9.

Watson MJ (1997) Evidence for 'significant' late-stage motor recovery in patients with severe traumatic brain injury: a literature review with relevance for neurological physiotherapy. Physical Therapy Reviews 2: 93-106.

Watson M (1995) Review of Motor Assessments in Head Injury Synapse: abstract of presentation at 'Update on Management of Head Injury', ACPIN National Conference; Birmingham (March).

Weinstein CJ (1983) Neurogenic dysphagia: frequency, progression and outcome in adults following head injury. Physical Therapist 12: 1992-3.

Williams PE (1990) Use of intermittent stretch in the prevention of serial sarcomere loss in immobilized muscles. Annals of Rheumatological Disease 49: 316.

Yorkston KM, Honsinger MJ, Mitsuda PM, Hammen V (1989) The relationship between speech and swallowing disorders in head injured patients. Journal of Head Trauma Rehabilitation 4: 1-16.

CHAPTER 4

Cognition

JUSTINE FAWCETT, ROGER JOHNSON

Introduction

Cognition is an active process involving thinking, language, memory, perception and attention. The areas of the brain involved in controlling cognitive functions are diffuse. As head injuries commonly cause damage to many different parts of the brain, they tend to result in multiple cognitive deficits. This means no two clients will present with exactly the same pattern of cognitive problems and there can be no one 'recipe' to rehabilitate clients with cognitive impairments. This makes rehabilitation in this area a complex and challenging subject but enormously rewarding for those who work in it. This chapter will introduce the basic principles in order to give the reader an understanding of the common problems and issues that arise. It will also suggest a variety of treatment approaches, options and ideas.

The areas covered will include memory, attention, executive skills and visual perception. Gross visual skills, such as visual fields, diplopia, and scanning, have been addressed in Chapter 3 and language is covered in Chapter 6. There is a vast literature relating to cognition and it is outside the scope of this chapter to go into the various theoretical debates in any great depth. Readers are advised to investigate other sources for more detailed information such as McCarthy (1990) or Walsh and Darby (1999). Models and theories that may have clinical application in a community rehabilitation setting will be discussed, although the relationship between neuropsychological theory and rehabilitation in practice is complex (Shallice, 2000).

It may be useful as a starting point, to consider how individuals with cognitive impairments present, and what it is that leads a clinician to suspect there are cognitive issues that need to be addressed.

Presentation of the cognitive problems

A client with cognitive or perceptual deficit in the early stages may fail to acknowledge any issues relating to impairment or handicap. Even at the community stage of rehabilitation he may describe the handicap he faces, but not understand the real impairment issues behind it. This is because it is the handicap that is meaningful and important to him. For example, he may describe how he uses a shopping list but always arrives home without several items; how he often misses the table when putting down a cup; or the fact that he does not 'get round' to doing certain tasks as he used to. Some aspects of cognition are easier than others for clients to appreciate and this means that while they may talk about their difficulties with memory or concentration, they will rarely be able to discuss other cognitive impairments, such as failures in planning or self-monitoring. Much of rehabilitation is focused around improving clients' understanding of the underlying impairment, so that they can minimize the handicap. For example, GT was a client, with frontal lobe damage, who tended to be impulsive and would arrive home from a shopping trip with many unwanted items. She was taught about the relationship between frontal damage and impulsivity, how impairment in planning skills can be implicated in impulsivity, and the impact of this on her lifestyle. She was then taught various strategies involving planning skills and structure, such as planning a shopping list and using it as a checklist when shopping, to minimize the handicap caused by the impulsivity.

Attention deficits tend to be described by clients in terms of not being able to concentrate. A client may comment that he can no longer settle to watch a whole film or describe how he gets easily distracted if reading or writing a letter. He may complain of not being able to deal with several things at once, such as doing domestic tasks with the radio on or joining in group conversations, or half completing tasks, or of poor noise tolerance. When talking to people, he may play with objects on the table in front of him or be easily distracted by noises or visual stimuli inside or outside the room. Chapter 6 considers how attention may affect communication in more detail. Often the client will attribute these behaviours to other causes – perhaps memory loss – not realizing that the underlying issue is to do with attention.

True memory problems are more readily recognized by clients and those in contact with them. The client may describe how he forgets to do things or express embarrassment at failing to remember conversations. He may be vague or inaccurate in his reporting of the situation. He may also repeat information over a relatively short period of time. Sometimes the client and family will seem puzzled by the fact that he can recall his childhood in great detail yet he is unable to remember a simple date or message. Typically, recent memory is impaired but working memory and remote memory are relatively intact following head injury. Skills and past knowledge are usually preserved too. In the early stages after a traumatic brain injury (TBI), clients may deny any difficulty with memory or rationalize poor performance on tests by stating that the tasks are irrelevant to their lifestyle and that they will be fine once they return to a familiar lifestyle. Even with reasonable insight, if demands placed on the client's memory are low, such as when first arriving home from hospital or in completing everyday household tasks, the client may indeed be unaware that he has any problems with memory. A client who is highly aware that he has memory problems may present with anxiety. In general, a person with mild memory problems is likely to have more insight and be able to describe the implications to his lifestyle more specifically. Occasionally TBI causes a severe amnesic syndrome where the client is unable to recall from one minute to the next.

Clients with executive problems may present very differently, depending on the site and severity of the injury, their level of activity and degree of insight. Some clients may present very well socially, reporting nothing wrong, and problems may not be apparent in conversation. In other cases, behaviour could be so disrupted that it would be difficult to hold a conversation at all. Sometimes the client may be overly talkative and it may be difficult to keep him to a conversation topic. In extreme cases he may have inappropriate behaviour and could be sexually disinhibited. However, the client may often feel that he has no problems, despite having what has been classified as a moderate or severe head injury, and in these cases it may be the family who highlight the difficulties.

The presentation of underlying perceptual impairments can be varied. The client may drop things or bump into things, he may be puzzled as to why he cannot do a familiar task or he may complain that he takes longer to do tasks or to find things. Other clients may initially present normally, and it may only be possible to define the problem by observing specific functional activities.

Assessment

Assessment is important for many reasons. It aims to identify the cognitive problems and areas for rehabilitation, and aspects of the individual's lifestyle that have been affected. It can be used to ascertain the level of insight and to clarify the client's own concerns and needs. In the light of the information obtained, realistic goals (including those related to insight) can be established. Assessment findings are also useful for informing clients about the nature of their disability.

Many clients find the assessment process very traumatic, so it is imperative to present the assessment in a positive way, identifying cognitive strengths as well as limitations. To obtain the best level of functioning and to see the true extent of skills and deficits, it is important to build rapport and trust, and create a non-threatening environment in which to assess the client. Launching in with difficult cognitive tests at a first meeting may put the client off the entire process. It is therefore important to consider carefully how to approach the assessment. There is much overlap between professions when it comes to the assessment of cognitive functions and a team approach is needed to obtain a complete picture. However, care must also be taken to avoid duplication.

The first task is to observe how the client presents and provide an opportunity for him to describe his symptoms. These more informal contacts can lead up to formal functional and psychometric assessments. Each stage of the process will be considered in turn.

Observation

The most important skill any therapist has is the skill of observation, particularly perhaps in normal contexts, such as over a coffee, finding the toilet, sitting in the waiting room, or arriving for an appointment. Opportunities for observation thus occur naturally and provide the fundamental first step in assessing the client's cognitive skills. Does he spill his coffee? Can he find the toilet and the way back? Can he communicate with strangers in a waiting room? Does he arrive late? The information gained from first observations begins to give a picture of areas that need to be investigated in more detail. It will also give clues to the level of assessment required and how best to approach the client.

How the client presents in other settings will also provide information on cognitive limitations, as these skills affect a person's ability to function both generally and physically. For example, in physiotherapy it is useful to note whether the client can remember the instructions to follow and if he is able effectively to concentrate when performing tasks. Evidence of perceptual deficits for body schema or neglect is much more noticeable within the physical assessment. This is a good example as to the importance of team communication.

Interview

Much information can be obtained from sources such as the referral and previous assessments from therapists and other professionals involved, for example the GP or mental health team. Before any functional or standardized assessments are completed it is also important to interview both the client and the next of kin/carer. Information can then be obtained on their current situation and level of activity, to compare with pre-morbid ability and lifestyle. Information can also be obtained about cognitive problems and how these affect performance of activities of daily living, and about clients' wishes regarding cognitive rehabilitation.

If the client agrees, it is useful to interview the client and carer separately to ascertain issues from a cognitive viewpoint, as both will have different needs, concerns, and wishes. By interviewing separately the therapist can also obtain an accurate picture of the situation. Clients with traumatic brain injury can have cognitive limitations that might mean their account of the situation is inaccurate (such as poor memory for events, confabulation, poor insight, poor autobiographical memory), or difficulty perceiving their carer's needs, perhaps because of rigidity or concrete thinking.

As was stated earlier, both client and family will usually describe the cognitive problems in functional terms, so the therapist may need to question in functional terms too. Thus, rather than asking if there is a 'problem with attention' it is better to use open questions that do not lead the client to a particular response. Asking 'How do you get on with watching television or films?' or 'How do you manage cooking?' may elicit more than leading questions do.

Functional errors commonly described by both client and carers are listed in Table 4.1, under the headings of attention, memory, executive dysfunction and perception, although, as has been said, the client himself will not always appreciate the underlying impairment.

Checklists can be used to ascertain practical areas of difficulty and the severity of the cognitive problems in everyday functioning, although certain issues must be borne in mind. Sunderland, Harris and Gleave (1984) found that, for example, self-questionnaires for memory had little validity, possibly because clients could not reliably recall their own memory failures, but questionnaires completed by relatives did provide an accurate measure of the actual incidence of memory failures. Using checklists with clients with executive dysfunction or with language disorders may be difficult, as they may not have the skills to process the question adequately enough to arrive at an accurate response. Literacy issues should also be borne in mind, as must ethnic differences, when considering the way in which information is presented.

Appendices 4.1 and 4.2 offer examples of checklists for memory failures and attentional difficulties.

Functional assessment

A client's strengths and limitations may be clarified by observation of performance in a practical setting ('functional assessment'). The assessment must be pitched at the right level to challenge the client, so that cognitive deficits will be highlighted, but it must not be so hard that the client cannot even start. The initial observations and discussions give the therapist information about the client's problems, skills and current level of activity. Physical limitations,

Table 4.1. Functional difficulties following head injury

Deficit	Functional error
Attention	Being unable to do two tasks at once.
	Intolerance of crowds or noise, leading to irritability.
	Finding it hard to watch a film or read a book.
	Disliking being in group conversations due to losing track, resulting in social isolation.
	Being distracted – for example, half doing tasks and not returning to complete them.
	Regularly burning food when cooking.
Memory	Repeating information in conversation or requests.
	Not remembering to do things.
	Failure to remember conversations or messages.
	Puzzlement at why childhood memories can be recalled yet all else is vague.
	Not passing on telephone messages.
Executive dysfunction	Being overtalkative.
	Being egocentric or selfish, not seeing other people's points of view.
	Becoming more irritable when out or asked to do things.
	Described as being 'lazy' and no longer doing the activities previously done.
	Frequently arriving late or running out of time to do tasks.
	Lacking concern, motivation, or being more easy-going.
	Concrete thinking, becoming fixed on ideas.
	Being untidy.
Perception	Being slower or unable to find objects.
	Misjudging putting a mug on a table.
	Being awkward and clumsy when using objects.
	Perseveration when starting an activity.
	Puzzlement at why unroutine tasks cannot be completed.
	Difficulty dressing.
	Knocking into doorways or furniture on the left.
	Ignoring one's affected upper limb.
	Difficulty telling the time or reading.
	Only dressing or shaving one side of the body.
	Poor objects selection for the task at hand.

language problems or the complexity of deficits will all influence assessment decisions. This information can be used to determine the level of assessment and an appropriate assessment tool, such as cooking, DIY tasks, shopping or computer use.

In assessing the client's function it is important to be flexible to his needs and not to have a 'one assessment fits all' approach. Many clinicians adopt an eclectic approach. Using activity analysis, tasks can be graded and adapted to address different issues. For example, the client with memory problems will need a relatively structured assessment to clarify the strengths and limitations in memory. The therapist may ensure the client plans a meal before shopping, to test everyday verbal memory for a list of items and topographical orientation. The client with suspected attentional deficits should be encouraged to prepare a meal involving three different items as a one-dish meal will tell you very little about the specifics of their attention deficits. The client with executive dysfunction will need an unstructured and novel assessment or the problems may not be apparent at all. For some clients with possible executive dysfunction the functional assessment will not highlight any issues as he may be able to live independently and it may be the organizational aspects or novel situations occurring in everyday life or work with which the client struggles. For some clients it may be impossible to make the functional assessment complex enough to identify problems, particularly if they live independently anyway. A task involving planning skills might be more likely to highlight their difficulties.

Table 4.2 suggests a hierarchy of assessment options, which can be used flexibly to provide different mediums and complexity of tasks. The first four tasks do not particularly address executive functioning, but are useful with other clients. Some tasks are traditional, daily activities, but others have been specifically devised, such as planning a trip to London, or constructing a form on the computer. The 'making a coat hanger' subtest from the Chessington Occupational Therapy Neurological Battery (Tyerman et al., 1986) is a useful way of assessing ability to follow complex instructions.

The Multiple Errands Task (Shallice and Burgess, 1991) was developed to assess the Supervisory Attention System. It tests the non-routine, problem solving, planning, organization and initiation required in everyday

Table 4.2. Assessment

---

1. Making a cup of tea.
2. Making a snack meal from the cupboard.
3. Making a coat-hanger
4. Making a cake from packet mix or a model from a kit.
5. Creating a form on the computer for use in a library music loaning section.
6. Planning how to make a birdbox.
7. Multiple errands task
8. Planning a day trip to London, including the schedule for the day and transport.
9. Making an unfamiliar meal, including all preparation and shopping.

---

functioning. The client is given a list of tasks to do, in the order they prefer, or feel would be best, including purchasing certain items, finding out specified information, and following certain rules within a set time period.

Making an unfamiliar meal is a useful exercise to assess skills in executive functioning and can include planning and implementing the task. This might involve getting to the shops, preparing and then making the meal, staying within a budget, completing the task within a time limit, and clearing up.

Within the assessment it is important to obtain a balance between ensuring that the client is successful in the task but not intervening too quickly as this will interfere with the client's thought processing and assessment of performance. Prompting should only occur if the client is unsafe or at the point where, if the client continues, it will not be possible to salvage the situation to prevent complete failure. Through experience it is possible to begin to identify common errors that are suggestive of cognitive deficits – for instance, the client who over-focuses on stirring the cheese sauce, despite the pasta boiling over, could be suggestive of problems with rigidity and/or attention. Overfilling or missing the mug when pouring tea could be evidence of problems with spatial perception or attention.

The limitation of functional assessment is that there is no normative data by which to predict the expected level of performance. For example a younger male may have few skills on tasks of this sort in the first place whereas an older woman may be able to complete the same task much more easily because it is so familiar. It is therefore important to correlate findings from a functional assessment with results of psychometric testing.

Psychometric testing

Psychometric tests form one part of the assessment. The strengths of tests are that they measure different aspects of cognition objectively and can be related to normative data that may take into account age, previous abilities and educational level. Various members of the team may complete psychometric assessments but eligibility to administer certain tests is restricted. This depends on the level of expertise that is required to interpret the results. Many tests require a training course to be completed to establish registration as an approved test user. Table 4.3 lists the main elements that must be covered in screening for cognitive deficits. In addition, measures of speed and estimates of previous ability will be useful.

Information about specific tests is outside the scope of this chapter. Texts such as Lezak and Spreen and Strauss (1998) (1995) are good sources for details about the range of tests available and their administration, and for normative and research data.

Standardized assessments are only as good as their interpretation. Clinicians need to be confident that tests are valid and reliable, and that

Table 4.3. The main elements that must be covered in screening for cognitive defects

MEMORY	FRONTAL LOBE FUNCTION
1. Orientation and recent events	1. Ability to monitor and correct errors
2. Immediate recall	2. Attention and distractibility
3. Ability to retain verbal and	3. Insight, behaviour, perseveration
visual recognition	4. Problem solving and reasoning
4. Long-term memory	
LANGUAGE	**SPATIAL AND PERCEPTUAL SKILLS**
1. Naming objects	1. Measures of spatial relationships
2. Ability to express ideas and proverbs	2. Drawing and copying
3. Verbal fluency	3. Visual recognition and analysis
4. Ability to follow instructions	4. Evidence of visual neglect or
5. Writing and reading	dyspraxia

norms are relevant (for example, for age, educational level, diagnostic group) to individual clients. Levels of intelligence may need to be taken into account – very high or very low premorbid intelligence may make test interpretation difficult. Anxiety and stress may reduce the level of a client's performance Results can therefore be unreliable with a margin of error reflected by statistical analysis.

Deficits in one area of cognition may interfere with performance in another; therefore the validity of the results may be affected. For instance, impairments in attention affect memory performance, language deficits interfere with those tests that depend on skills of verbal expression or understanding, and dysexecutive problems interfere with ability in problem solving tasks such as visual-spatial tests. In these cases, interpretation of results will be aided by careful observation and by information from a functional assessment.

Psychometric tests give an objective baseline from which to work, and help to clarify and categorize the nature of the problem. However, it is important to remember that the results of these tests will not necessarily give an accurate prediction about practical handicap. To obtain a picture of how deficits impact on everyday life, it is important to relate the results to outcomes on functional assessments and to the descriptions of problems identified by the client and family.

No one professional can assess all the areas that may be affected following head injury. Each profession tends to have a specific role and approach that will often overlap with other therapies. The neuropsychologist would use interview and psychometric testing to ascertain pre-morbid and post-injury cognitive, intellectual and perceptual skills. The occupational therapist may complete basic psychometric tests assessing memory, attention, perception and executive dysfunction but the approach would predominantly involve ascertaining levels of independence and the functional consequences of cognitive problems. The speech and language therapist may use interview and psychometric testing to assess language and cognitive neurolinguistics and look at the functional implications of cognitive deficits on communication skills in general. The physiotherapist would observe clients' cognitive and perceptual skills within their physical functioning – for instance, their ability to follow, remember or pay attention to instructions, or how they manage neglect of a limb. It is important that staff accept the overlap and avoid being territorial about their own specialist knowledge. The conclusion from their combined information ensures that the best rehabilitation is provided for clients.

Goal setting

Appropriate goals for cognitive rehabilitation depend on some idea of what long-term goals might be. For instance, will the client need memory strategies to enable him to achieve a long-term goal of living with a spouse or for the more exacting demands of a return to work? Long-term goals will need to be realistically estimated by the team. The discussions around goal setting with the client and carer can be a useful medium for improving insight and may contribute to the process of adaptation to disability.

Cognitive and perceptual problems cannot be seen in the same way as a physical disability – they are, as Chapter 1 stated, a 'hidden disability'. It is common for the client and family to be over-focused on the physical aspects of the disability and to overlook the cognitive problems, even when they are severe. Both community workers and relatives may think the client is well recovered because he looks 'normal'. This can put pressure on a client to return to previous activities, such as work or college, and cause conflict between family and the rehabilitation staff, who may perceive more clearly that this is premature. A careful return to activities such as work or college is usually necessary because of the demand made on cognitive skills and the need for time to adjust and learn appropriate strategies. A client's judgement about improvements may not be reliable and it is important to obtain objective evidence of progress. This could be in the form of feedback from relatives or an employer, or from functional tasks they have achieved, such as test results on a college course, evidence from entries in a diary, or other performance measures

As cognition impacts on every part of the rehabilitation process it is important to listen to the whole team's perspective. Working as a team will also help to establish priorities in rehabilitation. It may be that certain cognitive deficits will need to be addressed first for any rehabilitation to be of benefit – for example, the client with memory problems will require a memory strategy in order to get to appointments or to remember information given to him by other therapists. The client who lacks insight and awareness into the extent of his limitations will need rehabilitation to focus on this before he will accept that other interventions are beneficial. It is common for a client with obvious cognitive impairments only to acknowledge his physical deficits and to believe that if he receives enough physiotherapy then he will be all right. Intervention may have to be carefully timed for the client to accept it or for it to be beneficial. Therapists may have to begin by looking at physical issues first, and through building rapport and providing elements of education about head injury they can facilitate clients' understanding so that they are able to identify that cognitive issues exist too.

When addressing cognitive deficits it is important to have goals that are meaningful to the client. If the client struggles with initiation, motivation, attention and memory problems, these deficits may be increased if he cannot see the point of certain goals. Goals, initially, could be focused around specific tasks that the client needs to perform, such as being able to pass on a telephone message. Later, the goals may be focused on generalizing strategies to other situations or the client being able to formulate his own strategies for new situations that arise.

If a client has a low level of activity then he may have limited insight into his cognitive deficits as he has not yet been challenged in a way that helps him to realize that a problem exists. This is particularly true for those with executive dysfunction where a client may have been coping well with the structured routine of the hospital, so deficits are not apparent to the client or relatives. Once at home, in an unstructured setting and with an increase in his level of activity, issues may then come to light. Sometimes goals may need to be focused around increasing the level of activity and testing out cognition in a step-by-step manner.

Depending on cognitive limitations, clients may be unable to set goals realistically and they often find it hard to translate problems into goals. The therapist may then need to be more directive. Although people will set themselves targets, these are not normally specific or cognitively based. Goals may need to be precisely defined – for example, being able to read a book for 15 minutes rather than the broader target of improving concentration span to 15 minutes. An individual might set a target of completing all the decorating to be done in his house within three months, whereas a therapist would break this down into smaller, more manageable steps.

Goals therefore need to be specific; to relate to tasks that are realistic for the client, and, ideally, it should be easy to measure change.

Management

Cognitive rehabilitation is an approach that aims to enable the client to cope with the impairments they have as a result of brain injury. It is a long, slow, teaching process, which involves improving understanding of the cognitive deficits, together with skill re-learning and perhaps some restoration of function. However, the approach predominately focuses on helping the client to manage his problems by adapting or compensating through the use of strategies. This chapter will consider three approaches to the remediation of cognitive deficits, namely cognitive retraining, compensatory strategies and functional therapy.

Cognitive retraining

Cognitive retraining involves the practice, through therapy exercises, of specific cognitive skills in the belief that it will restore the lost function. Deelman, Saan and Van Zomeren (1990) stated that 'many people regard cognitive rehabilitation as a means of exercising impaired cognitive skills in the hope that they will improve'. There are many exercise books, remedial activities, and computer programmes on the market, which are based on this theory. The emphasis is on working on impaired function *in vitro* as a means of facilitating a more general recovery. However, it is controversial as to whether such an approach is of benefit. There are two main issues – whether repeated practice can lead to recovery and whether any gains achieved in carrying out the practice task can generalize to other activities. A further problem with this method is that practising a particular skill in therapy may only serve to highlight the deficit further with an adverse effect on mood or motivation. There is much research into the subject and although improvements in performance can be demonstrated on the exercise tasks, there is general agreement that training of this kind does not generalize to other settings.

Functional therapy

The functional approach involves the practice of the skills that clients need in order to re-establish their independence or their ability to pursue other activities. The emphasis is on working *in vivo* and training is focused directly on real life skills. This method can lead to improvement in basic practical skills such as the ability to dress despite physical handicap or to organize cooking tasks. It can also improve cognitive function providing practice is on a real life task rather than an artificial one. For example, improvements in attentional skills have been demonstrated following treatments of this kind (Sohlberg and Mateer, 1987; Robertson, 1990).

Compensatory strategies

A compensatory approach is based on the concept that clients with acquired brain injury must learn to circumvent their problems in order to achieve functional independence. The most obvious example is a client who is trained to use a notebook in order to deal with a memory impairment. These strategies might involve using strengths to compensate for weaknesses. For example, an individual with good visual memory but impaired verbal memory can be trained to exploit visual cues and mnemonics to memorize verbal information. The client must be able to generalize strategies to the environment away from the rehabilitation centre and the strategies need to predict the uncertain elements that could occur and lead to failure. For instance, if a client is being trained to use a diary, the strategy must also take into account where he will keep it so that, for example, it is not lost the moment he arrives home and changes his trousers!

The relative benefits of these different approaches to treatment are unclear although there have been many studies on the efficacy of cognitive therapies (for reviews see Cope, 1995; Malec and Basford, 1996; Cicerone et al., 2000). Improvements are probably more likely to follow efforts to develop residual skills (functional therapy) or compensatory strategies rather than cognitive retraining aimed at restoration of deficits, but there is little clear evidence on this point. Nevertheless there is consensus that clients can benefit from cognitive therapies in a number of ways. Integrated programmes of therapy that encourage active involvement from the client, and which are continued over a lengthy period of time, are most likely to be effective. Attention to establishing generalization of skills is also clearly important if the benefits of therapy are to endure and be of practical value to the client. Cicerone et al. (2000) have suggested that cognitive rehabilitation should always be directed towards everyday functioning and they recommend working in those areas of activity which are personally relevant to the client. Thus, cognitive therapy that is applied *in vivo,* or in circumstances closely resembling real life situations, and with priority given to skills which harness the client's motivation, will probably achieve the best progress.

Not all clients will prove amenable to or compliant with cognitive retraining. It is not always possible to achieve a positive impact on their lives. Various barriers that may affect the client's ability to benefit from rehabilitation are listed in Table 4.4. Shortcomings in support networks can undermine therapy strategies – rehabilitation should never be in isolation; team communication and family involvement are crucial to good cognitive rehabilitation. To ensure the development of skills, everyone around needs to be aware of the strategies being used by the clients so that they can support them.

So far, this chapter has adopted a descriptive, clinical approach in outlining how clients with cognitive deficits present and how to set about

Table 4.4. Barriers to intervention

Client based
Lack of insight and awareness of problems and consequences to lifestyle.
Poor motivation.
Poor initiation.
Lacking understanding of the problem.
Existence of multiple cognitive, perceptual or language impairments.
Severe memory deficits.

Support or activity based
Poor environmental and support networks.
Low level of activity so cognitive demands are too low.
The cognitive demands of an activity are too high resulting in continual failure, for example at work.

assessing and setting goals. However, understanding the theory behind the cognitive problems a client has, will enable the therapist to underpin her work and can suggest appropriate therapeutic techniques.

In order to discuss the theoretical basis of cognitive rehabilitation, it is necessary to consider the separate elements. To an extent such a separation is artificial, as cognitive skills interact and interrelate in complex ways. Few clients will have deficits in only one area of cognitive functioning. However, for the purposes of this discussion, attention, memory, executive functioning and perception will be considered individually. As stated previously, this is not intended to be a detailed review of theories and models, but rather offers an outline that explains why certain management approaches work.

Attention theory and management

Attention incorporates many aspects, including the ability to focus on and select relevant or interesting aspects of the environment, the ability to be alert and monitor the task in hand, and the ability to discriminate between competing demands. Attention is thought to be associated with frontal lobe damage and consequently some theorists conceptualize that attention is part of executive dysfunction. There are many models of attention. Sohlberg and Mateer (1989), for example, developed a model that perceives attention as a multidimensional cognitive capacity that is critical for new learning and all other aspects of cognition. This model is particularly useful within rehabilitation to break down the skill for both assessment and treatment purposes. It divides attention into five aspects, which are illustrated in Table 4.5. Sohlberg intended this model to form a foundation for retraining.

To explain the ability to complete two tasks simultaneously, Shiffrin and Schneider (1977) developed a two-way processing model. This theory

Table 4.5. Sohlberg's model of attention (1989)

1. Focused attention	The ability to respond discreetly to specific stimuli; visual, auditory or tactile; to focus on the task at hand.
2. Sustained attention	The ability to maintain attention on stimuli for a period of time (often called concentration). Behaviour should be at a consistent level during a continuous and repetitive activity.
3. Selective attention	The ability to avoid distractions, by ignoring internal stimuli (worries, pain, hunger) or external stimuli (noise, people, activities).
4. Alternation, 'attention switching'	The mental flexibility to enable shifting of the focus of attention between more than one task.
5. Dividing attention	The ability to respond to multiple tasks or multiple task demands. This performance may reflect rapid alternating attention or that one of the tasks can be processed more automatically.

suggests that within any mental activity there is a mixture of automatic and controlled processing. The former is fast and does not require attention, while controlled processes are slower and do place demands on attention. The processes are responsive to changing circumstances, so that if one of the tasks is highly automatic, there is spare processing to attend consciously to the other task. For example, when driving a car, automatic processes are used to operate the car while conscious attention can focus on the road ahead.

Shallice (1982) developed an information-processing model called the supervisory attention system (SAS). In brief, the SAS monitors behaviours that are routine or specific, and the model explains how processing changes from controlled to automatic mode as a result of practice. When a routine activity is rehearsed, the memories of the activity are stored as 'schemata'. These schemata are activated in response to stimuli from the environment – for example, the schema for turning off the alarm clock and getting out of bed is activated by the sound of the alarm. These routine activities come to be performed automatically and a procedure called 'contention scheduling' quickly selects the most appropriate actions in response to the stimulus. With a novel situation or problem, when the demands on attention are greater, the selection of the correct schema is controlled by the SAS. Following brain injury, the SAS may not function properly. The loss of control may mean that automatic processing chooses incorrect schemata and this can lead to distractibility. In illustration, RF, a client who sustained a mild head injury, made frequent errors in carrying out routine tasks – such as putting ice-cream away in a cupboard instead of the freezer.

Many extraneous factors will affect attention. These include those relevant to the person, task or environment. Mood states, such as depression, anxiety, fatigue, stress, and level of interest or motivation will all influence attention. Within the task, familiarity, complexity, duration, and understanding are also relevant factors.

Without attention there can be no further information processing. Attention allows certain information to be taken in and processed by memory. As we have seen, a client may complain of problems with memory when these may be the consequence of impaired attention. It is important not to miss this issue as rehabilitation would need a different focus according to whether the problem is one of attention or memory.

It is possible to analyse attention function and dysfunction in relation to the interaction of characteristics of the environment, the task and the individual. As has been stated, demands placed on attention can differ depending on the task familiarity and complexity. For example, JM was a client who sustained severe frontal lobe damage and had major problems with attention. He could focus and sustain his attention on a computer game of solitaire for 15 minutes, yet within a woodwork task he required constant supervision, as he was much more easily distracted. When using a fretsaw he could only sustain his attention for a few minutes. Unless prompted to return his attention to the task his performance was ineffective. He had interest and past experience in both computers and woodwork, yet his response to the tasks was different – probably reflecting differences in complexity or motivation.

Having briefly outlined some pertinent theories, how do they influence management?

Cognitive training and functional therapy

There is a wide range of computer software and pen and paper exercises available to enable clients to practise attention. These can be given to the clients as 'homework' so that they can practise these activities regularly. Exercises can be designed to target different elements of attention – for example, for focused and sustained attention, reading comprehension, letter-cancellation exercises, or telephone directory searches might be used. For alternating attention, crosswords or activities such as writing a letter while being responsible for answering the telephone are more suitable. If selective attention is impaired it may be useful to practise doing different activities with differing levels of background noise, for example. It is important that exercise tasks are meaningful activities for the client so that skills are improved in everyday activities. This will also increase motivation. It is common for clients to watch a lot of television, particularly if other activities are restricted due to their injury. Television will not improve their skills of attention and clients may need help to find new activities that exercise their attentional skills.

Compensatory strategies

Checklists, such as those discussed in the assessment section, can be used to identify key areas where attention reduces performance. Different areas may overlap or demand specific tasks. Various compensatory strategies are suggested in Appendix 4.3.

It is important to educate relatives, in order to increase their understanding of the nature of attentional problems. It is common for relatives to misinterpret the issues and to believe the client's inattentiveness is deliberate. Suitable advice, depending on the client's problems, might include speaking more slowly to him, reinforcing key issues, using short simple sentences, and demonstrating what needs to be done. It may be suggested that carers give a warning of issues that are about to arise (for example, 'it's five minutes before tea'). Carers may not be aware of the need to give cues, such as pointing, touching the client or saying his name, before giving instructions, for example in order to increase arousal and to make it clear when something is important. Factors such as tone of voice and eye contact can also prove important. Creating incentives and using spot checks to see if the client is still doing what he is supposed to, can be useful strategies for carers.

Memory theory and management

Memory is defined by Malia and Brannagan (1997) as a mental power by which information is kept in mind and can be recalled when required at some point in the future. There is still much controversy about the workings of the human memory. There are many theories and it is easy to be confused by terms, which are not always used in the same way. For example 'short-term memory' may be used to mean memory for events of a few minutes, hours or days ago but it can also describe immediate recall or 'working memory'. Figure 4.1 incorporates commonly used principles to explain the memory process. It provides a framework by which breakdown in the process following brain injury may be identified.

The link between attention and memory is a close one. Selective attention to information must occur as the first stage in the memory process. Sensory memory refers to this selection of information through the senses. Once the information is taken in, it is held in working memory just long enough for it to be processed. This may not involve transfer to a permanent store – for example, when looking for a telephone number, it is retained long enough for it to be used and then it is forgotten. There is still much controversy about the length of time for which information remains in working memory, it is probably a matter of seconds. Atkinson and Shiffrin (1971) state that, unaided, the duration is between 15 and 30 seconds. The capacity of working

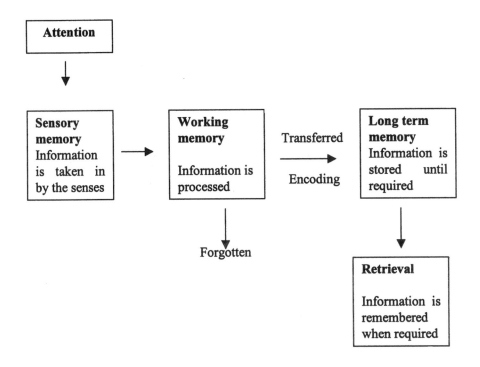

Figure 4.1. Memory process.

memory is also limited and is usually described as being approximately seven (plus or minus two) numbers or bits of information. There are ways of increasing the capacity of working memory, for example, through techniques such as 'chunking' (linking information) or repetition and rehearsal.

The term 'encoding' is used to describe the process by which information is categorized or organized according to meaning, so that it may be stored in long-term memory. The strength of this coding, and the ease with which the information will be recorded later, depend on the depth of processing at the time of learning. Craik and Lockhart (1972) stated that the greater the amount of processing, the more enduring the memory will be. The client's motivation, and the degree of importance placed on the information, are fundamental elements in determining the strength of the encoding process. The mechanisms of transfer from working memory to long-term memory are not fully understood.

The way in which memories are stored may be likened to a library where information is organized and categorized so that information can be found when required. Storage of information is believed to involve many areas of the brain and different types of information may be stored at different locations. Wilson and Moffat (1992) stated that, consequently, brain-injured people may have differing abilities according to the location of the damage. For example, memory for visual information may be preserved while verbal memory is impaired. This is illustrated by SW. He could recall the location of all his belongings in his home and could find his way around both familiar and strange locations, yet he was unable to recall a simple telephone message or the content of conversations as this required verbal memory.

Other categories of information, which appear to involve separate stores, are memory for knowledge and facts (semantic memory), autobiographical information (episodic memory), and memory for established skills, both mental and physical (procedural memory).

Retrieval involves recalling the information from memory when required. There are many reasons why recall may fail. Some theories are based on the concept that learning leaves a 'trace' (a physical or chemical change) in the brain and that, with time, this trace may fade or decay unless it is rehearsed. Ellis and Young (1990) identified three reasons for failure to recall information: failures of registration or attention; failures of retention; and failures of retrieval.

The process of retrieval is thought to be automatic, hence it is common to forget a new person's name but it may suddenly come back a short period later. This is why conscious efforts to recall facts are not always successful. Tulving (1983) states that retrieval will be optimal when it occurs in the same context as the original learning. He developed the concept of retrieval cues, whereby fragments of the original learning experience can prompt recall or recognition. Recognition is thought to be a superior form of recall where contextual cues are not required (Berryman et al., 1989). Thus, a person seen out of context, such as bumping into a local shopkeeper on a train, is recognized but it may be impossible to immediately recall where he has been seen before.

Deficits in memory after brain injury may therefore be due to problems with attention, resulting in failure to register information, or due to difficulty in processing or understanding information, resulting in failure to encode information; or to poor storage characteristics, perhaps including reduced capacity, resulting in poor retention of information; or to difficulty in retrieving information.

Specific memory disorders associated with head injury are retrograde and post-traumatic amnesia. Commonly people lose the last few minutes or hours before the event but will have relatively normal recall for other past memories. Occasionally clients may have a retrograde amnesia affecting many years. Sometimes clients will be unaware of their amnesia and this can lead to inappropriate actions. For example, HY had an amnesia affecting 20 years prior to his head injury, and in consequence tried to contact friends from that period, believing that he had seen them recently and that they would want to know about his accident. This caused friction between the client and his wife as he believed she was trying to stop him seeing his friends.

Post-traumatic amnesia (PTA) is a transient condition that is the final stage of the altered state of consciousness following head injury. There is some controversy about the definition of PTA and how it should be measured (Ahmed et al., 2000). For clinical purposes it can be defined as the time interval between the injury and the reinstatement of continuous day-to-day memory. Clients who are in PTA are disorientated and unable to retain any new information. They fail to retain facts such as the date or where they are, and cannot remember recent events. Post-traumatic amnesia ends when there is evidence of retention of any information that involves new learning. Occasionally, a client who is out of PTA may have persisting problems with orientation, which specifically affect their ability to keep track of time. Chapter 2 considers the measurement of PTA and depth of unconsciousness.

Cognitive training and functional therapy

There is much evidence that suggests that training memory by doing artificial exercises does not improve it. Schacter and Glisky (1986) reviewed the literature on memory rehabilitation and concluded that there was no evidence to support the effectiveness of repeated drill training with amnesic clients. Nevertheless, there are many commercially available computer programmes and exercise books available based on this approach. Clients and families often like this approach as it has high face validity and they feel that they are doing something to help.

Certain skills may be more effectively acquired by the use of specific learning strategies. Backwards chaining is an approach where the steps needed to complete a task successfully are demonstrated and the client starts by taking responsibility for just the last step. Once this ability is established the client takes responsibility for completing the last two steps, and so on until they can successfully complete the entire task. This might be applied to retraining dressing skills for a client with spatial impairments and physical disability following a head injury. Another training strategy is errorless learning (Baddeley and Wilson, 1994; Wilson et al., 1994). The client learns by repetition of correct responses or information and without introducing errors through guesses or premature reliance on memory alone. The theory is that an incorrect response may be assimilated as easily as correct ones and thus inhibit learning. The information is rehearsed with gradually vanishing prompts or cues.

Helping disorientated patients re-establish an understanding of their circumstances also requires a special approach. Deitz et al. (1992) outlined the common sequence of recovery of orientation as information about personal detail, followed by understanding of location and finally orientation to time. Disorientation with regard to time is the most resistant because of the larger component of new learning. Treatment requires consistent and structured individual reality orientation. The therapist needs to work with the family to gain an accurate account of facts and to ensure consistency. The use of family pictures and written information, or calendars, to prompt orientation to time and place may be beneficial. Families may reinforce confabulations for fear of upsetting the individual and they may need information and support about giving accurate feedback. An adaptive approach can be taken alongside this, such as labelling pictures, or providing written information.

Therapists should bear in mind the effects of distribution of practice in learning (Wilson and Moffat, 1992). Little and often is the recommended approach, rather than attempting to pack too much into a session. Testing the information after a delay of a few minutes, not immediately or after a long delay, will enhance learning. Learning in one context does not always generalize to other situations. This has important implications for therapy. Ideally, learning should take place in the client's own environment but, if this is not possible, then the therapist should teach the information in several settings. For example, the therapist may teach use of a diary in treatment sessions, but must encourage practice elsewhere – in the kitchen, in physiotherapy or out in the community.

When clients struggle to recall information, providing them with a carefully chosen prompt, which is in context with the original learning, may enable better retrieval. This is based on Tulving's theory of retrieval cues (1983). It is important for therapists to develop prompting skills that enable the client to arrive at the correct answer for himself. For example, if the client asks 'What am I doing this afternoon?' appropriate prompts might be 'Where can you find this information?' or 'What about looking in your diary?' It takes time and practice to develop skills in prompting and it is often difficult to strike a balance between giving the client time before stepping in with a cue or providing the answer before frustration develops. Table 4.6 offers examples of prompts.

According to Gross (1987) it is easier to relearn old information that has been lost than new information. Therefore, therapists should encourage clients to stick to what they know or build on existing information in their occupational pursuits. For example, clients should be helped to develop the work skills they had previously or pursue a course of study that they already have some knowledge about, rather than changing tack and starting something brand new.

Table 4.6. Examples of prompts

PROMPT	EXAMPLE
Asking questions	The cheese sauce is too runny and the client has gone to throw it away. PROMPT: 'What else could you do?'
Giving first letter cues	The client has memory problems and has forgotten your name. PROMPT: 'It begins with a J.'
Make suggestions on the next step or component of the task	The client is gardening and is unsure what to do next. It is obvious that if the tomatoes are not watered they will die. PROMPT: 'If I was you I would look at the tomatoes.'
Giving choices	The client cannot decide on what to cook. PROMPT: 'Maybe you could look in a recipe book or cook your favourite meal.'
Providing partial answers	In completing a DIY task of wallpaper stripping, the plaster has come off the wall in several areas. The client is unsure what to do. PROMPT 'You could clear it up with a . . .' 'You could look in yellow pages for a . . .'

Compensatory strategies

Many strategies to compensate for poor memory are commonly used in everyday life, such as diaries and calendars. This can be a 'selling point' because clients may accept 'normal' activities more readily. They are a way of compensating for the impairment, or managing it, to lessen the handicap. The best strategies to use will depend on what clients need to recall, and what their strengths and weaknesses are. A questionnaire can be used to determine the areas in which the client is experiencing practical problems (Appendix 4.1). As previously mentioned, this is best filled in by both client and carer, to obtain an accurate picture.

There is no rule as to who would benefit from which strategy – the therapist must ensure the strategy is designed to meet individual needs. Table 4.7, based on Greenwood et al. (1997), suggests factors that should be considered. To ensure that a strategy proves effective, training must be given in its use, and this should include when and where it might be used. Using role-play or practice in real life settings can encourage habit formation and generalization of skills. Strategies are most likely to be effective if the person used them pre-injury. Strategies may be based on external aids, such as diaries and lists, or be internalized (see Appendix 4.4).

Table 4.7. Factors in selecting memory strategies

- Nature and type of memory impairment.
- What does the client want to remember?
- What other cognitive deficits does the client have?
- What is the client's level of insight?
- What systems did the client use premorbidly?
- What is the client's attention like?
- Does the client have difficulties relating to executive functioning - initiation, planning, motivation?
- Has the client come to terms with his disability and is he looking for a solution?
- Will the approach be too demanding on the client and/or his family?
- Is the strategy maintainable?
- What are the client's strengths in memory – does the strategy use these?
- Will the strategy fit into the client's lifestyle, roles, habits and routines?
- What is the client's attitude towards the strategy?
- Is the client's mind already set?
- What does the client want to improve on first?
- Is support available to reinforce the strategy?

Internal techniques may be difficult to use after brain injury because of the mental flexibility and creativity required to invent these strategies. Using strategies that encourage processing of the information will enhance recall. For example, writing things down or forming tree diagrams means recall is more likely without reference to the record made.

Rehearsal and planning of what to say, or do, before doing it, will aid recall. Grouping items into categories can increase the number of items learnt. For example on a shopping trip a client may be asked to remember two dairy products and three vegetables. First letter cues may also help recall. The first letters might then be made into a mnemonic that is more easily recalled – for instance, the sentence Richard Of York Gave Battle In Vain can be used to cue the names and order of the colours of the rainbow. To remember a shopping list of milk, peas, oranges, flour, bread, and cheese, a sentence could be created such as Many People Often Feed Baby Chicks. This strategy is useful for lists or names, but it is not particularly powerful and clients may find mnemonic sentences as difficult to learn as the original items.

Visual imagery or visual associations will often prove more effective. Visualizing a picture will often help recall, particularly if it is amusing. For example, a person's name and facial characteristics might be linked to aid recall. The name Elizabeth Green could be associated with a visual image involving a crown and green hair. Alternatively, verbal associations might be used. For example, to remember a person's name, a verbal link could be made with a famous person who has the same name.

Place mnemonics make a visual link between items to be remembered and a series of places in a room. Thus, a list of jobs to do – pay the bills, phone a friend, wash the car – might be represented by the images of the television screen papered over with bills to pay, the friend sitting in the armchair, and the car wedged in the doorway. Recall is facilitated by checking each place to 'see' what needs to be done. A habit of always using the same locations makes the system easier to use.

The PQRST strategy is particularly useful for study skills - the letters stand for Preview, Question, Read, State and Test. Thus the client is encouraged first to preview the information by scanning it to get a general idea of the subject, then to identify and write down key questions which can be answered from the content. The material is read and the main points formulated by being stated in a written or verbalized summary. Finally, what has been learned is tested by seeing if the questions can be answered (Wilson and Wilson, 1997).

Many compensatory strategies can be practised during functional tasks. For example, VG attended a gardening group as gardening was an activity he enjoyed at home. His goals were focused around using a diary to remember to do things. He practised writing summaries of what he had done, so that he could recall activities for the next week. He was given homework to practise writing reminders in his diary and to make use of those reminders. He also used his diary as a prospective planner of tasks to be done in future weeks.

Executive skills theory and management

Frontal lobe brain injury results in an array of impairments that have been labelled the 'dysexecutive syndrome' (Baddeley, 1986). They may be likened to the skills used by a management executive, hence the origins of the term. Luria (1966) defined the frontal lobes as responsible for the programming, regulation and verification of action. Jouandet and Gazzaniga (1979) described frontal lobe function as a system that sequences or guides behaviour towards the attainment of desired goals. Cognitive deficits after frontal lobe damage included poor planning skills, reduced speed or efficiency with tasks of information processing, failure to initiate activities, perseverative responses, and a poor ability to monitor performance and respond to errors. Malia and Brannagan (1997) defined areas of behaviour or cognitive skill that are commonly associated with frontal lobe damage (Table 4.8). Behavioural changes, such as disinhibition, loss of concern and reduced motivation, are also associated with frontal lobe brain injury (see Chapter 5).

There is a general consensus that the frontal lobes are responsible for assessing response options, selecting an appropriate one, monitoring performance and outcome, and the correction of errors. These skills relate to intel-

Table 4.8. Frontal lobe skills and behaviours (based on Malia and Brannagan, 1997)

1. Self-awareness	Having an accurate idea of one's strengths and weaknesses.
2. Goal setting	Being able to set realistic goals that relate to one's skills.
3. Inhibition	Being able to stop a behaviour or action appropriately.
4. Initiation	Being able to start a behaviour or action appropriately.
5. Flexible problem solving	Having flexibility of thought.
6. Planning and organization	Being able to prioritize and organize one's actions.
7. Creativity	Being able to generate ideas.
8. Self-monitoring	Being able to monitor one's actions and make adjustments as appropriate.

lectual activities, language or behaviour. For example, in conversation a client with frontal lobe brain injury may fail to select appropriate ideas or responses, or monitor his language, as well as normal. As a result his discourse may be rambling and off the point. In another context, such as a visit to the pub, the same client may overlook the fact that a friend has inadvertently picked up his drink and immediately assumes that the barman must have taken it. He may impulsively storm to the bar and aggressively demand a replacement without evaluating the situation further or moderating his irritation. Moreover, he may fail to adapt his inappropriate behaviour when the barman fails to respond as he expects and his error is pointed out to him. These difficulties are often compounded by a lack of insight, which is commonly associated with executive dysfunction.

It should be noted that the nature of frontal lobe brain function is not well understood. Some authors define the cognitive skills the frontal lobe controls as problem-solving impairments. Other models emphasize the importance of frontal lobe function in goal directed behaviour or possibly in underlying intelligence itself. It can be difficult to diagnose executive dysfunction, as the impairments are neither task specific nor domain specific. A client with frontal-lobe injury may perform well on one problem-solving task but do poorly on another. Psychometric tests, even when designed to tap 'frontal lobe' skills, will often prove unreliable (Rabbitt, 1993). A series of tests, combined with observations on practical abilities and behaviour, may elicit symptoms consistent with frontal-lobe dysfunction.

Different tasks make different demands on the use of executive skills. During the initial stages of learning a novel, complex task, frontal lobe functions are critical, but as the skill is learned habits are strengthened and less frontal lobe involvement is required (Sohlberg, Mateer and Stuss, 1993). Therefore routine, familiar tasks place low demands on executive functioning, whereas novel, complex ones require high levels of executive skill.

In a structured hospital environment, the impairments relating to frontal lobe injuries can be easily missed and the therapist will need to challenge the client in an unstructured way in order for her and the client to begin to recognize the deficits. Some clients will prove to be difficult to treat as they fail to recognize their deficits. This may happen gradually once they have returned home and been given the time and opportunity to get back to normal activities. When the client meets obstacles or fails in some respect, he may be better able to realize that he has problems and he then becomes more amenable to a rehabilitation programme.

Clients with only a mild degree of frontal lobe damage can easily be overlooked for rehabilitation. Relatives may report that there are subtle changes in the client's 'personality' but they are often unable to define what these are. If the client believes that there is nothing wrong, then it may be decided that rehabilitation is not warranted. Sometimes, increasing the client's level of activity, or the demands and complexity of tasks, will highlight impairments for the client. For instance, TD was a 17-year-old boy who, on testing, was found to have frontal-lobe type impairments. The client was not back to work and his level of activity was low. His parents completed domestic chores and socializing with his friends placed little demand on his cognitive skills. Neither family nor client could identify any changes. TD was encouraged to return to work in a staged and supervised way. It quickly became apparent to everyone, including TD, that he was not completing the number of tasks he would have previously done each day. He was then better able to accept intervention aimed at exploring the causes of his reduced performance and advice on appropriate strategies to overcome the problems.

Cognitive training and functional therapy

There is no evidence that the many workbooks available, aimed at practising aspects of problem solving and reasoning, have any beneficial effect. It is therefore essential to take a functional approach in therapy for this type of disorder.

The focus of therapy needs to be on the practice of specific skills using a functional task that relates to the client's normal activities. According to Sohlberg, Mateer and Stuss (1993) it is possible to teach a client a specific skill or sequence of skills that involve conscious planning and monitoring. They postulate that with time and repetition these skills can become automatic in certain circumstances. Burke et al. (1991) described strategies for clients who had impairments in either problem solving, self-initiation or self-regulation. In each case, training in the use of checklist strategies reduced the amount of prompting and increased the number of tasks completed correctly. When the checklists were withdrawn there was no deterioration in performance. This suggested that performance had become routine or internalized and this enabled the learned skill to become established.

Clients who have sustained a head injury typically show deficits in several areas of cognition, perception and language, and these problems may be compounded by executive dysfunction. It is often difficult to disentangle the specific impairments that they have. The emphasis therefore needs to be on a functional approach. To illustrate this, DH was a client who had severe problems with executive dysfunction, particularly planning, organization, and self-monitoring. He was also unconcerned and euphoric. In addition he had an expressive dysphasia and a dyspraxia, but he was physically fit. He was unable to perform tasks such as cooking or his previous gardening and DIY activities. It was impossible to isolate specific deficits for treatment. A functional approach was taken and over a period of a year he re-learned both domestic and leisure tasks through practising the specific activities themselves, in his home environment. He became independent but remained chaotic in his time management and needed some external support.

Compensatory strategies

Clients will have differing levels of awareness but for compensatory techniques to work some degree of insight is essential. Crosson et al. (1989) identified three levels of awareness – intellectual, emergent, and anticipatory. Intellectual awareness is the ability to show some understanding that a particular function is impaired. At the lowest level this may mean that the individual is aware that he has difficulty with some activities. At a higher level, he may be able to understand the implication of the deficit for his lifestyle. With emergent awareness the client is able to recognize there is a problem and act accordingly. Anticipatory awareness is when a person is able to anticipate that a problem will arise as a result of his deficit and act to prevent it occurring.

Sohlberg and Mateer (1989) emphasize that providing structure should be the guiding principle in treating clients with executive dysfunction. They identified two approaches – specific exercises to enhance processing (for example, task verbalization, planning steps), and restructuring the environment (for example, alarms to cue checks on performance). Various techniques that can be applied are illustrated in Appendix 4.5.

Figure 4.2 highlights the necessary steps for successful problem solving. This can be used to help identify where the process has broken down for a client with executive dysfunction and therefore how to rebuild that process. Sohlberg, Mateer and Stuss (1993) describe a three-phase behavioural approach to training, in which the first stage consists of increasing the client's knowledge on how the strategy works; the second stage involves practising the use of the strategy; and stage three is generalization of the strategy to novel, real world contexts.

Cicerone and Wood (1987) developed a self-instructional training approach that involved four stages – first the client verbalizes the plan, and reasons for it, out loud, then he verbalizes each move while carrying it out, thirdly he whispers each move, and finally he converts this into internalized self-monitoring. The authors stress the importance of applying the training to everyday activities.

Evans, Emslie and Wilson (1998) found that external cueing systems, for example, provided by an electronic pager where specific messages can be received at certain times of the day ('neuropage'), were helpful with clients with problems of impulsivity, poor planning, and poor initiation. Many commercially available electronic organizers can provide a similar function. Simple written plans and activity charts can also be effective as external cues to compensate for executive dysfunction.

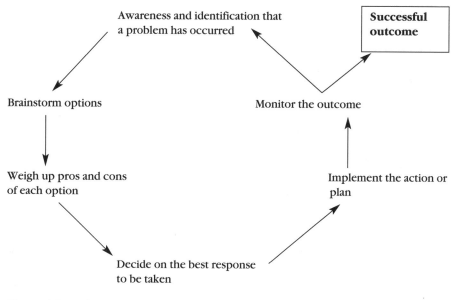

Figure 4.2. Problem solving.

Visual and spatial perception theory and management

The way in which people monitor what is happening around them, through the senses, is termed perception (Berryman et al., 1989). It is an active process of selecting, interpreting, and attempting to understand what is happening. Coon (1983) defined perception as the process of assembling sensations into a useable mental representation of the world. The perceptual process begins with the stimulation of the sense organs and ends with the brain interpreting and using the information it receives. The area of the brain responsible for interpretation of the visual stimuli is the occipital cortex at the rear of the brain, assisted by the coordinating function of the parietal lobe.

Visual perception is complex, involving many aspects such as judgement of depth, distance and movement, size constancy, closure, and figure-ground relationships. To illustrate this: when a person is reaching to pick up a mug, the brain has to interpret the stimuli it receives in terms of textures, shadows, contours, size and background in order to judge how far away the mug is, where the mug begins and the table ends, where to hold it as the contours of the mug turn into the handle.

Perceptual deficits after head injury may be highlighted by psychometric tests, but relatively few people will experience or describe practical problems in their everyday life. This is because the tests look at specific aspects of perception in isolation and in reality the brain uses many different cues by which to interpret the world. The brain can therefore compensate relatively easily for certain perceptual impairments. However, if a task places high demands on perceptual skills, such as assembly work, then perceptual problems may handicap a client more obviously. If a person has impairments in figure-ground discrimination, he may be slow to pick out a tool lying on a workbench amongst several others, or he may be unable to pick a knife out of a drawer full of cutlery. Even when a practical problem due to perceptual deficit can be observed, it may be very difficult to categorize the impairment and hence to select a specific treatment.

The principal deficits of visual-spatial and perceptual function are listed in Table 4.9 and described briefly below. For further reading in this area see Ellis and Young (1990); Grieve (1993); Zoltan (1996); Walsh and Darby (1999).

Apraxia

Apraxia is the inability to plan or sequence certain purposeful and voluntary actions. This may be in the absence of paralysis or motor weakness, and where there is no sensory loss or failure to comprehend what to do. Apraxias can be subdivided into motor apraxia and ideational apraxia. Motor apraxia is a disorder that affects the ability to carry out purposeful activities. It is thought to be caused by the loss of kinaesthetic memory for patterns of motor activity. Thus, use of everyday objects, such as a knife or fork or a hammer and nail, may become disorganized or impossible for the client to start. Routine or familiar activities may be completed automatically but with an element of clumsiness. Involuntary or automatic movement patterns, such as walking, should not be affected at all. Deficits are most often evident in upper limb activities but this reflects the complexity of tasks involving the arms and hands and dyspraxia may also affect lower limb actions. For example, AE was a client with motor apraxia

Table 4.9. Perceptual deficits

Apraxia	Motor
	Ideational
	Constructional
	Dressing
Body scheme disorders	Somatognosia
	Unilateral neglect
	Anosognosia
	Left/right discrimination
Agnosia	Visual object
	Prosopagnosia
	Astereognosis
	Auditory agnosia
	Colour agnosia
Spatial relations	Figure-ground
	Form constancy
	Depth/distance
	Positional

whose upper limb would not perform desired functional movements but who also struggled to move his foot in the patterns required to get shoes on easily.

Ideational apraxia is a disorder at the planning or conceptual stage of purposeful movement. The client is unable to 'think how' to organize an activity. He may be able to carry it out successfully without thinking about it, but will be unable to do so on command. Thus, a dyspraxic client may be quite unable to put on his reading glasses when asked to do so, but will put them on automatically, without difficulty, when given something to read. The client with ideational apraxia is likely to show particular difficulties with mimed activites and will struggle to imitate gestures. For example, if asked to demonstrate how they would stir an imaginary cup of tea or seal and stamp an imaginary envelope clients might complain that they cannot think how to start or perform actions bearing little relationship to the request. Sometimes they will use part of their bodies to represent the object – using a finger as if it were the spoon or a hand as if it were the envelope.

Constructional apraxia is an inability to deal with spatial relationships. The client will struggle to put the parts of a puzzle or assembly task together – particularly where the task is a novel one. Drawing or copying designs is likely to be affected and so too will be his attempt to draw a map of the rehabilitation centre. Typically left parietal lobe damage will lead to simplified drawings whereas right parietal problems result in fragmented or disjointed drawings (Figure 4.3).

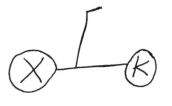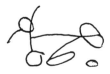

Left parietal lobe damage
- simplified drawings

Right parietal lobe damage
- disjointed/fragmented drawings

Figure 4.3. Client is asked to draw a bicycle – demonstrating constructional apraxia.

Dressing apraxia is a specific inability to dress, although it is likely to be associated with other apraxic difficulties. Dressing apraxia is thought to be due to a combination of disorders of body scheme and spatial relations. Mistakes are made in sorting the clothes out and orientating them appropriately. Thus, the client may struggle to work out how to get an arm into the sleeve of a coat or may end up with it on back to front.

Body scheme disorders

Somatognosia is a disturbance of body scheme, where the client is unaware of certain body parts or the relationship between them. Unilateral neglect is a failure to take in or use information from one side of the body. This can occur in the absence of visual field deficit or sensory loss. Clients commonly ignore the left half of their bodies and the condition appears associated with right hemisphere damage. This deficit is also associated with a spatial disorder as it does not just relate to the body. For example, if the client is asked to do some drawing, the left half of a flower (Figure 4.4) may be omitted or a man may be

Figure 4.4. A 48-year-old male, right-hemisphere brain injury with unilateral neglect ('copy what you see on the side of the page [the left] here [onto the right side of the page]').

drawn without a left arm or leg. If a client with spatial neglect is asked to imagine standing at one end of the main square in the town where he lives, and to describe what he would see, he may report only what would be on the right-hand side and report nothing that would be on his left. If he is then asked to report the scene as if he was standing at the other end of the square, he will now describe what he previously ignored and omit what he previously reported. Typically, such clients seem unaware of this anomaly and it demonstrates clearly that neglect can be conceptual in nature and is not due to sensory deficits. In practice, neglect affects a wide range of everyday activities such as reading, shaving, eating, dressing and negotiating objects on the affected side.

Anosognosia means a failure to perceive illness and is commonly associated with neglect phenomena. Clients with this disorder may rationalize their failure to use an affected limb, claim that they are using it when they are not, or sometimes delusions will be reported to the effect that the limb does not belong to them.

Agnosia

Agnosia is an inability to recognize or identify familiar objects despite intact sensory function and normal visual acuity. It is distinct from word- finding difficulties because the client will typically show no difficulty in naming body parts when touched and the ability to recognize and name objects through touch remains intact. Object agnosia is associated with a loss of the 'concept' for the object and this can be demonstrated by the client's difficulties in describing the use or characteristics of a named object. Moreover, while the ability to make copy drawings of objects will be intact, an attempt to draw them from imagination is likely to produce bizarre results (Figure 4.5).

Prosopagnosia is a specific inability to recognize faces. The client knows what a face is but has difficulty in recognizing to whom it belongs, even if it is a close relative or a famous person. The client may use other cues to recognize the person such as their voice, context, and clothing.

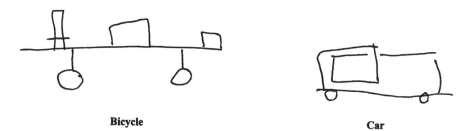

Bicycle   **Car**

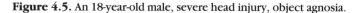

Figure 4.5. An 18-year-old male, severe head injury, object agnosia.

Astereognosis is an inability to recognize objects by touch with vision occluded, despite sensation and proprioception being intact and in the absence of a word-finding problem. A client with this disorder will be unable to identify objects given to him to handle while he is blindfolded. In practice, this would mean a client might have difficulty picking out something he required from his pocket, or be unable to find objects in the dark, for example.

Auditory agnosia is the inability to recognize speech or non-verbal sounds. Thus, the client may be unable to recognize the sound of a lawnmower, jangling keys or a bell.

Colour agnosia involves two separate entities – difficulty in discriminating between colours, so that a client may be unable to match or group colours, and being unable to identify them.

Cognitive retraining and functional therapy

The traditional cognitive retraining approach assumes that if a client practises a spatial or perceptual task his performance on similar activities will also improve. Thus, a client with dressing apraxia might practise spatial skills via a task such as building blocks in the hope that it will improve functional independence in dressing. However, there is little evidence that this is an effective treatment method (Robertson, 1990; Greenwood et al., 1997). A study by Edmans and Lincoln (1988) showed little or no benefit from training perceptual skills along these lines. They suggested that if clients showed no signs of benefit from treatments of this kind after six weeks then no gains would be made and the method should be changed. With some activities the client can improve at the specific task but there is usually no apparent generalization to real life activities and therefore the benefits are very limited.

Rehabilitation of perceptual and spatial deficits should therefore be functional in nature, and aim to practise the tasks the client needs to do. For instance, if spatial awareness and body image problems prevent a client from completing self-care tasks, then washing and dressing may be practised to achieve independence.

Compensatory strategies

Compensatory strategies, such as always laying clothes out and cueing orientation by finding the neck label, for example, may be included in training activities. Appendix 4.6 provides examples of compensatory strategies for perceptual and spatial deficits. Functional re-training of clients with spatial and perceptual deficits is a long and slow process but, with perseverance and consistency, gains can be made and independence at specific tasks achieved.

Evaluation and outcome

Evaluation of outcomes is crucial in determining whether the client is benefiting from rehabilitation. Compared to physical deficits, cognitive impairments are relatively hard to see and measure. Psychometric tests can be used to measure recovery but many tests lose their reliability if used too soon or too often. Some tests, such as certain measures of executive function, lose their novelty value and may not be usefully repeated at all. Lack of improvement on formal psychometric testing may not be reflected in the client's abilities in everyday activities. They may have progressed via the use of compensatory strategies. Functional measures are therefore likely to be the best criteria by which to measure progress towards short-term or long-term goals. Goal setting is an important part of rehabilitation planning but it is also an important basis for measurement of outcome.

After discharge from a rehabilitation programme, follow-up at three to six months is important to determine whether clients have continued to use strategies they have been taught and have maintained the same level of skill. Further rehabilitation may not be required if cognitive deficits are well managed or it may prove possible to build on the skills or level at which the client is functioning. If the client has not maintained the gains made, then the therapist should question whether further rehabilitation along the same lines is appropriate – is a different approach indicated? Were the original goals realistic?

In a community setting it is very difficult to get good outcome measures for cognitive rehabilitation that are sensitive to cognitive change and that are not subjective in their application. Presentation can be very different for each client as the personality and life experiences of each vary, as does the environment clients live in and how the problem affects them. A standard measure of outcome that would reliably and objectively demonstrate change in performance would have to be so flexible, and at the same time sensitive to change, that it does not yet exist. Wade (1992) is an excellent reference for details on various outcome measures.

Measures used to assess cognitive change might include specific tests, such as the Short Orientation Memory and Concentration Test (Katzman et al., 1983), or the Mini Mental State Examination (Dick et al., 1984). Such measures tend to be short and are therefore useful as screening measures but they fail to cover the full range of cognitive skill and, particularly, do not address executive dysfunction or perception for example. Alternatively, questionnaires might be employed, such as the Cognitive Failures Questionnaire (Broadbent et al., 1982), or the Memory Failures Questionnaire (Sunderland, Harris and Gleave, 1984). However, self-rating forms and satisfaction measures are of limited use in determining outcome for cognition, as memory deficits and poor insight can affect the way the client responds. Clients with executive problems have particular problems in completing self-report questionnaires because of their difficulties with self-monitoring and reflection, and their poor ability to make decisions.

Other measures, such as the Bartel ADL Index (Wade and Collin, 1988); Rivermead ADL Index (Whiting and Lincoln, 1980); Frenchay Activities Index (Holbrook and Skilbeck, 1983), and Nottingham Extended ADL Index (Nouri and Lincoln, 1987) are excellent measures of functional independence but are not sensitive to changes in cognitive skills. Many clients with cognitive impairments, but no other disabilities, will score 100% on entrance to a community rehabilitation programme on some functional measures such as the Bartel ADL Index. Measures have been developed to address a multidisciplinary team approach to outcome, such as the Functional Independence Measure (FIM) (Hamilton et al., 1987) and the Functional Assessment Measure, which was developed specifically for use in brain injury and adds a further 12 items to the FIM. (Hall et al., 1993). These measures have little content relating to cognitive disabilities likely to be encountered in a community-based rehabilitation programme.

Overall there is a general lack of outcome measures suited to measurement of cognitive changes. Many rehabilitation centres therefore attempt to use 'home-made' measures or else use nothing at all.

Conclusion

The processes controlling cognition and perception usually function in a smooth, synchronized and subconscious manner to enable individuals to interpret, respond and function within the environment around them. Following a brain injury the harmony of this process is disrupted to create a confusing and complex world, where the subconscious processes used to complete everyday tasks can no longer be taken for granted and novel activities may be overwhelming.

Cognitive impairments encompass a wide range of disabilities, which often present very differently in each client according to pre-morbid skills and experience, and the severity and type of injury. Only rarely are specific cognitive deficits found in isolation and the presentation is usually one of complex and diverse deficits. This means that it is essential to have a range of resources for both assessment and treatment and that there is no one right way. The cognitive therapist in community rehabilitation must work flexibly in order to respond to changing needs. She must also focus on goals that are meaningful to the client. They must work as part of a team of people with different skills in which every member has a role to play in cognitive rehabilitation.

Appendix 4.1: Memory Failures Questionnaire (based on Sunderland, Harris and Gleave, 1984)

Please rate the following questions according to the scale below:

A   Not at all in the last three months.
B   About once in the last three months.
C   More than once in the last three months but less than once a month.
D   About once a month.
E   More than once a month but less than once a week.
F   About once a week.
G   More than once a week but less than once a day.
H   About once a day.
I   More than once a day.

1   Forgetting where you have put something. Losing things around the house.
2   Failing to recognize places that you are told you have often been to before.
3   Not remembering a change in your daily routine - for example, a change in the time that something happens.
4   Having to go back to check whether you have done something you meant to do.
5   Forgetting that you were told something yesterday or a few days ago, and maybe having to be reminded about it.
6   Letting yourself ramble on to speak about unimportant or irrelevant things.
7   Having difficulty picking up a new skill. For example, a new game or gadget.
8   Finding that a word is on the tip of your tongue. You know what it is but you cannot quite find it.
9   Completely forgetting to do things you said you would do.
10   Forgetting important details of what you did or what happened yesterday.
11   When talking to someone, forgetting what you have just said.
12   When reading, being unable to follow the thread of a story, or losing track of what it is about.
13   Forgetting to tell someone something important. For example, a telephone message.
14   Getting the details of what someone has told you mixed up and confused.
15   Telling someone a joke or story that you have already told him once before.

16 Getting lost or turning in the wrong direction on a walk or journey
    where you have only been once before.
17 Repeating to someone what you have just told them or asking the same
    question twice.

Appendix 4.2: Attention Questionnaire (Malia and Brannagan, 1997)

Recognizing if you have a problem with attention

Rate the following statements according to the scale below.

5   I find this a very severe problem.
4   I find this a severe problem.
3   I find this a moderate problem.
2   I find this a mild problem.
1   This is not a problem.

1. Being easily distracted.
2. Concentrating for long periods of time.
3. Confusion if there is a lot going on.
4. Dealing with more than one thing at a time.
5. Making mistakes because of thinking of something else.
6. Finding your attention wanders more easily.
7. Getting mentally tired more easily.
8. Needing prompting to get things done.
9. Slowness in responding.
10. Spending time daydreaming.
11. Missing important details in tasks.
12. Feeling restless.
13. Difficulty sticking to a task. Jumping from one task to another without
    completing any.
14. Feeling 'spaced out' or blank.
15. Losing track in the middle of a conversation.

Appendix 4.3: Attention Strategies

To help maintain attention

• Adapt the external environment to reduce noise. For example, turn off the
  television, face a blank wall, get earplugs, go to a quiet room.

- Manipulate the information by writing it down, repeating or building visual or verbal associations.
- Encourage clients to pace themselves with regular breaks to get the best out of their sustained attention.
- Do one task at a time to ensure successful completion.
- Facilitate clients to break down tasks into components so they can simplify them. For example, cook with two or three items but use the oven and microwave and only keep one thing on the hob or grill that requires frequent attention.
- Plan ahead and get everything out for the task at hand, to avoid becoming distracted in the middle.
- Plan a schedule of the day or week to facilitate maintaining attention on priority tasks.
- Adapt internal wellbeing to reduce distractions from internal worries – for example reduce pain, hunger, anger. Write down internal thoughts to be dealt with later and to unload before commencing task.
- Use rehearsal techniques – for example, listen to a message and repeat it back immediately.
- Use a bookmark when reading to block off text that might distract, or to help maintain a focus on the line being read.
- Emphasize complete closure of an activity. Be organized and get into the habit of putting everything away before starting a new activity.
- Highlight key words in your diary, instructions or text notes when studying.
- Use self-instruction techniques (Webster and Scott, 1983). For example, ask someone to repeat the information, vocalize step-by-step performance of a task. Ask someone to slow down. Question yourself 'What should I be doing now?' Note that some clients find internal strategies very difficult following traumatic brain injury.

To bring attention back after a distraction

- Use checklists or diary planners and refer back to them at specific points in the day.
- Use alarms or electronic organizers to bleep and return attention to the task. E.g. when cooking use a timer or microwave oven. Build up an association between the alarm and taking medication.
- Use self-instructional techniques: 'Now what was I doing before the phone went?'
- Increase awareness of the problem so distractions are gradually less likely to occur.

Appendix 4.4: Internal and External Memory Strategies and Training

Internal

Repetition, rehearsal, grouping, first letter cues, visual imagery, visual association, mental tracing, verbal association, place mnemonics, PQRST.

External

Diary

Training could include:

- Storage.
- Reinforcement to carry it at all times.
- Help to get into a routine of looking in it at specific times of the day.
- What is intended to be written in it? For example appointments, things to do, birthdays, social events, household tasks.
- To write in before events take place.
- Practise planning skills and breaking tasks down into memorable components; for example when writing in someone's birthday also write in to buy a card, to ring them, to purchase a present etc.
- Whether abbreviations enable the client to recall the message or if full sentences are required to avoid misinterpretation.

Lists

For shopping, things to do. More efficient if a note book is consistently used rather than scraps of paper.

Wall planners

With a structured week of activities to be achieved. To enable clients to form a routine which reduces demands on memory.

Structure the environment

- Be organized, keep items in certain places – for example, purse always in a handbag, keys on a hook.
- Label cupboards or drawers.
- Get into a routine of putting items back after use.
- A written list of storage places may be required to ensure consistency from other members of the household and to help remember places until they are learnt.

Alarms

- To cue the client back to looking in the diary.
- To remember to take medication.
- To remember to get food out of the oven.

Note book

For lists. To write messages from conversations which are too long to put in a diary.

- Remember to date entries.
- Practise summarizing skills and picking out key points.

Electronic organizers

The cheaper the product, generally, the harder it is to learn to use, as the digital display may only fit a limited number of characters or be equal to a three-word message. The buzzer may only bleep for one item before requiring reprogramming. More expensive organizers sometimes have a feature so entries can be repeated.

They are complex to understand and so it is difficult to learn how to use them. Palm tops are expensive but easier to learn and to use. The alarms can be programmed to bleep repeatedly over weeks and months.

Cue stickers

Messages in strategic places. Beware they are soon ignored!

Appendix 4.5: Examples of Compensatory Strategies for Executive Dysfunction

Area	Examples of compensatory strategies
Self-awareness	Initially work on the impairments the client is able to recognize.
	Give accurate feedback on performance, negative and then positive.
	Convey the message about the problems in a way that is meaningful to the client.
	Carefully balance feedback versus reducing self-esteem, confidence or mood further.
	Use of discussion, video or self-evaluation through recording specific behaviours

	in a diary, with rating scales. Educate to increase understanding.
Goal setting	Break down tasks into appropriate manageable sized goals. Build on awareness of strengths and limitations to encourage appropriate goal setting. In a 'safe' setting use non-achievement of goals to increase insight and awareness followed by discussion. Create a careful balance between failure and damaging mood.
Inhibition	Feedback to increase awareness of the problem. Social skills training to re-learn appropriate behaviour. Positive reinforcement of appropriate behaviour. Strategies to encourage putting on the 'brakes'.
Initiation	Encourage initiation through use of checklists, structured routines, written programmes of activity, goal setting, creating incentives, verbal prompting, neuropager, alarms, electronic organizers. Behavioural techniques such as token economy, positive reinforcement can encourage motivation/initiation. Give sole responsibility for certain achievable tasks.
Flexible problem solving	Increase awareness as to how it affects performance and lifestyle. Strategies that encourage conscious problem solving. Use of a problem-solving model. Break down tasks into simple steps to eliminate problem-solving behaviour. Use of checklists.

Provide routines, structure and consistence
to overcome difficulty with managing
change.
Give time and prompts to encourage
alternative thought processing.

Planning   Strategies to encourage conscious
planning, for example meal organization-
planners, checklists with step-by-step
instructions – for instance for when
shopping.
Consciously learn the process of
prioritization.
Improve time management via
structuring week.
Break down tasks into steps to increase
awareness of correct stages of a task.

Creativity   Generation of ideas via a checklist, resource
books, brainstorming techniques, tree
diagrams.
Encourage structured routines to reduce
the need to generate ideas.

Self-monitoring   Learn to double check tasks consciously.
Video, feedback, discussion and self-
monitoring using diaries to increase
awareness of errors related to specific
behaviours.
Learn about problems in relation to
problem-solving model
Social skills training to increase awareness
and learn how to double-check, pick up
on cues.

Appendix 4.6: Examples of Compensatory Strategies for Perceptual Deficits

Area   Examples of compensatory strategies

Ideomotor   Encourage use of upper limb in appropriate
'safe' tasks.

	Stop conscious thinking and encourage automatic use – for example, DL was a client whose motor apraxia impeded dressing. She was encouraged to put her hand on the waistband and then told to just 'pull up'.
Ideational, constructional apraxia	Break down tasks into simple achievable steps. Use backward-chaining techniques. Be consistent in your approach to the task.
Dressing apraxia	Break task down into simple consistent steps. Lay item out first, use labels as cues for front/back. Wear easy clothes, for example T-shirts, tracksuits, jumpers.
Unilateral neglect	Increase awareness of the problem. Provide cues so the client learns to double check neglected side. For example a red line depicts the edge of the page for reading. Train client to self-monitor. Use checklists, mirrors to look in to check, verbal prompts.
L/R discrimination	Point rather than say left/right. Label or mark items requiring left/right discrimination. For example: shoes – red mark means right and blue is left.
Object agnosia	Practise use of objects in context.
Form constancy	Be consistent in the use of certain items for a particular task. Encourage manipulation of objects. Label where necessary. Organize and unclutter the environment.

Prosopagnosia	Label pictures, make a photo resource book or family tree.
	Encourage relatives to reinforce name and relationship.
Astereognosis	Encourage the client to look at the hand when using it.
	Increase awareness into the problem.
	Organize and unclutter cupboards so items are in view.
Figure-ground	Separate items and unclutter the environment. For example, hooks for keys or utensils.
	Organize cupboards and drawers so items have set 'homes'.
	Learn to scan systematically. Use cues such as: 'where am I likely to find the scissors?'
	Use red tape to distinguish between edges and certain items.
Depth/distance	Encourage client to feel the depth or distance with limb first. For example, to feel for the edge of the table with hand or to feel height of step by nudging with foot first.

References

Ahmed S, Bierley R, Sheikh JI, Date ES (2000) Post traumatic amnesia after closed head injury: a review of the literature and some suggestions for further research. Brain Injury 14: 765–80.

Atkinson RC, Shiffrin RM (1971) The control of short term memory. Scientific American 224: 82–90.

Baddeley AD (1986) Working Memory. Oxford: Clarendon Press.

Baddeley AD, Wilson BA (1994) When implicit learning fails: amnesia and the problem of error elimination. Neuropsychologia 32: 53–68.

Berryman J, Hargreaves D, Howell K, Holin C (1989) Psychology and You. Leicester: The British Psychological Society.

Broadbent DE, Cooper PF, Fitzgerald P, Parkes KR (1982) The Cognitive Failures Questionnaire and its correlates. British Journal of Clinical Psychology 21: 1–16.

Burke WH, Zencius MD, Wesolowskis MD, Doubleday F (1991) Improving executive function disorders in brain injured clients. Brain Injury 5: 241–52.

Cicerone KD, Wood JC (1987) Planning disorder after closed head injury. A case study. Archives of Physical Medicine and Rehabilitation 68: 111-15.

Cicerone KD, Dahlberg C, Kalmar K, Langenbahn DM, Malec JF, Bergquist TF, Felicetti T, Giacino JT, Harley JP, Harrington DE, Herzog J, Kneipp S, Laatsch L, Morse PA (2000). Evidence-based cognitive rehabilitation: recommendations for clinical practice. Archives of Physical Medicine and Rehabilitation 81: 1596-615.

Coon D (1983) Introduction to Psychology – Exploration and Application. 3 edn. St Paul MN: West Publishing Company.

Cope DN (1995) The effectiveness of traumatic brain injury rehabilitation: a review. Brain Injury 9: 649-70.

Craik FIM, Lockhart RS (1972) Levels of processing: a framework for memory research. Journal of Verbal Learning and Verbal Behaviour 11: 671-84.

Crosson B, Barco PP, Velozo CA, Bolesta MM, Cooper PV, Werts D, Brobeck TC (1989) Awareness and compensation in post acute head injury rehabilitation. Journal of Head Trauma 4: 46-54.

Deelman BG, Saan RJ, Van Zomeren AH (1990) Traumatic Brain Injury – Clinical, Social and Rehabilitation Aspects. Amsterdam: Swets & Zeitlinger.

Deitz J, Tovar VS, Beeman C, Thorn DW, Trevisan MS (1992) The test of orientation for rehabilitation; test re-test reliability. The Occupational Journal of Research 12: 173-85.

Dick JPR, Guiloff RJ, Stewart A, Blackstock J, Bielawska C, Paul EA. Marsden CD (1984) Mini-mental state examination in neurological patients. Journal of Neurology, Neurosurgery and Psychiatry 47: 496-9.

Edmans JA, Lincoln NB (1988) Treatment of visual perceptual deficits after stroke: four single case studies. International Disability Studies 11: 25-33.

Ellis AW, Young AW (1990) Human Cognitive Neuropsychology. Hove and London: Lawrence Erlbaum Associates.

Evans JJ, Emslie H, Wilson B (1998) External cueing systems in the rehabilitation of executive impairment of action. Journal of the International Neuropsychological Society 4: 399-408.

Greenwood R, Barnes MP, McMillan TM, Ward CD (1997) Neurological rehabilitation. Hove: Psychology Press.

Grieve J (1993) Neuropsychology for Occupational Therapists. Oxford: Blackwell Science.

Gross RD (1987) Psychology, the Science of Mind and Behaviour. London: Hodder & Stoughton.

Hall KM, Hamilton BB, Gordon WA, Zasler ND (1993) Characteristics and comparisons of functional assessment indices: Disability Rating Scale, Functional Independence Measure and Functional Assessment Measure. Journal of Head Trauma Rehabilitation 8: 60-74.

Hamilton BB, Granger CV, Sherwin FS, Zielezny M, Tashman JS (1987) A uniform national data system for medical rehabilitation. In Fuhrer JM (ed.) Rehabilitation Outcomes, Analysis and Measurement. Baltimore: Brookes, pp. 137-47.

Holbrook M, Skilbeck CE (1983) An activities index for use with stroke patients. Age and Ageing 12: 166-70.

Jouandet M, Gazzaniga MS (1979) The frontal lobes. In Gazzaniga MS (ed.) The Handbook of Behavioural Neurobiology. Vol. 2. New York: Plenum.

Katzman R, Brown T, Fuld P, Peck A, Schechter R, Schimmel H (1983) Validation of a short orientation – memory – concentration test of cognitive impairment. American Journal of Psychiatry 140: 734-9.

Lezak MD (1995) Neuropsychological Assessment. 3 edn. New York: Oxford University Press.

Luria AR (1966) Higher Cortical Functions in Man. New York: Plenum Press.

Malec JF, Basford JS (1996) Post-acute brain injury rehabilitation. Archives of Physical Medicine and Rehabilitation 77: 198-207.

Malia K, Brannagan B (1997) Caring for Carers Handbook. Chessington: Cognitive Functions Workshop.

McCarthy RA (1990) Cognitive Neuropsychology: A Clinical Introduction. London: Academic Press.

Nouri FM, Lincoln NB (1987) An extended activity of daily living scale for stroke patients. Clinical Rehabilitation 1: 301-5.

Rabbitt P (1993) Methodology of Frontal and Executive Function. Hove: Psychology Press.

Robertson I (1990) Does computerised cognitive rehabilitation work? A review. Aphasiology 4: 381-405.

Schacter D, Glisky E (1986) Memory rehabilitation: restoration, alleviation and the acquisition of domain-specific knowledge. In Uzzell B, Gross M. Clinical Neuropsychology of Intervention. New York: Martinus Nijhoff, pp. 257-82.

Shallice T (1982) Specific impairments of planning. Philosophical Transactions of the Royal Society of London (B) 298: 199-209.

Shallice T (2000) Cognitive neuropsychology and rehabilitation: is pessimism justified? Neuropsychological Rehabilitation 10: 209-17.

Shallice T, Burgess P (1991) Deficits in strategy application following frontal lobe damage in man. Brain 114: 727-41.

Shiffrin RM, Schneider W (1977) Controlled and automatic human processing. II: Perceptual learning, automatic attending and a general theory. Psychology Review 84: 127-90.

Sohlberg MM, Mateer CA (1987) Effectiveness of an attentional training programme. Journal of Clinical and Experimental Neuropsychology 9: 117-30.

Sohlberg MM, Mateer CA (1989) Introduction to Cognitive Rehabilitation. New York and London: The Guilford Press.

Sohlberg MM, Mateer CA, Stuss DT (1993) Contemporary approaches to the management of executive control dysfunction. Journal of Head Trauma 8: 45-58.

Spreen O, Strauss E (1998) A Compendium of Neuropsychological Tests (2 edn). New York: Oxford University Press.

Sunderland A, Harris JE, Gleave J (1984) Memory failures in everyday life following severe head injury. Journal of Clinical Neuropsychology 6: 127-42.

Tulving E (1983) Elements of Episodic Memory. Oxford: Oxford University Press.

Tyerman R, Tyerman A, Howard P, Hadfield C (1986) The Chessington Occupational Therapy Neurological Assessment Battery. Aylesbury: Nottingham Rehabilitation Ltd.

Wade DT (1992) Measurement in Neurological Rehabilitation. Oxford: Oxford Medical Publications.

Wade DT, Collin C (1988) The Bartel ADL index: a standard measure of physical disability? International Disability Studies 10: 64-7.

Walsh KW, Darby D (1999) Neuropsychology. A clinical approach. Edinburgh: Churchill Livingstone.

Webster J, Scott R (1983) The effects of self-instructional training on attentional deficits following head injury. Clinical Neuropsychology 5: 69-74.

Wilson BA, Baddeley A, Evans J, Shiel A (1994) Errorless learning in the rehabilitation of memory impaired people. Neuropsychological Rehabilitation 4: 307-26.

Whiting S, Lincoln N (1980) An ADL assessment for stroke patients. British Journal of Occupational Therapy 43: 44-6.

Wilson BA, Moffat N (1992) Clinical Management of Memory Problems. London: Chapman & Hall.

Wilson BA, Wilson LC (1997) Coping with memory problems. Bury St Edmunds: Thames Valley Test Company.

Zoltan B (1996) Vision, Perception and Cognition (3 edn) Thorofare, NJ: Slack Incorporated.

CHAPTER **5**

Behaviour problems

Roger Johnson, Julie O'Brien

Introduction

Behaviour changes after severe traumatic brain injury are commonplace. They can constitute significant handicaps in themselves but will also compound the problems an individual may have due to other disabilities. It is difficult to quantify the behavioural consequences of brain injury in any objective way. It may be impossible to disentangle changes in behaviour that have arisen as a direct result of the brain injury itself from those that are the consequences of stress or mood disturbance associated with the experience of trauma and disability. Moreover, it is often difficult to treat people with behavioural disturbances successfully because many show poor insight and a poor ability to comply with treatment. Behaviour disturbance is therefore complex to understand and difficult to manage.

Sometimes, early on in the course of recovery, problems such as aggressive behaviour may be extreme and lead to considerable disruption. However, serious difficulties of this kind rarely persist and the common presentation is of more moderate changes in behaviour such as some increase in irritability or a tendency to react more impulsively. These symptoms may not prevent individuals returning to live at home and resuming some of their previous social activities or even getting back to work. The main impact of behaviour changes after acquired brain injury is felt by families and within the community. Changes that are quite subtle in nature can lead to considerable stress and friction in social relationships and may interfere with the individual's ability to cope successfully with many aspects of his previous life.

Behaviour problems will frequently interfere with rehabilitation efforts and those with acquired brain injury therefore represent a particularly challenging group of patients. This chapter provides:

- an outline of the nature of the problem;
- an account of how behavioural symptoms can be assessed; and
- guidelines about approaches to management and treatment in a community rehabilitation setting.

The problems

The fact that behaviour may change following injury to the brain has been recognized for a long time. The classic account is that of Phineas Gage whose frontal lobe brain injury in 1848 has already been described in Chapter 2. The doctor who treated him, Dr Harlow, noticed that his personality had changed. He recorded that Mr Gage was 'exceedingly capricious and childish, but with a will as indomitable as ever; is particularly obstinate; will not yield to restraint when it conflicts with his desires.' His employers would not employ him again because whereas before he had been 'efficient and capable' he was now 'fitful, irreverent, indulging at times in the grossest profanity (which was not previously his custom), manifesting but little deference to his fellows . . . his friends and acquaintances said he was 'no longer Gage' (Harlow, 1848).

The changes which followed Phineas Gage's accident are all too often repeated following severe head injuries sustained in road traffic accidents or other traumatic injuries. Take the case of a young woman who sustained a severe head injury with a post-traumatic amnesia of two or three weeks and evidence from a brain scan of right frontal lobe brain injury. Nine months after the injury she was able to present herself very well at a neurosurgery outpatient clinic. It was noted that her intellect and affect appeared to be normal and there were no neurological signs. She had no complaints and believed she had made a full recovery. Nevertheless, a few months later, after she had returned to her work as an assistant manager with an insurance company, a rather different account emerged from her employers. They said that she had become immature in her manner and that she tended to talk excessively with customers. In staff meetings she was inclined to agree with whatever was said to her and showed an inability to weigh up issues or arrive at her own opinions. When her parents were asked for their comments they listed considerable changes. Previously she had been a quiet and careful person but since her injury she had become garrulous and noisy. Her sense of humour had become much more childish; she had become careless and untidy and she no longer showed the same concern about her appearance or about personal hygiene, sometimes even sleeping in her clothes. She was less reliable and had become haphazard over matters such as paying her bills or managing her money sensibly. Her parents described her as showing a lack of appropriate concern about such matters and she appeared to have no insight into what had happened to her. If questioned about these problems she was likely to lose her temper in a way that was very much out of character with her previous disposition.

This account illustrates a common pattern of behaviour change after brain injury. It also shows how disturbed behaviour can follow brain injury with little sign of other disability. This lady had made a full physical recovery from her injury; she showed few signs of intellectual difficulties, and she was able to present herself, at least on brief encounter, extremely well.

The behaviour changes following brain injury are well documented (see for example Wood, 1990 or Lishman, 1998). The symptoms can be divided into two broad categories: underactive and overactive behaviours (Table 5.1).

Underactive behaviours

Underactive behaviours include inertia, lack of motivation and lack of spontaneity. For example, a young woman who had sustained a severe head injury spent a lot time in bed after she had returned home. When she did get up she was quite capable of sitting about and doing nothing. She needed prompting to persevere with even the simplest of tasks, such as getting dressed. She did not initiate any conversation and would often ignore the telephone ringing or the front door bell. On one occasion she had stood and watched the toast catch fire in the toaster but had made no effort to do anything about it. If her husband tried to persuade her to do more or to go out then she tended to become verbally abusive. In other situations that might evoke an emotional response she seemed impassive.

Overactive behaviours

Overactive behaviours are typically those of disinhibition. Such individuals may be hyperactive and restless, always doing something, and often interfering with what others are doing. They are more likely to be aggressive in

Table 5.1. Underactive and overactive behaviours following brain injury.

Underactive behaviours	Overactive behaviours
Apathy, inertia	Restless
Loss of concern	Impulsive
Lack of drive or motivation	Aggressive, irritable
Lack of emotional response	Outspoken, rude, facetious
Poor initiation, no spontaneity	Euphoric

their manner and perhaps sexually disinhibited too so that they become promiscuous or show ill-judged sexual behaviour. People showing changes of this sort have typically become more impulsive and more outspoken. They may tell strangers in the street what they think of the clothes they are wearing for example, or push someone out of the way in a shop queue. A lack of awareness or concern is often evident. For example, a man of about 30 showed changes of this sort following a head injury in a car accident. A typical instance related to his enjoyment of growing his own vegetables in his garden. After the injury, he would survey not only his own back garden for the best cabbage for his tea but his neighbours' gardens too. He would happily hop over the fence and take something from one of their gardens if it seemed better. When confronted by his wife over these activities he showed no concern and denied that this was an unusual thing to do. Moreover, he was quick to lose his temper with her and insisted that it was her attitude that had changed since the accident and not his.

Sometimes loss of inhibitions will result in more extreme forms of behaviour disturbance. For example, following a severe head injury, a man showed violent aggressive outbursts. In hospital he frequently threatened violence and occasionally hit out at nurses and therapists. He was equally aggressive towards his family and other visitors and he was noted to be particularly abusive towards his wife. There was some improvement so a discharge home became possible. However, within a few days he had threatened his wife with a knife and she had felt it necessary to escape via a window. She went to live with relatives because she did not feel safe to be alone with her husband.

Identifying problems

Symptoms such as those described in these examples will not be evident all the time. There may be episodes or long periods when the brain-injured person will appear entirely normal in his behaviour. Features from the different categories of behaviour described here may often be observed in the same patient on different occasions. This is particularly likely following concussion because the injury to the brain is typically diffuse and a variety of functions may be affected. There may be a fluctuation between periods of normal manner, episodes of overactive or impulsive behaviour, and times when the person becomes inert and apathetic.

In each of the examples of behaviour change described above, the question is how can we be sure that the behaviours observed are the direct result of the brain injury? In the first case the young woman who stayed in bed may simply have become depressed as a consequence of the trauma she had experienced. The man taking his neighbour's vegetables might be right when he said that it was not he who had changed. Even in the last example, the violent behaviour the individual showed could be to do with previous characteristics or previous problems in the relationship between him and his wife rather than a result of the head injury. In addition, such behaviours might well be aggravated by frustrations, or perhaps confusion, about what has happened and might not be wholly accounted for by the direct effect of altered brain function.

Definition of behaviour change after brain injury is therefore difficult and cannot be objective (Eames, 1990). It depends on the account of others, or possibly the judgement of the individual himself, to substantiate that behaviour has changed. The recognition of symptoms may depend on the context. For example, in hospital it is unlikely that there will be any complaints about a patient who is passive and compliant. However, once they are at home the same symptoms may be seen as clearly out of character and can lead to considerable problems within the family. There is therefore an important distinction to be made between behaviour change and behaviour problems. Whether a change in behaviour becomes a problem or not depends on the context and on the consequences. In a study of the incidence of behavioural symptoms following severe head injury (Johnson and Balleny, 1996), a comparison was made between difficulties reported at different stages in recovery. While patients were still in hospital care, within a few weeks of their injuries, therapy and nursing staff identified behaviour problems in about 30% of them. The most frequent problems were irritability together with disinhibited and disruptive behaviours. Once patients had returned home, partners or parents recognized symptoms in about 80% of cases, the commonest complaints being apathy and irritability. Aggressive behaviour was more commonly reported at home than in hospital, as were disinhibition and reduced social skills. The differences probably reflect the difficulties in identifying behaviour change in hospital in the absence of information about previous character. Only just over half (58%) of the families who identified behaviour change in their relatives perceived these changes as amounting to a problem. For example, a mild increase in outspokenness following a head injury was seen as no problem, and possibly as an improvement, by the spouse of a previously taciturn man. Yet, in another case, similar symptoms were disturbing to the partner and a source of embarrassment.

Many of the changes that occur following brain injury are quite subtle and may not be outside the range of normal behaviours. Thus, loss of temper, which is so frequently reported after traumatic brain injury, does not usually mean that the person will show violent rages or outbursts of physical aggression. More typically, individuals will have become more likely to snap in conversation or perhaps assert their views more strongly and more aggressively. This may be significantly different to their previous disposition but is not necessarily any worse than the level of irritability some other people might show normally.

Sexual and emotional changes

Loss of sexual interest or motivation, and sexual dysfunctions, are common-place following acquired brain injury (Kreutzer and Zasler, 1989), particularly during the early stages of recovery. Overactive sexual behaviour associated with disinhibition, or, more rarely, changes in sexual preference, may also arise as a direct result of brain injury (Miller et al., 1986). However, Aloni and Katz (1999) have pointed out the difficulties in separating changes in sexual behaviour that may be primary effects of a brain injury from those that are secondary to trauma and the emotional consequences of a serious injury. Sexual issues are discussed further in Chapter 8.

Changes in emotional responsiveness will be associated with a brain injury. Symptoms of anxiety and depression are commonplace but whether they are direct or indirect effects of brain injury is often unclear. Apathy, inertia and sleepiness are frequently observed in the early stages of recovery following concussion but they are not necessarily symptomatic of depression – although they are often mistaken for it. Anxieties, even panic reactions, are common in response to the experience of cognitive deficit and failure. Mistakes due to defective memory, or other intellectual shortcomings, can lead the person to withdraw from situations they feel unable to manage. This may progress to a point where they avoid contact with other people and may be reluctant even to go outside their homes. The person may feel unable to deal with any pressure or to make decisions, and they may show angry reactions or withdraw from company if such demands are made on them.

Other patients may show a more abnormal pattern of emotional response and one that is more clearly associated with the brain injury itself. Emotional responses may be exaggerated and perhaps triggered at inappropriate times. For example, following a stroke an elderly man found himself laughing at situations that were not funny. This was his response when he was told that his brother-in-law had died. He was aware of what he was doing but said he felt unable to control his behaviour and once he started to laugh he found it very difficult to stop. He was troubled by this problem and it inevitably caused embarrassment for his family too. Other patients will show emotional lability, quickly switching between laughing and crying with neither being appropriate to the situation. It is common for people with this kind of problem to retain insight and matters will then be aggravated by their awareness that they have lost emotional control and by feelings of distress and embarrassment about it.

Mental health problems

Obsessional disorders occasionally develop following brain injury (Kant, Smith-Seemiller and Duffy, 1996; Tallis, 1997), and more serious mental health problems, such as paranoid thinking or schizophrenia-like disorders may arise but there is little evidence of any direct link between brain injury and the onset of these disorders. It is perhaps more likely that the stress associated with a traumatic accident precipitates a psychiatric illness in patients who are already vulnerable to develop one. Changes of these kinds after traumatic brain injury are described by Lishman (1998). They belong more clearly than other behavioural symptoms to the field of psychiatry and are outside the scope of this chapter. When mental illness and brain injury are present together, joint working between a brain injury rehabilitation team and a mental health team is likely to be essential.

Incidence

The literature about the consequences of severe head injury has many references to the high frequency of behavioural disturbance although estimates vary widely. This is often because sample populations differ on measures such as severity of injury or the stage in recovery when they are assessed. In addition, different criteria are used to judge whether behaviour change is present or absent. Some authors suggest that behaviour changes occur in less than 30% of cases while others place the incidence as high as 90% (see Jacobs, 1990). It might be supposed that the frequency of behaviour problems would relate to severity of injury but there is no clear relationship between severity of the damage sustained and behavioural symptoms (Johnson and Balleny, 1996). The most likely explanation for this is that the location of the damage is much more significant than its extent in determining whether behaviour problems will follow. Behavioural change probably rarely arises as a direct result of minor head injury where there is only a short period of unconsciousness and a post-traumatic amnesia of no more than 24 hours. Studies of patients of this sort occasionally report some increase in irritability but disruptive behaviour disorders are absent (Jones, 1974; Rutherford, Merrett and McDonald, 1979).

In the study by Johnson and Balleny, behaviour change was identified in 80% of those sustaining severe head injuries. In about half of these cases the changes were rated as causing significant practical problems by relatives or carers. However, this study also showed that both incidence and severity of symptoms varied quite considerably at different stages in recovery. Early on, while the individual is still an inpatient in hospital or a rehabilitation unit, behaviour problems can be quite extreme. This may be because at this stage clients are still confused and in an amnesic state. They may have no understanding of where they are or what has happened. They can become violent when thwarted in their attempt to leave the hospital ward or when some nursing procedure is initiated that is incomprehensible to them. For example, a lady still confused by the effects of a recent head injury, appeared to be under the impression that she was visiting the hospital for a health and safety course. She became agitated that she would be late to pick her children up from school and then physically aggressive when staff felt it necessary to restrain her in her efforts to leave the acute care ward.

Alternatively, extremes of sexual disinhibition may be displayed under such circumstances. In one instance, a man in the early stages of recovery from a severe head injury, tried to make a sexual assault on a nurse. This appeared to be the consequence of his failure to understand where he was or what was going on and he therefore misinterpreted what he had been told to do. The nurse had instructed him to wait in his bed for her, although she had perhaps not made clear that this was for the purpose of taking a blood sample. Once confusion clears and individuals start to understand their circumstances better, behavioural episodes of this sort become unlikely or they moderate dramatically. Once through the acute phase, extreme behaviours are unusual.

Most often, only minor signs of disinhibition will be seen during the acute phase of recovery. The individual may be a little irritable or argumentative and relatives will perhaps report more swearing than usual, or they say they feel embarrassed at some of the comments he is making to the nurses. Within a few weeks of injury the person may appear to have returned to normal with perhaps minor changes that can be perceived only by close family members. Interestingly, a number of studies (for example McKinlay et al., 1981; Brooks et al., 1986) have noticed that this may be followed by a later deterioration in behaviour. In the study by Johnson and Balleny (1996) only 13% of those with behaviour problems showed physical aggression during the first 18 months following severe head injury but at more than 18 months post injury this proportion had risen to 55%. The most likely explanation for this deterioration in behaviour is that it is only at this late stage of recovery that the person is becoming fully aware of the limitations and frustrations imposed by the injury. It may be that by this time the person has tried and failed to return to work; he may have failed to cope with previous hobbies so well, and he may be experiencing difficulties in maintaining social relationships. Realization is beginning to dawn that a full recovery might never be possible. Thus, it may be a combination of aggravations of this sort, together with some direct effect of the brain injury on the ability to control temper, which leads to worsening symptoms.

Incidence of emotional disturbance

Depression and anxiety are common after brain injury but there are wide variations between different estimates of frequency (McCleary et al., 1998). For example, one study that investigated a series of patients one year after traumatic brain injury found that 13.9% were suffering from significant depressive symptoms (compared to 2.1% in an uninjured population) and 9.0% were suffering from panic disorders (compared to 0.8% in a control group; Deb et al., 1999). Other studies have suggested much more frequent problems of emotional distress. Tyerman and Humphrey (1984) looked at a series of patients seven months after head injury. They reported that more than half were suffering from clinical depression and just under half showed severe anxiety symptoms. The problem is that the incidence of emotional disturbance may be linked in a complex way to severity of the brain injury, the nature of the recovery that is made, and to the length of time since the injury. Few studies have looked at changes in mood over time (McCleary et al., 1998).

Mild levels of injury are associated with high incidence of depression and anxiety from an early stage – which may then moderate. In contrast, these symptoms are absent or very rare to begin with after more severe brain injuries (Bond, 1984). This is because considerable recovery in cognitive function and insight may be necessary before there is sufficient awareness for depression to develop. It is usually some time before severely brain-injured people realize the extent to which their work prospects and other capabilities may have been lost and only then is depression likely to develop. Bowen et al. (1999) found that depression following brain injury showed little change between six months and 12 months post injury but they provide some further discussion about changes in emotional disturbance over time.

Anxiety problems are also likely to develop as clients become aware of their vulnerability to forgetfulness and other errors. This means that signs of increased depression and worry relatively late on, can, paradoxically, indicate that progress has taken place in other respects. The problem for many of those with severe brain injury is that once anxiety and depression start they may prove persistent. This is particularly likely for individuals who have to contend with permanent disabilities that limit what they are able to achieve.

Causes

Changes in behaviour following brain injury are most often associated with damage to anterior aspects of the cerebral cortex. The 'overactive' types of behavioural disturbance appear to be associated with fronto-orbital lesions. Patients with damage here are likely to be disinhibited, impulsive, euphoric or emotionally labile and show poor judgement. With dorso-lateral lesions in the frontal lobes there is likely to be an underactive pattern of behaviour. These patients are typically apathetic, slow in their responses and emotionally indifferent although they may show occasional angry outbursts. A third group are sometimes described as 'akinetic'. They show a lack of spontaneity and may also show motor weakness including incontinence. In these cases it is the medio-basal aspects of the frontal lobes that are implicated. These distinctions were first made by Kretschmer (1956; see Parker and Crawford, 1992), although the nature of the link between location of damage and behaviour changes observed is still not entirely clear.

The disturbance of intellectual function, which is typically seen after frontal lobe brain injury, may also be the basis for some aspects of behaviour disturbance such as disinhibition and loss of judgement. For these patients, problem solving may fail due to an inability to assess the possible options available, or to an inability to chose between them. There may be poor attention to performance and to feedback about outcome (Duncan et al., 1996). This can lead to impulsiveness and inappropriate responses to mistakes. For example, a young man endeavoured to return to work in a vehicle repair workshop following a severe head injury. His work was sometimes normal but he was vulnerable to serious errors. On one occasion he was respraying the paint work on a red car. Halfway through the task the paint ran out so he picked up a nearby spray gun and finished the job with blue paint. He showed no signs of noticing the unusual colour scheme and expressed little concern when his foreman objected. This single-minded approach to the task, with little attention to outcome, could also be seen in his behaviour. He had become argumentative and would persist with his own point even when this was not achieving what he wanted. He was then quick to become angry and outspoken. Thus, inappropriate behavioural responses and deficits in problem solving may reflect the same failure to judge the situation properly or attend to the consequences.

Patients with this pattern of impairment will typically deny their symptoms. Lack of insight, together with emotional indifference or apathy, is associated with right anterior brain injury. The patients who show behaviour disturbance will often also show difficulties in recognizing the nature of their own deficits and this represents a particular problem in treatment. They are likely to dispute that their behaviour is any different or be quick to rationalize loss of temper or other behavioural symptoms. Some people are adamant that it is not they that have changed but their family or friends. This can develop into a paranoid style of thinking. In a majority of cases, denial of symptoms after acquired brain injury seems to be a genuine failure to perceive change rather than a defensive reaction to unacceptable information. If confronted about their misperceptions then this will often aggravate aggression and hostility.

Behaviour change associated with epilepsy

Rarely, episodes of behavioural disturbance may be associated with seizures. There can be a link between temporal lobe epilepsy and aggressive outbursts. Fugue states are very occasionally observed following head injury. For example, a year after a severe head injury a man started to wander away from his home from time to time and become lost. Hours later he would turn up some miles away with no recollection of how he got there or what had happened. Partial seizures can lead to brief episodes of confusion, loss of attention or unresponsiveness. Auras associated with seizure activity may take many forms. They can have transitory effects on emotion, leading to sudden feelings of anxiety or fear, for example, or cause the person's sense of reality to be disturbed (Lishman, 1998). One individual, who had partial seizures following a head injury, suffered from an aura during which he became quite certain that someone was standing just behind him.

Aggressive behaviour, and other behavioural phenomena, may be recognized as epileptiform because the behaviour shows no relationship to events or circumstances but seems to occur at random. Onset is likely to be sudden, with little or no warning other than perhaps a change in demeanour immediately beforehand. Moreover, there are likely to be other signs of seizure activity and often the patient is unable to remember what happened after the event. In between seizures the patient's behaviour may be entirely normal (Fenwick, 1989).

Behaviour change associated with emotional disturbance

Emotional distress may arise as a reaction to the trauma of injury or symptoms of this sort may be direct consequences of the brain injury itself. Discriminating between the two must be approached with caution (Aloia, Long and Allen, 1995). In a study of patients who had suffered a stroke, Starkstein, Robinson and Honig (1989) suggested that depressed mood was more likely in patients with left frontal lobe damage but he noted a link between low mood and basal ganglion damage too. If the right hemisphere had been damaged then posterior lesions were most often associated with depression. However caution is needed in interpreting these observations because the nature of the link between mood and location of damage is unclear. Raised irritability, inertia, and loss of motivation are associated with both brain injury and depression. Increased talkativeness may be symptomatic of disinhibition. Alternatively it can reflect raised anxiety. Tearfulness may be due to an emotional lability caused by brain injury or may indicate depression. Clues to help discriminate between different causes for emotional disturbance after brain injury can sometimes be found in the nature of what the individual says. Depressed or anxious people are more likely to talk coherently about their concerns, with evidence of awareness and understanding about their situation. Their expression of emotional distress is likely to match what they are saying. On the other hand, brain-injured individuals may be unable to account for their tearfulness, their loss of motivation or for feelings of irritation. Emotional responses arise less predictably and may seem at odds with the circumstances. Typically, they may show a marked lack of appropriate concern.

Post-traumatic stress disorder

A common confusion about the origin of behavioural symptoms after serious injury arises where someone is suffering from a post-traumatic stress disorder (PTSD). Symptoms include flashbacks and intrusive thinking about frightening aspects of an accident. It is recognized that impairments of memory and concentration are common with this condition. People suffering from PTSD may also appear to show behavioural change because they will make great efforts to avoid talking about their injury and to avoid reminders about what happened. They often show increased irritability and anger. They are reluctant to admit to their symptoms not least because to talk about what happened is upsetting for them. Thus, if there is also some possibility that they suffered a concussion, it may be wrongly supposed that behavioural changes are indicative of brain injury.

In fact, if there was sufficient concussion to cause brain injury then there will be amnesia for the circumstances of the injury such that symptoms of PTSD will be relatively unlikely. By definition, a diagnosis of PTSD depends on the client having a specific and frightening recollection of the trauma itself. Post-traumatic stress and severe concussion are therefore unlikely to occur together (Sbordone and Liter, 1995) although there is controversy about this (Bryant and Harvey, 1999). There are clearly some people who sustain a head injury but nevertheless show symptoms of PTSD. Figures for the incidence of such cases vary widely but there is evidence that it can occur even where there has been a severe concussion (McMillan, 2001). This may be either because some limited memory for the circumstances of the injury has been retained or symptoms may develop because of imagined experience of the trauma after they have learnt what happened.

Stress disorders may be quite common in association with minor head injury where the amnesia is not so extensive as to exclude all memory of the accident (McMillan, 1996). Clients may be able to remember realizing a serious accident was about to happen or they may be able to recall other frightening events a short while afterwards – such as being trapped in their cars for example.

It is important to keep in mind the possibility of PTSD symptoms for all head injuries, irrespective of the severity of concussion. However, it is particularly important to do so when assessing those whose accidents appear to have resulted in only a mild degree of concussion. Some people may describe symptoms suggestive of head injury, including even a very short amnesia, but the cause can be the fear and emotional trauma of the accident rather than a blow to the head.

Previous disposition

There are a number of other factors, which may prove relevant when considering the causes of behaviour change after brain injury. There is some evidence that brain injury has the effect of aggravating previous characteristics and is rather unlikely to lead to completely new behaviours. This idea applies particularly to the development of antisocial or criminal behaviours. It is almost unknown for a brain injury to be followed by problems of theft or fraud, for example, in a previously law-abiding citizen. What does happen is that the person who was previously inclined to minor misdemeanours may embark on more serious offences after brain injury. Thus, one individual who had a record of car theft and motoring offences, graduated to robbing post offices at gunpoint following a severe head injury. Of course a direct link between these events cannot be proven but the injury seemed to make him bolder and less concerned about the consequences of his actions in both his criminal behaviour and in other activities. Moreover, his greater recklessness and reduced judgement appeared to have the effect of making it easier for the police to catch up with him.

Previous disposition is also relevant because it is recognized that there is a slightly greater chance that those people with pre-existing behavioural and emotional problems will sustain head injuries (Tobis, Puri and Sheridan, 1982; Weller, 1985). This may be because these people are more likely to take risks or make poor judgements. It may also be the case that people with emotional troubles are more likely to be distracted or inattentive and therefore more vulnerable to accidents.

Other causal factors

Age may play some part in the development of behavioural problems after brain injury. Young males are more likely to sustain head injuries through car accidents and through fights, compared to females or older age groups, and they are more likely to be of an aggressive disposition compared to older people. It may be the case that younger people have fewer resources and less experience to help them cope with stress and so they are less well equipped than older people to deal with disability and frustration. Thus, younger people may be more likely to show aggression and other disruptive behaviour after traumatic brain injury.

Other factors that may result in behaviour disturbance without there being a direct link with brain injury are the effects of alcohol consumption and taking drugs. It is recognized that brain injury can leave the individual more sensitive to the effects of alcohol. Thus, a small quantity of drink can lead to quite a significant aggravation of behaviour problems. The interaction between drugs and brain injury is less well known but increases in aggression or other disruptive behaviour are probably less likely under these circumstances although effects on cognitive function may be more marked (Julien, 1996).

Pain or fatigue can also lead to an increase in irritability. Other environmental influences may stem from changes in social relationships that are not themselves the direct effects of the brain injury. For example, a grown-up son or daughter, who has left home, may be obliged to return following an injury. A mother may respond by being overprotective, too restrictive and controlling. This inevitably leads to friction and behavioural problems - but ones that may have no direct link with the brain injury sustained.

There are therefore several factors to consider in judging the causes of behaviour change after traumatic brain injury. It is likely that in many instances behaviour problems are a product of altered behavioural control as a direct result of the brain injury itself, but adverse environmental factors will often exacerbate matters. Thus, when things are going well there may be little sign of abnormal behaviour. When things become stressful, or there is some other source of aggravation, then inappropriate responses may quickly become evident and they may be more extreme than normal. An unusually clear-cut example of this was provided by a young man called Jack. He initially showed no signs of behaviour problems following a severe head injury. He returned to live with his wife and things seemed to settle down well, apart from some problems with memory and minor physical disability. Some months later his brother-in-law moved into the house. Jack had never got on particularly well with him but this had not been a significant problem. However, within a week or two of this event Jack was showing extreme temper outbursts towards his brother-in-law and threatening physical assault. His only comment was to say that he found it irritating to have someone else living in their small house. By all accounts this behaviour was completely at odds with his previous disposition. Once the brother-in-law moved out things settled down and Jack's wife reported that his behaviour appeared normal again. This illustrates how sometimes both the effects of a brain injury and a source of stress are necessary for behaviour problems to be expressed. This is an important consideration when it comes to treatment because sometimes tackling the sources of stress can prove as successful as treating the behaviour problem directly.

Assessment

Assessment of behaviour disorder will be limited by the difficulties already described in defining and identifying behaviour problems in an objective way. In a majority of cases behaviour changes will not be apparent when the client is interviewed in an outpatient clinic. Behaviour cannot be tested in the same way as a complaint of poor memory might be measured by setting the person an appropriate task. Behaviours that might be objectively rated, such as physical aggression, are usually too infrequent to be observed during an interview. For much of the time, brain-injured individuals may appear entirely normal in their behaviour with perhaps only a hint of uninhibited conversation in the form of the occasional personal comment or the use of bad language. On this basis more significant behaviour change might be suspected but it can only be confirmed by a relative or partner. Of course, behaviours may be reported that are extreme enough, or sufficiently unusual, to mean that there is little doubt that they are abnormal and the result of brain injury, but caution must be exercised in making these judgements and it is always important to seek the views of family members or close friends.

The evaluation of behavioural problems in a community setting must take several issues into account if the nature of the difficulties and potential for treatment are to be correctly identified. An account of the behaviour problems needs to be obtained from both the client and from a partner or family member. They may give different stories. The person who has suffered the brain injury may have little insight or their judgement may be impaired due to poor memory or other intellectual difficulties. The relative's account is not necessarily reliable either. Relatives may prefer to rationalize or diminish the problem (Romano, 1974) or they may be slow to recognize the nature of the change or even fail to perceive it at all (Thomsen, 1974; Brooks et al., 1986). Symptom ratings made by relatives can also be biased by the level of stress and anxiety they are experiencing (McKinlay et al., 1986).

It is important to find out about the severity and location of the brain injury, and about other symptoms the client may be experiencing. For example, if there has been a severe concussion and a brain scan shows evidence of right frontal lobe brain injury, then it might be suspected that a report of irritability reflects the brain damage sustained. On the other hand, in the case of someone with a left hemisphere stroke, who has very little speech as a result, and a right-sided paralysis, it is perhaps more likely that frustration is the cause of irritability. In the latter case the approach to treatment may need to focus on efforts to circumvent communication difficulties, for example, with little to be gained by trying to tackle the irritability directly.

Not all behaviour change following a traumatic accident is caused by head injury. Sometimes, behavioural symptoms show a variability that suggests some other factor may be their basis, such as depression or anger about what has happened. Clients may describe periods of days or weeks when there are no symptoms but say that things seem to worsen when something goes wrong or when they start to feel low in mood. For example, a man expressed anger and distress at the nature of a road traffic accident, which had occurred through no fault of his own, and had caused him various troubles. His outbursts of temper seemed to coincide with events that reminded him of what had happened, such as meetings with the lawyer pursuing his claim for damages or being driven somewhere because his disabilities prevented him from driving himself. Other stressful events, which were unrelated to the accident, did not lead to the same angry reactions. This pattern suggested anger with a realistic focus and perhaps a stress disorder rather than the effects of a brain injury. In fact, irritability can arise for so many reasons after a traumatic accident or illness that it is essential to have a wider range of symptoms than irritability alone to support a diagnosis of behaviour change due to brain injury. Where this is the case then poor temper is usually associated with other signs of disinhibition such as outspokenness or impulsive actions.

The need for careful evaluation of the evidence before concluding that behaviour change is a direct consequence of a concussion is illustrated by comparison of two patients, both seen about one year post injury, who presented with complaints of increased irritability. Both also described symptoms of depression and anxiety and complained of mild absent mindedness and poor concentration. Neither showed any clear evidence of significant intellectual impairments when formally assessed. In the first case (BB) there was considerable memory disturbance for a period of 24 hours after the injury although complete amnesia probably affected only about one hour. His outbursts of anger occurred in response to things going wrong for him, and were usually directed at other people, but reminders about the accident most often precipitated them. He was clearly very angry about the circumstances of his accident and said himself that 'he had become rather obsessed about it'. Neither he nor his partner reported any other changes in behaviour although he was much more nervous in a car and had shown some symptoms suggestive of a stress disorder earlier on in the course of his recovery. In the second case (TD) the initial injury was a probably more severe because there was a complete amnesia for a period of about 24 hours. Moreover, unlike BB, problems with aggression and agitation had been noted by nursing staff in the first few days after the injury. TD was similar to BB in that he expressed a lot of anger about the circumstances of his accident. However, his partner observed that he easily became angry at other times too, and often over trivial matters. Moreover, she noted other subtle changes in behaviour. She thought TD was generally a little more impulsive in his reactions, rather less concerned about things, and more rigid in his style of argument. Some word-finding difficulties were also described although these were not evident on formal tests.

Thus these two patients make very similar presentations, with reports of an increase in aggressive behaviour, but they probably suffer from different problems. The difficulties BB shows appear to be emotional, with no indications of organic damage, whereas TD's aggressive behaviour may well be due to a brain injury. His head injury was more severe, with early signs of poor behavioural control; his partner noticed other changes in his manner, and described a mild dysphasia.

What to record

Caution is needed about interpreting the nature of behaviour problems. It is essential to be objective and to document behaviours only in terms of what can be observed. For example, if a patient is frequently hitting out at his carers, and shouting and swearing, then these are the behaviours to record. If they are documented as 'aggressive behaviour' or as 'attention seeking' then this is making assumptions about the emotions or motivation underlying the behaviour. Moreover, it labels the patient in a way that may bias the perceptions or expectations of others. If a successful behavioural training plan is to be made it is necessary to define the behaviour in terms that lend themselves to treatment aims (for example: 'discourage hitting out at the carers' or 'reduce the frequency of swearing'). There is a danger that if things are not done in this way then bias may interfere with devising a good treatment plan. A detailed analysis of the problem as a part of the assessment process will enable errors of this kind to be avoided.

It is important to obtain a history of the symptoms, starting with the client's characteristics before the injury. Previous disposition may provide some clues to understanding current symptoms. Obviously aggressive outbursts are of greater significance in someone reported to be passive and easy-going previously, compared to the person who is described as 'having a bit of a temper' before. Behaviour during the early stages of recovery may also provide clues. Agitated behaviour when someone is first coming round after a period of unconsciousness is quite often the precursor to later behaviour disturbance (Levin and Grossman, 1978). If an apparently mild problem of being a little outspoken and talkative is first described one year post head injury, then it might be questioned whether this is because of brain injury or whether some other change underlies the problem. If questioning, or the clinical record, shows that the symptom was evident early on in the course of recovery, but has since improved, then brain injury may be the cause.

Frequency recording

It is useful to get an idea of the frequency and pattern of behavioural difficulties. Is it possible to identify what sets things off? How long do episodes last? Are there any factors that seem to help settle things down again? Information of this kind can be obtained by asking a client and his partner or carer to keep a record of behavioural symptoms. This is best done by the use of an 'ABC chart' (originally described by Yule and Carr, 1987). Apart from recording time and date there are three columns. A is for antecedents – what happened just before an incident; B is for behaviour – in other words a brief description of the event itself, and C is for the consequences – that is, what the outcome was or what happened to settle things down again.

Once one or more target behaviours have been identified, a formal record of the frequency with which the behaviour occurs may be made (event recording). This can provide a baseline against which subsequent change can be judged. A frequency record may be a matter of simply counting the number of episodes – such as the number of times swear words are used or the noting of each occasion when the person is heard shouting inappropriately. This works for brief, circumscribed events, or for a measure such as total time engaged in therapy without becoming distracted. It does not apply so well to persistent behaviour problems such as staying in bed or perhaps a frequent but less well-defined behaviour such as 'complaining'. In these circumstances some form of time sampling is the best index of frequency. For example, a record could be made every 10 minutes and the behaviour observed at that point is recorded. In this way the proportion of time for which the person stays in bed, or engages in complaining behaviour, can be documented. There are no exact rules about how these measurements should be made – they need to be adapted according to circumstances.

In clinical practice a baseline record may prove to be something of a luxury. If a client presents with a significant problem that is causing a good deal of distress and disruption at home then there may be a need to initiate a plan for appropriate management without delay. Baseline measures can also be self-defeating in another way and this perhaps applies particularly to working with people within the context of their homes and family. Quite often the instruction to record behaviour, without any suggestions about treatment, is reported to result in a decrease in inappropriate behaviour. This is probably because, in his efforts to make a record, the client starts to monitor his performance better and is more motivated to try to moderate his behaviour. Clients will sometimes report that they are motivated to try to avoid entries being made by the knowledge that a partner or carer is also making a record of what happens. Of course, this is only likely to occur with relatively mild problems and where the client has some degree of insight and motivation already established.

Behaviour rating scales

There are a variety of standard assessments that may be used to aid identification of behavioural symptoms following brain injury. A number of these are reviewed by Pender and Fleminger (1999). The best ones for assessment in a community setting are probably rating scales, completed by a family member and/or the client, such as the Neurobehavioural Rating Scale (NRS; Levin et al., 1987) or the Katz Adjustment Scale (Katz and Lyerly, 1963).

The NRS was designed as a scale to be completed by clinicians or therapists working with patients in acute care or in rehabilitation settings. It therefore depends on rating observable behaviours and some training on use of the scale is recommended to ensure ratings are used in a consistent way. There are 27 items rated on a seven-point scale ranging from 'not present' to 'extremely severe'. In addition to behavioural criteria such as 'hostility/ uncooperativeness' or 'disinhibition' there is a wide range of other measures including cognitive measures such as 'memory deficit' or 'expressive deficit', and emotional factors such as 'depressive mood' or 'emotional withdrawal'. It can therefore provide only an overview of behavioural change.

The Katz Adjustment Scale includes 127 items and also covers a wide range of symptoms, many of which are about mood or personality rather than behaviour. However, it has a better range of behavioural variables than the NRS such as stubbornness, childish behaviour or talking too much. It also has the advantage that it is designed to be completed by a family member and by the client. Thus, a check on reliability of reports and particularly on the level of insight from the client can be made. Poor ability to recognize behavioural problems by clients will mean that their motivation and compliance with a treatment programme are likely to be low. Ratings for pre- and post-brain-injury variables can be made. A four-point scale is used ranging from 'almost never' to 'almost always'. Normative data, for an American population, have been published for the Katz scale (Hogarty and Katz, 1971) and a version adapted for those with brain injury was reported by Jackson et al. (1992).

The DEX questionnaire follows a similar design with 20 items rated on a five-point scale (Burgess et al., 1996). The items are much more focused than the NRS or Katz scales on behavioural changes and the associated cognitive and emotional symptoms that are likely to follow head injury. The DEX questionnaire, like the Katz scale, has the advantage of parallel forms to be completed by the client and by someone who knows him well, and it can be used to rate pre- and post-injury behaviour. Rating scales such as the Katz or DEX are subjective and they can therefore be unreliable. They give an overview of changes that have occurred rather than a detailed measurement of behavioural symptoms specific to a particular client. They are therefore useful in initial assessment but less relevant as measures made for the purposes of evaluating treatment and outcome.

The Overt Aggression Scale is, as the name suggests, specific to the measurement of aggression. Although originally designed for use with a psychiatric population it has been adapted for use with brain-injured clients by Alderman, Knight and Morgan (1997).

Summary of assessment methods

Accurate assessment must include consideration of several factors. There may be emotional problems such as stress or depression, which might account for behavioural symptoms. After an initial interview there may be a need to collect further information on a formal basis – such as a frequency record or an ABC chart. The information gleaned from an analysis of the behaviour problem should enable targets for treatment to be identified and an appropriate treatment programme can then be devised. The attitude of clients is very important. Are they aware there is a problem? Do they show some concern to try to tackle it? A principal consideration for treatment is whether clients are motivated to tackle the problem or not. If they are, then 'self-control' methods of treatment are possible. Helping individuals develop strategies to moderate their own behaviour is usually the most effective approach. Sometimes well-motivated clients may already be able to report some strategies they have tried to use in order to moderate their behaviour. However, all too often after brain injury there is inadequate insight or concern for this approach to be possible, in which case 'external control' methods are needed. These depend on training family members or carers to respond to the individual in such a way as to discourage and minimize behavioural outbursts. At the same time there is a need to try to encourage appropriate responses. These methods are more difficult to implement, particularly in a community rehabilitation setting. Treatment methods are discussed more fully in a later section.

Goal setting

Goals for progress in dealing with behavioural symptoms must be individually determined and will depend on the stage in recovery. While individuals are still in acute care, immediately following brain injury, it is likely that they will be confused and perhaps have little understanding of their circumstances. Once consciousness has been regained after severe head injury, there may be a long period when they are still amnesic and quite unable to grasp where they are or what has happened to them. Alternatively, as awareness is regained, the first reaction may be one of disbelief and fear. In either case this may lead to behavioural outbursts. These episodes may be caused by feelings of confusion and fear as much as by direct effects of brain injury. Sometimes the behaviour changes observed at this stage can be quite extreme or even bizarre in nature. For example, a 23-year-old patient denied that he was in hospital and insisted he was back at school. He substantiated this by claiming that several of the ward staff were teachers that he recognized. In such circumstances it is common for people to insist they be allowed to leave the hospital and for them to become physically aggressive if prevented from doing so. Similarly, aggression may be the response to treatment from a physiotherapist, or to a nursing procedure, because patients do not understand their circumstances. They may both misperceive what is happening and be frightened by events. At this early stage goals must therefore be limited in the sense that formal treatments are likely to have little impact and in any case problems may settle quite quickly as confusion clears. Time must be allowed for further recovery. The main needs are for an agreed policy of management; for repeated reassurance and explanation to patients aimed at improving their understanding and reducing their fears, and to ensure the safety of client, staff and other patients.

Once patients have progressed to an inpatient rehabilitation unit or have returned home, perhaps within a few weeks of injury, treatment goals will still need to be limited because patients' understanding and compliance may remain poor. Instigating detailed treatment plans may be superfluous because rapid progress is likely to continue at this stage and the circumstances usually change quite quickly. Goals are most likely to be determined by the effects behaviour problems may have on compliance with treatment and on enabling the person to be looked after safely at home.

The timing of behavioural interventions is important. If they are initiated too early in the recovery process then poor compliance may mean that little is achieved by a formal approach to treatment over and above the gains from the natural process of recovery. However, if behaviour problems are not addressed then they may be aggravated by inappropriate responses from family and others. For example, if irritability is dealt with by giving in too readily to the demands being made, then this will encourage further outbursts. A young man who started to make flippant sexual comments from time to time after a severe head injury provides another example of a way in which behaviour can become worse. These were responded to by teasing him in a similar vein and by treating the whole matter as a joke. The attention and social exchange gained in this way had the effect of encouraging him. The frequency of his comments went up and matters became increasingly out of hand. A habit of inappropriate behaviour may develop in this way, which can then prove difficult to reverse.

At a later stage, when recovery has slowed down or perhaps stopped, the nature and extent of persisting problems will be clearer. Goals will then need to relate to the consequences of the behaviour. The behavioural symptoms may be causing disruption to other family members or be putting the client at risk. Motivation and a realistic attitude partly determine what might be achieved and if these are absent then there may be limits to what can be done in a community setting. Behavioural problems that are a hazard to others (as might be the case with physical aggression) or that put clients themselves at risk (for example, through refusing necessary treatment or by making their proper care at home impossible) may be difficult to treat without imposing some direct controls on what the individual can and cannot do. Treatment by admission to a unit specializing in behavioural management might then be indicated, or the employment of specialist care staff to work with the client within a community setting might be needed. Treatments on this basis will be expensive and goals may have to be established with financial constraints in mind.

Goals for behavioural management need to be broken down into a series of steps. If there are a number of presenting problems then it is best to prioritize and focus on one or two goals initially. These are likely to be the ones that seem most urgent but sometimes it can be expedient to start with the ones the client is most concerned about or best prepared to accept. Also, it can be best to start with a relatively easy goal that might be achieved without too much difficulty. Success can then boost the motivation of client and therapists. For example, a client might be showing a generally more aggressive manner, tending to be impatient and argumentative for much of the time, which occasionally escalates to verbal abuse and swearing. The diffuse nature of the problem might suggest a good starting point would be to focus on outbursts of swearing and see if this could be reduced in the first instance.

It is particularly important when treating behavioural problems that there is consensus between everyone concerned about the goals to be achieved. Ideally this should include clients, but they may have limited insight or other intellectual problems that preclude this. Consensus about goals is important for two reasons. Firstly, if behavioural treatment is to be effective it is very important that family members, carers and therapists are all giving consistent responses to inappropriate behaviours. If a majority adopts a policy of ignoring angry outbursts but one or two others feel that it is better to talk to the client about his anger, this may actually encourage the behaviour and make the problems worse for those who are endeavouring to ignore it. The second reason is that there is sometimes disagreement about what constitutes a behaviour problem. For example, occasional and perhaps fairly mild comments of a sexual nature may be seen by one carer as offensive and by another as easily managed and not unreasonable in a seriously disabled man with little other outlet for his sexual feelings. Another possibility is that the client may have different views to everyone else about his behaviour. Perhaps he acknowledges a tendency to speak his mind but denies that the loss of temper, which others are concerned about, is any different from normal. On the one hand loss of temper may seem the priority because it is causing disruption but on the other it may be better to start with goals the client is prepared to work on. Therefore, there must be good communication and agreement about goals before treatment is initiated in order to maximize the chances of success.

Management

Treatment of behavioural problems cannot be carried out with the patient alone. It must necessarily include family members or carers, therapists who might be seeing the patient regularly for other purposes, and sometimes other people in the community who come into regular contact with them such as school staff or work colleagues. This is because managing the way *other people* respond to the patient's behaviour is as important, and often more important, than working with the client directly. Consistency of response is a key aspect of the effective management of behaviour problems.

Before considering methods of treatment for behavioural disorder it is useful to review guidelines about responding to unexpected 'acute' episodes, usually of aggression or other disruptive behaviour, which may arise in the course of rehabilitation or during care work. Some knowledge about how to deal with these situations is important because it will enable therapists and care staff to feel confident about managing clients with severe behaviour disturbance. Identifying appropriate responses to difficult behaviour may prevent things getting worse and help calm the client.

Guidelines for responding to behaviour outbursts

These ideas relate to 'one off' behavioural episodes that are specific to a context (such as a sudden outburst of temper after someone is told he must stay in hospital, or anger at being kept waiting in a clinic), and which require immediate management. The strategies address the issue of how to respond appropriately to a difficult situation as it arises so as to prevent it escalating and perhaps becoming dangerous. This approach is quite different from behavioural management methods, described later, where there is an established pattern of difficult behaviour and the best responses are often those that aim to pay no attention to inappropriate behaviour. The guidelines described for 'emergency' situations usually entail doing the opposite because ignoring the client may lead to escalation.

The guidelines laid down by the Health Service advise that if a client is behaving in a manner likely to be dangerous to himself or to others, the first priority is ensure the safety of other people. A common mistake is to confront someone who is threatening violence, or who is causing damage to property, when the best course is to withdraw and make sure other clients are safely out of the way. The next priority is to ensure that colleagues are aware of what is going on, and to gain back up before tackling the situation in any other way. In hospital settings this may include notifying a consultant or a psychiatrist and initiating procedures that should already be established for gaining help from male staff. Situations of this extremity are fairly rare or short-lived.

Negotiation

A majority of isolated episodes involving aggressive or difficult behaviour, particularly those occurring early on in the course of recovery and in the context of hospital ward or rehabilitation unit, may be defused by negotiation. The important point is to avoid confrontation or argument because this is likely to aggravate the situation. Many angry or uncooperative patients feel that they have real grievances and frustrations about their circumstances, or about the way they are being treated. The particular problem for many patients with brain injury is that poor memory or other intellectual impairments mean that they do not understand their situation well. They may also be feeling frightened and confused. Despite the best intentions, matters are often made worse by disputing what patients are saying and telling them what they should do. This is particularly likely in a busy ward or clinic. For example, the brain-injured patient who has little patience may be quick to complain about being kept waiting. The response from a busy nurse, to the effect that he hasn't had to wait long at all and must wait his turn the same as everyone else, may precipitate a more serious aggressive outburst. Problems can also arise because there is a tendency for professional staff to respond to an agitated or angry patient on the basis of what they think their concerns are rather than spending a little time learning what is actually on his mind. Asking about their concerns, listening, and acknowledging what they are saying are more likely to calm things down. It may be possible to introduce information about their situation that can inform and reassure them. This may be directly in response to what they are saying – reiterating information about when visitors are coming, for example, or giving an explanation about the nature of their therapy programme.

It is obvious, but easily overlooked, that patients with brain injury, while perhaps able to converse and function normally in many ways, may have great difficulty in remembering or understanding what is said to them. Information often needs to be given as simply as possible and perhaps frequently repeated. This is always necessary following head injury as long as the patient remains in post-traumatic amnesia. In other cases the problem may not be so much one of forgetfulness or confusion about their situation but rather that patients who are at an early stage in recovery may have no ability to understand the situation at all. Not surprisingly, they are therefore likely to become angry about an enforced stay in hospital or about efforts to treat them when neither seems necessary in their view. Sometimes, when patients have no insight and are adamant there is nothing wrong with them, they may listen to information about problems that can follow a head injury such as they have had, but only if it is presented in a way that does not state directly that they themselves have such symptoms.

A common problem in hospital or on a rehabilitation unit is aggressive patients who insist that they should be allowed to leave or perhaps pursue some other ill-advised course of action. In most cases it is inappropriate to try to detain a patient with brain injury forcibly, by sectioning them under the Mental Health Act. Apart from the fact that this can rarely be justified, it is likely to be counterproductive. Constraints will invariably lead to an increase in aggressive behaviour and in most hospital and rehabilitation settings the only method of restraining the patient is through medication. This will inevitably interfere with rehabilitation and perhaps with the process of recovery itself. If a situation of this sort cannot be defused by negotiation or reassurance, it may be possible to arrive at some compromise between the patient's own plans and the needs it is felt he has in terms of rehabilitation. For example, a young man who was an inpatient on a rehabilitation unit a few weeks after a severe head injury, was becoming increasingly aggressive and uncooperative towards therapy. He acknowledged some physical disabilities that affected the coordination of his left side, but would not recognize changes in either his behaviour or in his intellectual abilities. He was insistent that he should not only go home but that if he were back at work he would be able to cope perfectly well. Discussion with his parents established that they felt prepared to test out their ability to look after him at home. The client agreed to attend the unit as an outpatient but only because of his need for further physiotherapy. With this arrangement his aggressive outbursts quickly moderated and caused little trouble either at home or on his visits to the unit. He remained in good contact with the rehabilitation team and as his recovery progressed he gradually came to accept the need to engage in therapy aimed at helping other problems he had started to notice, such as poor memory. Similarly, it became possible to advise him on a more cautious plan about his work.

Distraction

Efforts to divert patients' attention away from the cause of their agitation can help. Suggestions for managing confused or agitated patients along these lines are described by Yeun and Benzing (1996). In some circumstances it may be possible to engage angry clients in some other activity or focus their attention on another topic. For example, asking about the nature of their work may distract patients who are irate about their need to leave hospital and get back to work. This can be a particularly important strategy where there is a frontal lobe brain injury. These patients are not only prone to aggressive outbursts, but a common intellectual difficulty for them is that they become more fixed or rigid in their thinking. They may become angry over some quite minor matter but then seem unable to let it drop. The more agitated they become the harder this seems to be for them. Distraction onto some other subject or activity is therefore often essential and once this has been achieved the original source of annoyance may seem to have lost its importance. For example, a patient became angry about being asked to walk across to a therapy department. His anger was focused on being told what to do and the fact that he preferred to watch television. Questioning him about what he liked to watch on television distracted him and, once calm, reintroducing the idea of going to therapy raised no objections!

Interpersonal skills

There are a number of guidelines about maintaining an awareness of appropriate interpersonal skills when dealing with an angry or agitated individual. Posture and manner are important. It is best to try to remain calm and appear relaxed. Sitting down is likely to be less threatening although sometimes it may be safer to remain standing if physical assault is a possibility. Personal safety should be maintained by keeping a little distance from someone who is threatening violence and by being aware of escape routes. Equally, it is important that the patient does not feel hemmed in by being detained in a small office, for example, or by the presence of too many people.

Dealing with angry or agitated patients depends on experience as much as on knowledge of strategies. For this reason the more senior members of a team must take the lead in dealing with such patients and less experienced staff should not do so on their own or without close supervision. Most units and rehabilitation services will have policies and rules about safeguards and protocols for responding to behavioural outbursts. This applies not only within rehabilitation units but particularly to community teams where patients may be visited in their homes. Although infrequent, the risk of assault may be higher here. It is essential that staff, particularly those new to a team or unit, know what the policies are and understand when to implement them.

The guidelines described so far are aimed specifically at behavioural outbursts that are isolated and unexpected. For many clients with brain injury a more persistent pattern of behavioural problems will be evident and there is a need for strategies that will reduce their frequency or severity. There are three principal headings under which the treatment of persistent behaviour problems might be considered. These are:

- The use of medication.
- Indirect methods of treatment – control of environmental triggers and strategies of reassurance.

• Treatment methods designed to improve behavioural control. These can involve either external controls (behavioural strategies imposed on the patient) or self-control methods (patients endeavour to establish their own methods of control).

Medication

The use of medication to manage behavioural difficulties should be approached with caution. There is some evidence that many drugs can have abnormal effects on someone with brain injury (Cantani, Gluck and McLean, 1992) and guidelines on appropriate drugs to use are given in the British Society of Rehabilitation Medicine Report (1998). However, medication cannot of itself lead to long-term resolution of behavioural difficulties. Drugs are most useful in two circumstances. Firstly, if clients are too agitated or irritable to benefit from negotiated methods of treatment, then medication may help them to become calmer and more likely to comply with other management strategies. Drugs can then be withdrawn. The second indication for use of medication is for clients who show such extreme behavioural outbursts that they are a danger to themselves or others. There may then be little scope to tackle the problem in any other way.

Medication is sometimes the appropriate treatment for emotional disturbance such as disabling levels of anxiety or depression but caution should be exercised to ensure that a correct diagnosis has been made and that the symptoms are not those of other changes following brain injury such as apathy or excitability. This should be managed by a psychiatrist with expertise in medication and brain injury.

Indirect methods of behavioural treatment

Indirect methods of treatment mean dealing with environmental or other factors that may be triggering disturbed behaviour. These methods of behavioural management are the weakest but can be particularly relevant during recovery from brain injury because behavioural difficulties are very often the result of an interaction between reduced control due to brain damage itself, and the stresses and difficulties that arise as secondary consequences of the injury. Analysis of the frequency and pattern of behavioural difficulties will often show that particular circumstances or concerns are likely to precipitate episodes. For example, someone with increased irritability may find noise and busy situations particularly aggravating. Once back with their family they can find young children very difficult to deal with. Things may be improved simply by identifying the occasions when this is most likely to cause conflict and by arranging to timetable activities with young children so that it does not exceed the client's tolerance. Identifying other activities to engage in at the most difficult points in the day may also help. Fatigue may be a major factor in precipitating angry outbursts and this may indicate that the client is trying to do too much during the day or not getting enough sleep. Suggesting changes in their timetable, and introducing better rest breaks, might be accepted by clients without their having to acknowledge the difficulties with their behaviour. An improvement in their behaviour may follow.

Sometimes, angry outbursts may be in response to mistakes the person makes, perhaps due to poor memory. Early on in the course of recovery this may be aggravated by a failure to understand the situation and errors of memory may be blamed on others. Thus something is lost because 'my partner has moved it', or a missed appointment is because 'no one told me about it'. Helping the person to understand the nature of their difficulty, and how it may relate to the injury they have sustained, can moderate outbursts. Reassurance and explanation, which may need to be repeated frequently because of poor memory or other cognitive difficulties, can be sufficient in some instances to calm things down and enable improvements.

Stress is a common basis for behaviour problems following brain injury. This may either interact with poor impulse control due to the effects of the injury, or give rise to behavioural problems quite independently. The person who is struggling to cope with routine tasks because of physical injuries sustained in a road traffic accident is inevitably frustrated and perhaps depressed. This may be expressed as impatience and irritability. If, in addition, they have sustained a brain injury with the effect of reducing the control that they have over their behaviour, then outbursts in response to frustration may be extreme. Some brain-injured patients are able to maintain normal, or near normal, levels of behavioural control providing there are no sources of stress and so long as they feel that they are able to cope with what they are doing. Behaviour problems can therefore be managed successfully in some instances by tackling the sources of stress. Alternatively, improving clients' ability to manage the stress they experience, through relaxation training, counselling or help from a specialist working in a psychiatric outpatient service, may also lead to moderation of behaviour problems.

Of course, many behaviour problems after brain injury do not lend themselves to approaches of this sort. If individuals are disinhibited so that they speak their mind or they are inappropriate with strangers when out in public, the triggers for these behaviours are likely to be unpredictable and therefore difficult to control. They may express no concern about their behaviour and show a marked lack of anxiety or distress.

External control methods of behavioural management

When behaviour problems prove persistent and the patient shows little awareness or motivation, then behavioural modification methods are indicated. This approach to treatment is based on learning theory. The principle is that inappropriate behaviour is the consequence of a learning process and can therefore be 'unlearned'. Many abnormal patterns of behaviour observed after brain injury are those that are learned as a result of subsequent events. For example, abnormal means of gaining attention may develop as a result of loss of independence or perhaps because of communication difficulties. Other disturbances of behaviour may be more clearly the direct result of the brain injury sustained, such as sudden and apparently unprovoked loss of temper. These may therefore prove less amenable to treatment although a process of learning will often maintain these behaviours. Thus, natural recovery should lead to better control of temper but if carers or family members develop a habit of responding in an inappropriate way (increased attention, the client getting what he wants immediately) then this may maintain the behaviour or make it worse.

Despite the effects of brain injury on cognition and memory the ability to learn and adapt may be well preserved albeit at a slower rate. This is because the capacity for association learning is largely unaffected by cortical damage (Goldstein and Oakley, 1985; Goldstein, 1997). Good reviews of the principles of behaviour modification and learning theory, in the context of neurological rehabilitation, are provided by Ward (1997) and by McGlynn (1990). It has been established that this is an appropriate theoretical basis for the treatment of behaviour disturbance after brain injury. The underlying premise is that behaviours that are consistently associated with reinforcement or encouragement will increase in frequency whereas if there is either no response or an unfavourable response then the frequency will decrease. For example, someone who shows loss of temper and disruptive behaviour, and gets what he wants as a result is likely to behave in this way with increasing frequency. If their behaviour is ignored and their inappropriate demands are denied then their disruptive behaviour should decrease. To be effective, responses of this sort must be immediate and consistent.

Treatment in specialist units

The difficulty with this approach to treatment is that it necessitates some degree of control over the client. A partner or other members of the family may find it very difficult to ignore their demands. This might be because of the nature of the previous relationship or because the person cannot be physically prevented from doing or getting what he wants. For example, a man who had sustained a severe head injury developed the habit of walking into town and picking fights with other people, often after he had been drinking. His partner had little influence over what he chose to do. She did not feel able to restrict the money he had to buy alcohol, nor was it appropriate to try to impose any physical restraint on him leaving the house. Sometimes it may therefore be necessary to consider seeking treatment for a client within the controlled environment of a specialist, inpatient behavioural treatment unit. If behaviour problems are extreme then this may be justified. However, units of this sort are few and far between. There are very few within the NHS for people with brain injury, and those in the private sector are expensive. It is therefore important that only those clients who cannot benefit from more cost-effective strategies are treated in this way and where benefit from an intensive programme of behavioural management can be expected. In practice, financial constraints mean that referral to specialist units may be something of a last resort. The consequence of this is that clients treated in such units have often shown persistent and severe behaviour problems for many months or years before being admitted and patterns of abnormal behaviour are well established and therefore more difficult to treat than they might have been earlier on.

Because the behaviour problems treated in specialist units are often severe, the methods can also seem quite severe. For example, disturbed behaviour may be managed by using a 'time out' strategy. There are a number of ways in which this can be done but one practice is for clients to be removed to a small bare room the moment rules of behaviour have been transgressed and they remain there for a short period, or until they have become calm. Control might also be imposed by withholding access to television or trips out unless behavioural targets are met. These methods can bring behaviour under control quickly. The client learns to avoid the adverse consequences of inappropriate behaviour. The strategies used in these settings are described in detail elsewhere (Eames and Wood, 1985; Wood, 1987; Wood, 1990). Some people may have ethical concerns about these methods. Access to television or trips out may be seen as something people should have by right. Excluding people by placing them in a time-out room usually has to be done without their consent and may therefore be seen as an infringement of their personal freedom. These constraints must therefore be used with careful consideration and where less restrictive treatments have proved unsuccessful or where it is thought likely that they will fail. When behaviour problems have proved intractable, and they either seriously interfere with the patient's rehabilitation and recovery, or they mean that the person is a potential danger to themselves or to others, then these methods may be justified.

Behaviour is often 'context dependent' and there can be problems with treatment in specialist units because behaviour may change once the person is placed in an artificial environment of this sort. For example, someone may show aggressive or disruptive behaviour at home with their family but in other locations, and in the company of friends or therapists, these behaviours may be rarely observed. Moreover, the behavioural control learnt by clients during their admission to a special unit may not carry over well to the circumstances they have to deal with in their normal environment at home. Thus, treatment in a unit can lead to significant improvements but sometimes the problem behaviour may develop again following discharge. If the behaviours and skills acquired during a period of treatment are not applied and maintained in the real world then the rehabilitation effort has failed (McGlynn, 1990).

Treatment in a community setting

Training in real life contexts (*in vivo*) is therefore preferable. In a community rehabilitation setting it is not possible to exercise the same level of control as in a specialist unit. Nevertheless, the same principles can be followed although methods may need to be less rigorous. Withholding a client's 'rights', such as access to television or restricting the number of cigarettes they have, can only be justified if this can be seen as essential to a behavioural training programme and if the problem behaviour is serious enough to warrant such a regime. Wherever possible, a contract with the client should be drawn up so that they are party to the plan, either in detail or at least in principle. Moreover, there may be a need for a considerable amount of education or training aimed at carers and family members, including perhaps children, about behavioural problems and the rationale for management.

Treatment along behavioural modification lines may prove difficult within the community but nevertheless some control can often still be applied. The principal strategy to be used, and the one that perhaps lends itself best to working with behaviourally disturbed patients in a community setting, is the control of attention. Most behaviours are less likely to continue if normal social interaction and responses are withdrawn. In everyday life, an outburst of temper or ill-judged comment is likely to elicit attention and thus the behaviour can be inadvertently encouraged. The important point to recognize is that a negative response (such as shouting back) or a response that may seem helpful (such as starting a discussion about the problem) may well reinforce the behaviour because the client gains attention in this way too. This is particularly likely for disabled people, in residential care, for example. Their activities may be very limited and they may be suffering from a general lack of stimulation. In this situation a good argument may relieve boredom and become something to be repeated! Making sure they receive attention when their behaviour is appropriate, and none when it is not, will promote the development of normal patterns of behaviour.

Reinforcement strategies

The selection and control of reinforcement or rewards in behavioural modification programmes is a complex subject. Reviews of the principles and various strategies, in the context of neuropsychological rehabilitation, are provided by Wood (1987), Giles and Clark-Wilson (1993) and Goldstein (1997). The control of attention through use of a time-out room, as used in a specialist unit, is unlikely to be possible or appropriate in community rehabilitation, but there are other ways of imposing time out. A well-motivated client, with some degree of control, may respond to encouragement to leave the situation that is provoking his inappropriate behaviour ('self-imposed time out'). For example, a period of seclusion in his own room for a patient living in a community home will allow time for the person to calm down and then perhaps tackle the situation that led to a behavioural outburst in a more constructive way. For a client who is less motivated and unlikely to comply with this plan, a similar effect may be achieved by the carer or partner withdrawing so that the person is left alone and gains no attention or other payoff. In some instances, it may be important to give the client clear but brief feedback about the nature of the behavioural transgression. For example, when what started as a complaint has progressed to becoming abusive, or when a patient starts to masturbate during a therapy session, apparently without awareness that this is inappropriate to the circumstances, then a short comment to draw attention to the inappropriate nature of the behaviour can be effective. If this 'warning' is not sufficient to stop the behaviour then the carer or therapist should withdraw. It is not necessary to leave the person on his own for more than a short period of time.

Of course, this is not always possible for safety reasons and it can also fail if, for them, being left alone is a favourable outcome. This strategy will fail too if the client simply follows the person attempting to withdraw and continues to act inappropriately. In these cases there are other ways of controlling attention. It can be sufficient to withdraw attention simply by ignoring what is said and making no response or eye contact ('time out on the spot'). This might be either for a short period of time or until inappropriate behaviour has stopped. This method can be used during the course of therapy or care procedures when it may not be safe to leave the client alone. For example, conversation and eye contact can be stopped at the point when a severely disabled patient has become verbally abusive while being assisted to wash and dress. The care activities can continue and the patient's safety is maintained. Once abuse stops, or if appropriate comments are made, then conversation and other social reinforcement can be reinstated. Over a period of a few days strategies of this sort can lead to significant improvement. Difficulties can arise if the behaviour is already well established and has perhaps been inadvertently encouraged by the nature of the response that has been given to outbursts previously. When the response policy is changed this may result in an initial increase in abusive behaviour because it does not command the same attention as it did before. This is particularly likely if previous reinforcement has been applied on an intermittent basis (Murphy and Oliver, 1987). This is quite commonly the situation where a family has been struggling to deal with inappropriate behaviour, sometimes giving in to demands but being firmer on other occasions. It is important when behavioural management programmes are planned that this possibility is recognized. Therapists or carers who implement the programme must not be deterred if behavioural difficulties initially deteriorate, but should persevere with the plan in a consistent manner.

The control of attention is only one option and in many circumstances it may not be useful. For instance, in the example above the withdrawal of social interaction can be a positive reinforcement for some patients if they have a preference for silence or for being on their own, and a quite different regime must be devised. Observation of behaviour before a treatment programme is planned will reveal what the preferred activities are for a particular individual. Factors that tend to maintain inappropriate behaviours may also be evident. There is a need to take care to identify appropriate reinforcement for each client and ensure that it is something that is valued by him.

Thus, for one client praise as a response to appropriate behaviour may prove sufficient to facilitate change. For someone else rewards may need to be more tangible and more motivating. For example, cigarettes might be used as a reward for completing a task without complaint. In principle, rewards need to be provided immediately and contingent on the expression of appropriate behaviour and this should occur every time ('continuous reinforcement'). In later stages of a treatment programme, schedules of intermittent reinforcement may be introduced to consolidate learning and establish skills that will prove more resistant to deterioration once the formal programme has ended. Remote rewards, such as a trip out at the end of the week, are generally ineffective because of the delay. They are particularly inappropriate for people with memory or other cognitive difficulties where a deferred reward may have little or no effect.

Rewards such as praise or cigarettes are described as 'primary' because they are of immediate value to the client. Charts or graphs of performance, although of no intrinsic value, can also act as primary rewards in themselves. For example, this might be used for a patient who finds it hard to tolerate a specific physiotherapy exercise for more than a short period. He can be encouraged to plot a daily graph of the length of time for which he has persevered with treatment. The goal of maintaining an upward trend in the graph can act as an effective form of feedback and positive reinforcement.

Under some circumstances secondary reinforcement can be particularly useful. In these cases the primary reward is deferred but a 'secondary' reward is contingent on appropriate behaviour. This is most often in the form of tokens or stars, although money is also a form of secondary reinforcement. These methods can work well to increase desired behaviours in a poorly motivated or unconcerned client. For example, a chart can be used to tick off completed tasks. A reward, such as watching a video, is gained when an agreed number of tasks have been completed. These methods depend on adequate memory and an ability to understand the system. Some people with brain injury find it difficult to sustain motivation for a reward that may only be obtained some time later. An alternative strategy can be applied in which tokens are lost when inappropriate behaviour occurs ('response cost'). The requirement to hand over tokens when they default can help clients to improve their awareness and self-evaluation. This method lends itself to programmes that aim to decrease an unwanted behaviour such as swearing. An illustration of a treatment of this kind is provided by Alderman and Ward (1991) in which a lady was successfully treated with a response-cost programme to reduce the frequency of repetitive speech.

Preferred activities can be used as a method of reinforcement. This is known as the 'Premack principle' – named after the person who originally defined it (Premack, 1971). An activity that the patient enjoys is made available as a reward for engaging in therapy or completing a task which is disliked or for which the patient has little motivation. Encouraging a behaviour that is incompatible with the inappropriate behaviour can also be an effective means of shaping more normal patterns of behaviour. For example, someone might be encouraged to play games with other clients if this was found to encourage cooperative interaction. This might then have the effect of moderating poor social skills or reducing angry outbursts when the client is with these same people in other contexts.

Care should be taken when designing a treatment programme along behavioural modification lines that the encouragement of appropriate behaviours is considered at least as much as the control of outcome following unwanted behaviours. The technique of rewarding appropriate or desired behaviours, while discouraging disturbed behaviour ('differential reinforcement'), is important in ensuring that not only are abnormal behaviours lost but that at the same time appropriate and adaptive behaviours are developed.

Limitations to behavioural treatments

It is often stated that behaviour modification programmes cannot be effective unless they are carried out in a controlled environment. Responses to abnormal behaviour need to be highly consistent from everyone working with the client and under all circumstances. These constraints suggest that a patient treated in this way must therefore be managed in a specialist in-patient unit with staff who are trained and experienced in these methods. While this may be true for more serious behavioural problems, and particularly those that are well established, the principles of behaviour modification can prove effective under less rigorous conditions (Peters, Gluck and McCormack, 1992). In particular, consideration of factors such as the pattern of attention clients may be receiving in response to their behaviour and looking at levels of occupation or social contact that may be incompatible with behavioural symptoms can prove beneficial. Behavioural modification methods also highlight the importance of good communication between all those working with a client with behavioural difficulties. Problems need to be evaluated carefully and a policy of management, which is agreed and understood by all those working with the client, should be drawn up. In community settings this should ideally include family members and others, such as home care workers or day centre staff, as well as therapy staff. Other clients in a rehabilitation facility or day centre cannot be party to the therapy programme and this can lead to difficulties. Sometimes a degree of control can be exercised by ensuring the client is separated, either geographically or in terms of the days of attendance, from others who are particularly likely to aggravate behavioural difficulties.

The commonest pattern of behavioural difficulty in community rehabilitation settings is for the problems to be confined to certain contexts for the most part – such as loss of temper at home with family members but for this to be rare with other people or outside the home. Moreover, in a majority of instances clients encountered through community rehabilitation services will show at least some degree of awareness and concern about behavioural symptoms and this means that a different approach can be pursued.

Self-control methods

Alternatives to externally enforced methods of behavioural control are strategies designed to help the individual gain better control of their own behaviour. These methods can be very effective. They depend on clients having some degree of insight and motivation to improve their behaviour although this does not necessarily have to be particularly good. Providing the client is able to acknowledge or recognize some aspect of the problem this is sufficient to initiate making a behavioural record. This can help to highlight the nature of the problem and improve insight. Sometimes a client may not agree that there is a problem with his behaviour but might acknowledge that a partner or parent is concerned. On this basis he may be prepared to keep a behavioural record – perhaps sometimes in the belief that this will show there is no problem. Discussion of the record, along with that made independently by a family member, can lead to gradual progress in insight and improved motivation to pursue treatment strategies.

Self-control treatments are based on the notion that clients fail to follow the normal process of evaluating their own behaviour but that they can re-establish this if they understand the nature of the process and have strategies to help them follow it. The first stage in the way we react to a source of irritation, or some other event requiring a behavioural response, is concerned with our perception or interpretation of what has happened. This may be accurate but it is easily biased by factors such as previous experience and preconceptions. Secondly, we make an evaluation (perhaps subconsciously) of the behavioural responses available to us and choose one we think is appropriate. We then attend to the consequences of our behaviour and, if necessary, adapt or moderate the response. Thus, under one set of circumstances we might feel annoyed with someone but judge it better not to express this, whereas on another occasion showing anger may seem to be the best course to take. If the latter choice is made we normally take note of the effect our angry response has. If there is a feeling that one has acted too hastily then some moderating response may follow.

The problem for the person who has sustained a brain injury is that this process breaks down. Clients may evaluate the situation poorly and react impulsively. They may make a poor decision about what sort of response is appropriate to the circumstances. They appear to pay little or no attention to whether their behaviour achieves what they want, and they will often seem unaware of the reactions of others. Each stage of this process needs to be strengthened to help someone with behavioural difficulties regain control.

If they have difficulty in recognizing that some of their responses are inappropriate then the first step may be to improve insight. One strategy is for both client and a partner or family member to keep independent records. Feedback from the two records can help clients gain a better understanding of their behaviour. Caution is needed to ensure that this does not lead to conflict between clients and their partners. The aim should be to establish a 'contract' between them about how feedback is best given. Certain times of day can be identified for feedback between them when a relaxed mood is likely. Ideally the pattern for these sessions should be for the client to take the lead in identifying any behavioural problems that have arisen and to seek elaboration or comment from his partner. This may be difficult to achieve but the important point is to ensure that the partner does not simply provide feedback as a list of criticisms and complaints but that the process is more positive. Family members are likely to need careful advice and some training in how they should manage the situation in a positive and supportive way.

A self-control training programme might include the following stages:

- In many instances, particularly when loss of temper is the main problem, clients may not be able to judge when their behaviour is inappropriate. Their first problem is often that they find they lose their temper very suddenly, with little warning, and therefore they have no time to think about trying to control it. Nevertheless most people can learn to recognize the first signs that they are becoming tense, excited or angry and with practice they can get better at anticipating their behaviour.

- The next step is to establish a means of inhibiting the impulsive and ill-considered responses that they are inclined to make. There is a need for a strategy in the style of 'counting from 1 to 10 before acting' but this is too weak because it does not counter the feelings of anger or arousal and most people find it too difficult to apply. An alternative is for the person to rehearse a specific idea or thought about an imagined adverse consequence of loss of behavioural control. This might be an image that generates an element of worry or concern for the client because this will tend to counter feelings of anger or other impulsive responses. The idea used will need to be specific to the client's particular circumstances. Thus, one individual might make effective use of an image of his wife and family leaving because of his behaviour. In another case, a man who admitted to particular fears about ending up in prison because of his aggressive behaviour found an image of being confined in a small cell helped him to gain control of his outbursts, although there was no likelihood of this actually happening. The most effective images are often those that are exaggerated in this way. The image selected also needs to be brief and well rehearsed so that it can be quickly and easily applied as soon as the first signs of rising tension are noticed.

- Once the tendency to make an immediate or impulsive response has been inhibited, the third stage in self-control training is for clients to recognize that they can make a choice about how they respond. They must be encouraged to attend to the likely outcomes of their behaviour and to the fact they can exert some control over these. Many people will need a standard strategy that they can apply to ensure that they maintain control. For example, they may find it best to leave the situation ('self-imposed time out') until they feel calmer or until the source of aggravation has dissipated.

A good illustration of a treatment of this sort is provided by McCullough et al. (1977). They describe a successful self-control treatment of severe temper outbursts in a 16-year-old, despite an 11-year history and initial difficulties because the client was reluctant to acknowledge the nature of his problem.

More recently, Medd and Tate (2000) have described cognitive behavioural strategies and shown that training brain-injured clients in their use can lead to a reduction in aggressive behaviour.

Self-control methods require motivation and effort on the part of the client but can be very effective for the management of behaviour problems of moderate severity and those that need to be tackled at home or at work. The ideas involved are very straightforward but they are not particularly easy for people to implement. There is a need for a period of training that allows clients to become familiar with the strategies they need to use. It is important that they are advised that progress may be slow so that they do not establish the wrong expectation and give up when this is not met. The possibilities for training and education in behavioural management aimed at clients and carers, have been described by Carnevale (1996) and by Iverson and Osman (1998).

Group work

One way of teaching self-control strategies is through group work. For example, problems with loss of temper can be tackled effectively through anger management groups (Medd and Tate, 2000). Problems with social skills are commonplace after brain injury and may be best treated in a social group. Disinhibition or poor judgement will lead to problems such as inappropriate comments, excessive talkativeness or not knowing when to end a conversation. Anxiety and low self-confidence will also have an adverse effect on a person's ability to deal with social interactions. Sometimes these symptoms arise because of worries or embarrassment about forgetfulness or because of difficulties with communication. Many clients therefore find it hard to maintain social relationships after brain injury and tend to become socially isolated.

Groups lend themselves to role playing and rehearsal. The principles, as in other self-control methods, are those of providing clear feedback about behaviour to the client, and encouraging appropriate responses. The advantage of group work is that both these aims can be achieved to good effect by the comments and social approval of the other group members. Social skills groups for those with brain injury are described elsewhere (Johnson and Newton, 1987). However, group work does not suit everyone and care should be exercised in selecting people to participate in treatment groups. In brain injury rehabilitation it is often the differences between two patients, with apparently similar injuries, that are more striking than the similarities. There is a danger for some that feedback about performance from their peers, or comparison of their abilities with others in the group, may misinform and may risk an increase in self-consciousness or undermining confidence.

Summary of approaches to treatment

Treatment of behaviour problems in a community setting must be flexible in order to accommodate the needs and circumstances of the individual. The treatments described here cannot be applied prescriptively. There is a need to adapt them according to particular needs. Moreover, they are not necessarily alternatives. Often the most effective treatments in community settings are based on an eclectic approach where appropriate ideas from different models are combined.

Many community rehabilitation services or care settings struggle to cope with behavioural problems because of a lack of training in how these problems should be tackled. Therapists or carers can find themselves dealing with a potentially violent individual, for example, or with someone who is capable of extremes of embarrassing behaviour when out with them in public places. Perhaps it is with this aspect of disability more than any other that it is essential for therapists and carers to feel confident in what they are doing. It is probable that a positive and confident relationship between therapist and behaviourally disturbed client will contribute to the success of the treatment (McGlynn, 1990).

Evaluation and outcomes

Evaluation of the outcome of behavioural treatment serves a number of purposes. Firstly, it is a necessary extension of the treatment itself. It has already been made clear that treatment methods need to be adapted according to events as treatment progresses. Sometimes, the initial strategies that are suggested do not work as well as they might. Clients, or their carers, may find them difficult to implement. For example, a man who was showing outbursts of temper agreed to a plan whereby his wife would give him feedback, as part of a record-keeping exercise, about her judgement of the frequency of these episodes. In fact, the man had also developed an acute awareness of the trouble his injuries had caused to his family and he would sometimes become distressed when events reminded him about this. Unfortunately, the reports his wife gave about his outbursts had exactly this effect and upset him considerably. This aspect of the treatment plan was therefore deemed inappropriate. Thus there is a need to monitor progress regularly and adapt the treatment plan according to outcome.

Secondly, a behaviour programme must be carefully evaluated in terms of the need for it to continue in the longer term. In some cases improvement is achieved and this is maintained when treatment is withdrawn. Longer term problems, and particularly those where brain injury is the direct cause of the symptoms, may require a good management programme over a much longer period or perhaps indefinitely. If a programme is instigated and behavioural difficulties quickly moderate, then there is a danger of concluding too quickly that therapy can be withdrawn.

Outcome measures

Outcome measures by which the effectiveness of the treatment might be determined are subject to a number of problems. Suitable criteria must be identified by which outcome should be judged. Standardized scales that might be used for this purpose may be of limited use because of their subjective nature. They may not lend themselves to frequent repetition because of length, because they are insufficiently specific to treatment targets, or because narrow scales can provide only a crude measure of change. This applies particularly when working with clients within the community where direct observation of behavioural symptoms by the therapist may not be possible. Formal records must therefore be made by the client or by family members and this is likely to be unreliable – particularly if rating scales are used. The best measure is often to look directly at changes in symptoms by measuring the frequency of the target behaviour. A measure of this type will be more likely to detect small changes. This may provide a reasonably objective and reliable measure of change that could, if necessary, be recorded by a family member or carer. For example, a simple written record of the number of aggressive outbursts, or a time sampling record of levels of activity is something a carer or partner can be trained to do.

In many instances outcome of behavioural treatment may be appropriately measured by functional criteria about changes that may follow moderation of behavioural symptoms. For example, clients' improved access to or compliance with other therapies, their level of independence, or perhaps the amount of care or supervision needed may be improved once behaviour problems are under better control. Criteria of this kind are limited by their vulnerability to subjective judgements but they are relevant because it is often the limitations in these activities that lead to recognition that there is a need for behavioural treatment in the first place. A client unable to benefit from physiotherapy because of disruptive behaviour, or someone who could not go out in public unsupervised because of disinhibited outbursts, can be seen to have achieved a good outcome from a behaviour programme if he has become more compliant with physiotherapy or has become safe to go into town on his own.

It is also possible for there to be a positive outcome where there may have been little or no significant change in behavioural symptoms. Family members or therapists who are trained to manage aggressive or disruptive behaviours may report reduction in their level of stress or improvement in their confidence about working with the client. This may not be reflected by any significant progress in the client's symptoms in response to the management plan but rather reflects the level of confidence of carers or therapists in dealing with the situation. On a similar basis, circumstances can arise where it is suspected that a behaviour management programme may be effective in preventing deterioration although progress may not be achievable. Thus, it can be possible to identify measures of successful outcome other than improvement in the patient's condition.

There are a variety of other methods that might be used to evaluate behavioural treatment and measure outcome. Some of those used in the context of specialist inpatient treatments are reviewed by Alderman, Bentley and Dawson (1999). The frequency of symptoms during the course of treatment is the most direct measure of change although this does not necessarily demonstrate what factors in the treatment have directly influenced outcome, or even that the changes observed relate to the therapy at all. The most obvious pitfall in this respect is that the benefits of treatments carried out in the earlier stages of recovery can be confused with improvements that are the result of natural recovery, resolution of confusion, or progress in other aspects of cognitive function.

Single case design

Where a more exacting investigation of outcome is wanted then probably the best methods are those of single case methodology (see Barlow and Hersen, 1984; Wilson 1987, for an overview of this approach). Repeated measurements are made over a period of time. This might be a daily record of the number of shouting episodes, for example. The basic strategy in single case design is to make a baseline measure of the symptoms before treatment with the aim of documenting the pattern of behaviour and to establish whether any changes might be occurring anyway. For example, progress might occur due to natural recovery or efforts already being made by a partner. This first phase of evaluation might last for two weeks. Treatment is then implemented and the daily record is maintained so as to plot changes in frequency. This is referred to as an 'A-B' design where A is the baseline and B is the treatment. This may be augmented by a period of no treatment with a further period of measurement to evaluate whether change can be sustained. This phase might also be used to test maintenance of improvement in different settings. For example a period in a day centre might be commenced but with continued measurement to ensure behaviour control is maintained in this new environment.

More sophisticated strategies enable the link between intervention and outcome to be more clearly demonstrated. For example, periods of treatment versus no treatment might be alternated (an 'A-B-A-B' design) to test the importance of the treatment itself or to measure the effect of varying elements of the treatment. A further strategy is to use multiple baseline measures. This might apply where several behaviours need to be tackled. After a baseline period measuring all target behaviours, treatment for one of them is initiated. After a period during which improvement may be demonstrated, treatment is started on the next target behaviour. In this way the link between introduction of treatment and change in behaviour can be demonstrated. (see, for example, Alderman and Knight, 1997). These methods may be less easily applied in a community rehabilitation setting because of the problems of carrying out consistent and frequent observation of behaviour. Nevertheless there is no reason why carers or family members should not be trained to keep records of this sort. Alternatively a record may be made by a therapist using time samples suited to the frequency with which visits and observations can be made.

Limitations to outcome measures

In a community setting it is often difficult to use good objective measures of symptoms or changes in the response to treatment because the client cannot be observed systematically and because environmental factors will be varied. Softer and more subjective measures may therefore be necessary. Rating scales completed by client and a family member, carer or partner, at stages during the course of treatment may give some indication of outcome. However, subjective measures are unreliable not least because a client's self-report may be biased by poor insight and poor judgement about his own behaviour. There may be a considerable disparity between a client's rating of behavioural symptoms and those reported by a partner or family member.

There can be no one method of measuring outcome applicable to all behavioural treatments. The diversity in the nature and severity of the symptoms, in the circumstances and characteristics of clients, and the method of treatment adopted means that outcome measures must be adapted accordingly. The choice of outcome measures may also be determined by the purpose of the exercise. Very different considerations may apply if the aim is to learn whether a particular method is successful and worth development for clinical purposes compared to a need to demonstrate to a fund holder that time spent on behavioural treatment is cost effective. The former might suggest a rigorous single case design that might help identify the link between treatment strategies and progress. The latter might be better served by looking at functional changes following from a period of treatment, the associated improvement in independence, and the reduced costs that follow.

Conclusion

Behaviour problems are particularly difficult consequences of brain injury. They can be personally threatening as well being complex in nature and difficult to evaluate and measure. Therapists and care staff from any professional background may complete their training with no first-hand experience of how to manage behavioural problems and few will feel that they have adequate resources to deal with them. As a result, behaviour problems may be given inadequate attention and this can result in symptoms becoming more entrenched and harder to treat. Sometimes this means that referral to specialist units may be the only option. Treatment of this sort is expensive and would often be unnecessary if good management strategies could be applied earlier and if community rehabilitation staff had more training. In many instances there is no need for specialists in behavioural management to be employed to apply these treatments. Quite straightforward management plans, carried out early on, and focusing on *in vivo* treatment strategies, are effective in moderating behavioural problems. The need is therefore for therapists and care staff who work with brain-injured patients to have training opportunities that provide the necessary skills and confidence. One estimate is that less than one person per million of the population per year (50 to 60 people in England and Wales) needs inpatient treatment for behavioural disorder following brain injury (McMillan and Greenwood, 1993). A very much larger number of clients and families need advice about behaviour management, or treatment, that could be successfully carried out within a community rehabilitation setting.

References

Alderman N, Knight C (1997) The effectiveness of DRL in the management and treatment of severe behaviour disorders following brain injury. Brain Injury 11: 79-101.

Alderman N, Ward A (1991) Behavioural treatment of the dysexecutive syndrome: reduction of repetitive speech using response cost and cognitive overlearning. Neuropsychological Rehabilitation 1: 65-80.

Alderman N, Bentley J, Dawson K (1999) Issues and practice regarding behavioural outcome measurement undertaken by specialised service provider. Neuropsychological Rehabilitation 9: 385-400.

Alderman N, Knight C, Morgan C (1997) Use of a modified version of the Overt Aggression Scale in the measurement and assessment of aggressive behaviours following brain injury. Brain Injury 11: 503-23.

Aloia MS, Long CJ, Allen JB (1995) Depression among the head injured and non-head-injured: a discriminant analysis. Brain Injury 9: 575-83.

Aloni R, Katz S (1999) A review of the effect of traumatic brain injury on the human sexual response. Brain Injury 13: 269-80.

Barlow DH, Hersen M (1984) Single case experimental design: strategies for studying behavioural change. Oxford: Pergamon Press.

Bond M (1984) The psychiatry of closed head injury. In Brooks N (ed.) Closed Head Injury: Psychological Social and Family Consequences. Oxford: Oxford University Press, pp. 148-78.

Bowen A, Chamberlain MA, Tennant A, Neumann V, Conner M (1999) The persistence of mood disorders following traumatic brain injury: a one year follow up. Brain Injury 13: 547-53.

British Society of Rehabilitation Medicine Report (1998) Rehabilitation after Traumatic Brain Injury. London: BSRM.

Brooks N, Campsie L, Symington C, Beattie A, McKinlay W (1986) The five year outcome of severe blunt head injury: a relative's view. Journal of Neurology, Neurosurgery and Psychiatry 49: 764-70.

Bryant RA, Harvey AG (1999) The influence of traumatic brain injury on acute stress disorder and post-traumatic stress disorder following motor vehicle accidents. Brain Injury 13: 15-22.

Burgess PW, Alderman N, Wilson BA, Evans JJ, Emslie H (1996). The dysexecutive questionnaire (DEX). In Wilson BA, Alderman N, Burgess PW, Emslie H, Evans JJ (eds) Behavioural Assessment of the Dysexecutive Syndrome. Bury St Edmunds: Thames Valley Test Company.

Cantani E, Gluck M, McLean A (1992) Psychotropic - absent behaviour improvement following severe traumatic brain injury. Brain Injury 6: 193-7.

Carnevale GJ (1996) Natural setting behavioural management for individuals with traumatic brain injury: results of a three year care giver training programme. Journal of Head Trauma Rehabilitation 11: 27-38.

Deb S, Lyons I, Koutzoukis C, Ali I, McCarthy G (1999) Rate of psychiatric illness 1 year after traumatic brain injury. American Journal of Psychiatry 156: 374-8.

Duncan J, Emslie H, Williams P, Johnson R, Freer C (1996) Intelligence and the frontal lobe: the organisation of goal directed behaviour. Cognitive Psychology 30: 257-303.

Eames P (1990) Organic bases of behaviour disorder after traumatic brain injury. In Woods R (ed.) Neurobehavioural Sequelae of Traumatic Brain Injury. London: Taylor & Francis.

Eames P, Wood RW (1985) Rehabilitation after severe brain injury: a special unit approach to behaviour disorder. International Rehabilitation Medicine 7: 130-3.

Fenwick P (1989) The nature and management of aggression in epilepsy. Journal of Neuropsychiatry 1: 418-25.

Giles GM, Clark-Wilson J (1993) Brain Injury Rehabilitation. A Neurofunctional Approach. London: Chapman & Hall.

Goldstein LH (1997) Behaviour Problems. In Greenwood R, Barnes MP, McMillan TM, Ward CD (eds) Neurological Rehabilitation. 2 edn. Psychology Press. Hove: Erlbaum.

Goldstein LH, Oakley DA (1985) Expected and actual behavioural capacity after diffuse reduction in cerebral cortex: a review and suggestions for rehabilitative techniques with the mentally handicapped and head injured. British Journal of Clinical Psychology 24: 13-24.

Harlow JM (1848) Passage of an iron rod through the head. Boston Medicine and Surgery Journal 39: 389-93. Cited in O'Driscoll L, Leach JP (1998) 'No longer Gage': an iron bar through the head. British Medical Journal 317: 1673-4.

Hogarty GE, Katz MM (1971) Norms of adjustment and social behaviour. Archives of General Psychiatry 25: 470-80.

Iverson G, Osman A (1998) Behavioural interventions for children and adults with brain injuries: a guide for families. Journal of Cognitive Rehabilitation 16: 14-23.

Jacobs HE (1990) Identifying post traumatic behaviour problems: data from psychosocial follow-up studies. In: Wood RL (ed.) Neurobehavioural Sequelae of Traumatic Brain Injury. London: Taylor & Francis, pp. 134-50.

Jackson HF, Hopewell CA, Glass CA, Warburg R, Dewey M, Ghadiali E (1992) The Katz adjustment scale: modification for use with victims of traumatic brain and spinal injury. Brain Injury 6: 109-27.

Johnson DA, Newton A (1987) Social adjustment and interaction after severe head injury: II rationale and bases for intervention. British Journal of Clinical Psychology 26: 289-98.

Johnson RP, Balleny H (1996) Behaviour problems after brain injury: incidence and need for treatment. Clinical Rehabilitation 10: 173-81.

Jones RK (1974) Assessment of minimal head injuries: indications for in-hospital care. Surgery and Neurology 2: 101-4.

Julien RM (1996) A Primer of Drug Action. New York: WH Freeman & Co.

Kant R, Smith-Seemiller L, Duffy JD (1996) Obsessive compulsive disorder after closed head injury: a review of the literature and report of four cases. Brain Injury 10: 55-63.

Katz MM, Lyerly SB (1963) Methods for measuring adjustment and social behaviour in the community. Psychological Reports 13: 503-35.

Kreutzer JS, Zasler ND (1989) Psychosexual consequences of traumatic brain injury: methodology and preliminary findings. Brain Injury 3: 177-86.

Levin HS, Grossman RG (1978) Behavioural sequelae of closed head injury. Archives of Neurology 35: 720-7.

Levin HS, High WM, Goethe KE, Sisson RA, Overall JE, Rhoades HM, Eisenberg HM, Kalisky Z, Gary HE (1987) The neurobehavioural rating scale: assessment of the behavioural sequelae of head injury by the clinician. Journal of Neurology, Neurosurgery and Psychiatry 50: 183-93.

Lishman WA (1998) Organic Psychiatry: the Psychological Consequences of Cerebral Disorder. 3 edn. Oxford: Blackwell Science.

McCleary C, Satz P, Forney D, Light R, Zaucha K, Asarnow R, Namerow N (1998) Depression after traumatic brain injury as a function of Glasgow Outcome score. Journal of Clinical and Experimental Psychology 20: 270-9

McCullough JP, Huntsinger GM, Nay WR (1977) Self control treatment of aggression in a 16 year old male. Journal of Consulting Clinical Psychology 45: 322-31.

McGlynn SM (1990) Behavioural approaches to neuropsychological rehabilitation. Psychological Bulletin 108: 420-41.

McKinlay W, Brooks N, Bond MR, Martinage DP, Marshall MM (1981) The short-term outcome of severe blunt head injury as reported by relatives of the injured persons. Journal of Neurology, Neurosurgery and Psychiatry 44: 527-33.

McMillan TM (1996) Post-traumatic stress disorder following minor and severe closed head injury: 10 single case studies. Brain Injury 10: 749-58.

McMillan TM (2001) Errors in diagnosing post-traumatic stress disorder after traumatic brain injury. Brain Injury 15: 39-46.

McMillan TM, Greenwood RJ (1993) Models of rehabilitation programmes for the brain injured adult. II. Model services and suggestions for change in the UK. Clinical Rehabilitation 7: 346-55.

Medd J, Tate RL (2000) Evaluation of an anger management therapy programme following acquired brain injury. Neuropsychological Rehabilitation 10: 185-201.

Miller BL, Cummings JL, McIntyre H, Ebers G, Grodes M (1986). Hypersexuality and altered sexual preference following brain injury. Journal of Neurology, Neurosurgery and Psychiatry 49: 867-73.

Murphy G, Oliver C (1987) Decreasing undesirable behaviours. In Yule W, Carr J (eds) Behaviour Modification for People with Mental Handicaps. 2 edn. London: Croom Helm.

Parker DM, Crawford JR. (1992) Assessment of frontal lobe dysfunction. In Crawford JR, Parker JR, McKinley WW (eds) A Handbook of Neuropsychological Assessment. Hove: Lawrence Erlbaum.

Pender N, Fleminger S (1999) Outcome measures on in-patient cognitive and behavioural units. Neuropsychological Rehabilitation 9: 345–61.

Peters MD, Gluck M, McCormack M (1992) Behaviour rehabilitation of the challenging client in less restrictive settings. Brain Injury 6: 229–314.

Premack D (1971) Language in chimpanzees. Science 172: 808–22.

Romano MD (1974) Family response to traumatic head injury. Scandanavian Journal of Rehabilitation Medicine 6: 1–4.

Rutherford WH, Merrett JD, McDonald JR (1979) Symptoms at one year following concussion from minor head injuries. Injury 10: 225–30.

Sbordone RJ, Liter JC (1995) Mild traumatic brain injury does not produce post traumatic stress disorder. Brain Injury 9: 405–17.

Starkstein SE, Robinson RG, Honig MA (1989) Mood changes after right hemisphere lesions. British Journal of Psychiatry 155: 79–85.

Tallis F (1997) The neuropsychology of obsessive-compulsive disorder: a review and consideration of clinical implications. British Journal of Clinical Psychology 36: 3–20.

Thomsen V (1974) The patient with severe head injury and his family. Scandanavian Journal of Rehabilitation Medicine 6: 180–3.

Tobis J, Puri K, Sheridan J (1982) Rehabilitation of the severely brain injured patient. Scandanavian Journal of Rehabilitation Medicine 13: 83–8.

Tyerman A, Humphrey M (1984) Changes in self concept following severe head injury. International Journal of Rehabilitation Research 7: 11–23.

Ward CD (1997) Learning and skill acquisition. In Greenwood R, Barnes MP, McMillan TM, Ward CD (eds) Neurological Rehabilitation. 2 edn. Hove: Psychology Press, Erlbaum.

Weller MP (1985) The sequelae of head injury and the post-concussion syndrome. In Granville-Grossman K (ed.) Recent advances in Clinical Psychiatry 5. Edinburgh: Churchill Livingstone.

Wilson B (1987) Single-case experimental designs in neuropsychological rehabilitation. Journal of Clinical and Experimental Neuropsychology 9: 527–44.

Wood RW (1987) Brain Injury Rehabilitation: A Neurobehavioural Approach. London: Croom Helm.

Wood RW (1990) (ed.) Neurobehavioural Sequelae of Traumatic Brain Injury. London: Taylor & Francis.

Yeun HK, Benzing P (1996) Treatment methodology. Guiding of behaviour through redirection in brain injury rehabilitation. Brain Injury 10: 229–38.

Yule W, Carr J (1987) (eds) Behavioural Modification for People with Mental Handicaps. 2 edn. London: Croom Helm.

CHAPTER 6
Communication

ROSEMARY GRAVELL

It is difficult to overstate the importance of communication. The ability to communicate effectively underlies all social interaction and is what enables people to build and maintain social relationships. This chapter will address the disorders of communication that may result from head injury and the assessment and management of those disorders. The complexity of the communication process makes it particularly vulnerable to the effects of a head injury. The fact that communication is such a complex process means that it is important to be aware of what is meant by the term before attempting to understand the nature of possible disorders. This discussion will therefore begin by describing communication in general.

What is communication?

Effective communication is the transmission of a message between sender and receiver within a social context. Specific abilities required for the process include sensori-perceptual, linguistic, cognitive and motor skills. In addition the individual must be able to take into account the particular social context in which an interaction occurs. In many ways it is artificial to attempt to separate the specific communicative abilities and the context, because it is those very abilities which enable a person to react appropriately to context. However, it is a useful way to describe the communicative process. Communication depends not only upon individual abilities but on motivation and opportunity to use those abilities, as can be seen in Figure 6.1.

Specific communicative abilities

A message may be received via any of the sensory pathways. The auditory route is used not just to receive spoken language, but also allows reception of non-verbal messages, such as environmental noise and tone of voice. The visual

Breakdown at any point along the chain may result in a communication disorder.

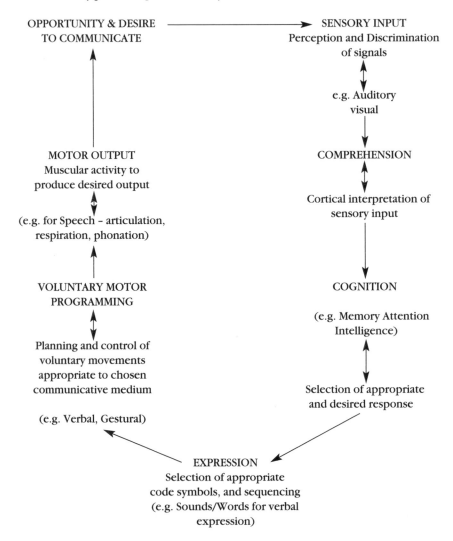

Figure 6.1. Communication chain.

channel is important in reading but also to take in many non-verbal behaviours from the sender, such as facial expression and gesture. Touch may communicate a variety of emotional messages and may also be used, as in Braille, as a symbolic language system. Even smell and taste can communicate something, as numerous scent and food adverts testify. Thus it is apparent that both verbal and non-verbal channels are of importance in the communication process.

A message that is taken in via any of the senses must be processed and understood. Intact linguistic and cognitive abilities are essential to the ability to make sense of the message and to formulate a response, and these are interrelated.

Linguistic ability is a cortical function by which the units of language can be understood and used expressively. Verbal language is a complex system, based on the 'building blocks' of sounds (phonemes) or written letters (graphemes). These are formed into words by the application of systematic rules, a process that is usually entirely automatic. The words are then linked by grammatical rules (syntax) to form phrases, sentences and longer units. The meaning of the words and longer units is referred to as the semantic content. Finally there is the pragmatic aspect, which is the way in which language is actually used in 'real life' and which takes the context into account.

To illustrate the semantic and pragmatic levels, Body, Perkins and MacDonald (1999) use the example of the word 'here' that has an explicit semantic meaning, but can only be understood if there is an ability to extract inferred meaning from the context in which it is used. That is, the command 'come here' depends on awareness of where the speaker is located. In addition, tone of voice, facial expression, body language and other non-verbal behaviours will vary according to the speaker's intent. 'Come here' may be uttered seductively or in anger, for example. The pragmatic level is not limited to language but encompasses both verbal and non-verbal aspects of what may be described as 'social communication' or interpersonal skills.

Language use at the discourse level – that is, beyond the sentence level – has been the focus of much interest recently. Different styles are apparent, dependent upon the purpose of discourse. For example, asking someone to relate an event or story would elicit a style described as 'narrative'; giving instructions or directions would be 'procedural'; and there is a distinct 'conversational' style. It is at this level that the cognitive skills, such as attention, self-monitoring, memory, organization and so on, most obviously interact with language skills, in order to produce logical and coherent output.

Cognitive abilities underlie communication in a variety of ways. Attention, perception, information processing, memory and executive functioning are all interrelated with linguistic and general communication skills. Attention, for example, is a prerequisite if language is to be taken in and processed. Not only are these cognitive processes critical to the ability to use specific linguistic skills, but at the pragmatic level they are important to the ability to take social context into account, as will be seen later in this chapter. The motivation to want to communicate is also a factor.

Having received and understood a message, and formulated a response, the receiver becomes the sender. Appropriate voluntary movements must be programmed to allow the new message to be sent verbally or non-verbally, and finally there is the actual physical expression of the message. This may be by speech, writing, or a variety of non-verbal means such as body movements, gesture, proximity, facial expression, appearance, drawing and so on. Indeed a message may be sent via any motor channel, just as it may be received by any of the senses. Those messages will usually be deliberate, but much may also be communicated non-intentionally.

The context

Communication does not occur in a vacuum. The context in which an interaction takes place will affect the linguistic and behavioural choices that are made. For example, two words or phrases may have much the same meaning but one may be deemed inappropriate in a particular situation because it is too formal or informal. For instance, using the terms 'geezer' or 'bird' may be acceptable in certain settings, but 'man' and 'woman' are the more likely selections in a formal meeting. Similarly, how physically close people stand to each other may depend on the degree of intimacy between them or on their sociocultural background, as different cultures have differing behavioural norms. These choices are generally automatic and it is only when the unwritten rules are violated that people become aware of them. Detailed discussion of the numerous theories concerning context is beyond the scope of this chapter, but it may be useful to illustrate one approach.

In 1995, Hartley outlined a model of social communication encompassing four 'contexts'. The social/cognitive context includes the relative roles of participants, relative status, the degree of intimacy of the relationship, cultural background, the emotional and cognitive status of the partner, shared knowledge, intentions and goals, and the overall purpose of the interaction. Socially accepted conventions to do with the interaction include taking turns as speaker/listener, knowing when information needs to be included or can be assumed to be shared, and topic selection. The purpose of the interaction may be to give or gain information, to express feelings, to control, as social ritual, or for story telling.

The physical context would refer to the surroundings, time, location of participants and the people present. Linguistic and non-verbal contexts refer to the continuous influence of these behaviours on the interaction. Non-verbal behaviours include paralinguistic aspects (such as intonation), gesture, body movements and proximity.

Hartley goes on to outline the central role of cognitive processes on the ability to take the context into account when making communicative choices. An individual must be motivated and alert in order to want to enter a social situation. Appropriate social behaviour will depend on stored knowledge, formed through experience, of linguistic forms and behaviour in different settings and for different purposes. This knowledge of social 'rules' will enable individuals to make socially acceptable choices of verbal and non-verbal behaviour (and appearance).

It is apparent that communication takes into account many factors in addition to language and speech. In order to discuss the possible ways in which communication can be affected by head injury, the simple model illustrated in Figure 6.1 will be followed. This chapter focuses on communication, but it is important not to lose sight of the fact that most people with head injury will have multiple impairments, albeit at differing levels of severity. Other influences will therefore interact with communication impairments in how each person presents and the outline offered here is no more than a general guide.

Communication disorders after head injury

Motivation and opportunity

Insight and motivation to communicate are critical considerations. Communication has been described as a two-way process and an impairment of communication, on any level, will not only affect the individual but will also place added burdens or responsibilities on the other person in an interaction. This can result in fewer opportunities being set up in which communication can occur. It can also mean that communication failure will create a vicious circle of decreased motivation to communicate, reduced opportunity and so on. The obvious example of this is in one of the recognized risks of institutional life, when communicative opportunity is restricted and gradually fewer efforts are made to seek social outlets. In addition, many of the general consequences of head injury can place restrictions on the person's lifestyle – for example, a physical disability may obviously restrict the opportunities for communication, as may perceptual or behavioural issues. This latter point is illustrated by the case of a 22-year-old accident victim, who became verbally sexually disinhibited, as a result of which women did not feel comfortable spending time with him.

Insight is a factor in motivation to communicate. Lack of insight often means the individual is quite happy to continue to communicate, without awareness of the inappropriateness of their efforts or of listeners' reactions, and this may cause others to lose motivation to communicate. The example above, of the young man who made sexual remarks, illustrates this. He had no insight into the effect of his comments on others and failed to understand why former female friends no longer visited him.

Motivation is a complex area as it relates both to cognition and to secondary psychosocial reactions to loss. Organic causes of lowered motivation will need to be addressed in a very different way from functional causes. While it is not uncommon for the person with a head injury to have reduced insight it is worth pointing out that this is not always the case. Some clients have excellent insight and may seem to over-attribute 'normal' behaviours to the head injury – for example, the occasional word loss that most people experience.

Sensory impairments

Although discussion of sensory impairments is outside the scope of this chapter, it is important at least to make reference to the likelihood of sensory impairment having an effect on communication skills. This may be in both obvious and subtle ways, whether due to peripheral or central damage. They will also impact on managerial decisions in rehabilitation. Obvious effects would include visual impairment affecting reading, hearing loss affecting the ability to take in messages, and loss of sensation leading to an inability to respond to touch. More subtle implications include difficulty taking in non-verbal clues as a result of visual impairment – thus, for instance, the facial expression accompanying words intended sarcastically may not be appreciated and the words taken literally. Similarly, hearing difficulty may mean intonational cues are missed.

Sensory impairments may be pre-existing, may be caused by the head injury or be due to other damage at the time of the injury. This issue is mentioned in Chapter 2.

Language disorder

Cognitive-communication disorder and aphasia

After head injury it is well established that linguistic changes, in relation to both comprehension and expression, do occur. These include reduced comprehension as the length, duration, complexity, rate of delivery or level of abstraction increases. More abstract language would include use of analogies and inferring, rather than stating, information. If people cannot understand more abstract comments, it will, for example, affect the ability to appreciate word-based humour. Clients may need very clear, concrete, literal statements. Thus, for example, saying 'It's like wading through treacle' may convey neither the intended meaning nor the empathy the phrase was meant to engender. An illustration of this can be seen in a young head-injured woman, who was asked to explain what was meant by a supervisor saying to an employee 'you can't climb a ladder with your hands in your pockets'. Her response was to interpret the utterance literally and say that you need your hands to hold on to the ladder.

Expressively, there may be a reduction in vocabulary and in naming skills, and poor verbal fluency. If word finding is affected there may be hesitations during speech, use of circumlocution (that is, attempting to convey the meaning of a lost word by talking around it), or inappropriate word use. Conversation may be disjointed and hard to follow, with little structure and a tendency to stray off the subject.

The nature of language disorder has been the subject of considerable debate in the literature. It is now generally accepted that there is a difference between people who have specific language disorder (aphasia) as a result of *focal* brain damage and those whose language skills are impaired as a result of the *diffuse* damage commonly found after traumatic head injury.

Focal brain damage to cortical speech-language centres leads to the specific language disorder referred to as aphasia (or dysphasia – the two terms signify degree of severity, but in practice are often used interchangeably). Aphasia is a condition that affects all aspects of language, via both the spoken and written channels. The exact nature and degree to which comprehension and expression in each channel is affected will 'vary as a function of the location and extent of brain damage' (Davis and Holland, 1981). For example, one person may have predominant difficulties in expressing himself through language, with halting speech as he struggles to find words, or he may be limited to repeated stereotyped utterances. Another may be more impaired in the ability to understand and, although able to speak fluently, may use inappropriate or nonsense words or phrases, with little awareness that the language is not normal. While there are typical patterns of impairment, it is no exaggeration to say that all clients with aphasia are unique in the overall way in which they present.

Historically, people with diffuse brain injury were given aphasia tests, on which they performed poorly, but those individuals did not show overt aphasic behaviours in everyday life. The language changes described at the beginning of this section are qualitatively and quantitatively different from those seen in aphasia. Holland (1982) nicely described the difference between head-injured people's communication skills and the communication of aphasic people, when she wrote that 'those with aphasia communicate better than they talk, while those with head injuries talk better than they communicate'.

The need to draw a distinction between aphasia and language changes due to diffuse head injury, together with increasing attention to the complex interplay between language and cognition, led to the term 'cognitive language disorder' (Hagan, 1984) being coined. The broader term 'cognitive communication disorder' recognizes that the underlying cognitive impairment does not specifically affect language, but the whole process of communication. Many references explicitly support this distinction (for example, Ellmo et al., 1995; Body and Parker, 1999) and McDonald, Togher and Code

(1999) point out 'it is now well recognised that communication problems following TBI are distinctly different to those subsequent to a more focal lesion such as occurs in a cerebrovascular accident or a penetrating head injury.' These broader communication issues will be discussed in greater detail later in this chapter.

However, in the field of head injury it is rarely that simple, and it is important to be aware that the two conditions can co-occur. Cherney and Miller (1991) diagnosed 6% of their sample of 360 head-injured patients as aphasic and point out that primary contusions may have localizing neurological signs such as aphasia. This may be more likely in the early stages – Groher (1977) found evidence that aphasia in the acute stage after head injury tends to resolve quickly in most cases, leaving this qualitatively different condition.

Aphasia is a massive subject and beyond the scope of this volume as it is not specific to traumatic, diffuse head injury. Many volumes exist describing the nature and management of aphasia and those interested should investigate these texts. What is important, however, is to stress that if aphasia does occur after closed head injury there are also likely to be other cognitive losses, so it is likely that the aphasic impairment will be complicated by cognitive-communication disorder.

Other language disorders

Specific reading and writing disorders after head injury have usually been looked at as part of aphasic syndromes. Although outside the scope of this chapter it is worth mentioning that reading techniques may be altered as a result of compensating for impairment of basic visual processes. It is therefore important to ensure a comprehensive analysis of basic visual function as well as considering whether there may be specific dyslexia or dysgraphia.

Snow, Douglas and Ponsford (1998) point out the similarity between right hemisphere and frontal lesions in their effect on language. Varley (1995) attributes right-hemisphere verbal-fluency deficit to underlying cognitive disruptions rather than a disturbance of lexical knowledge. Many right hemisphere language disturbances are also seen in diffuse closed head injury – such as difficulty using contextual information and with complex and abstract comprehension, altered discourse structure, confabulation (the production of 'memories' which have no basis in fact), dysprosody (impairment of intonation and stress) and pragmatic changes. Assessment may establish whether the linguistic impairments described as right hemisphere language disorder are disproportionate to any cognitive deficit or a general consequence of cognitive impairments resulting from diffuse damage. If it is felt there is a specific right hemisphere syndrome, again the diffuse damage following head injury will mean such disorders are complicated by cognitive communication impairments.

Cherney and Miller (1991) found 2% of their sample to have specific right-hemisphere communication disorder, but they also point out the similarity of functional presentation to those with diffuse damage. It is also worth noting that this differential diagnosis may not make a difference to management plans.

Samuel et al. (1998) describe a dysprosody after severe head injury as a specific disorder, not secondary to cognitive deficits. That is, a failure to process intonation and stress patterns and thus to recognize emotional features of language. They point out that this may 'dramatically alter communicative intent and accentuate social isolation'. A person thus affected may, for example, not be able to use intonation to know whether a comment is intended as a question or statement, or to know whether – to use the earlier illustration – the words 'come here' are uttered seductively or in anger.

Cognitive-communication disorder

Linguistic aspects of cognitive-communication disorder have been introduced in making the distinction between it and specific language disorder. In general after head injury, discourse level comprehension and production are affected rather than the phonological or syntactic levels. Thus, while sounds, words and sentences are structured normally, the content is not 'normal' in that there is a lack of cohesion and logic. The term 'cognitive-communication disorder' encompasses a wide range of communicative impairments that are attributable either directly to the effect of cognitive impairment on communication in its broadest sense or to the complex interplay between linguistic and cognitive skills. Cognition is discussed in greater depth in Chapter 4, but it may be useful briefly to consider how specific cognitive impairments may affect communication. Hartley (1995) offers a much more comprehensive discussion of this area and the following outline draws upon her comments.

Attention

Attention impairment may be on different levels, as has been discussed in Chapter 4. Difficulties at the level of arousal will be reflected in difficulty gaining clients' attention and actually orienting them to the topic. It may be that non-verbal behaviours, such as eye contact and facial expression, give the appearance of a lack of interest in the person with whom they are interacting (although it may reflect a genuine lack of interest!). If there is a problem maintaining attention both input and output may be affected – for example, the individual may miss words or sections of the conversation, giving the impression of misunderstanding or incompletely understanding information or may tend to jump between topics without warning.

Many head-injured people have difficulty filtering out redundant or distracting sensory input. Background noise, movement or group situations will be difficult to handle and result in a decreased ability to understand and follow conversation or written information, and in tangential or rambling discourse. This will affect many social and other situations – going to the pub or the gym, attending classes, working in an office environment and so on. Internal distractions may equally intrude. If shifting attention is an issue it may be revealed in difficulty switching between topics or indeed in adapting to the changing roles of speaker and listener within the interaction.

A 45-year-old man who had been in a road traffic accident, and had sustained attention impairments, had marked difficulty communicating with family and friends but appeared to cope well at the rehabilitation centre he attended. His wife described a man who never took on board the whole message, who seemed confused about information, and who continued to talk about subjects long after that conversation was over. A home visit revealed a constant barrage of noise at home, with three young children and a mixture of television and radio constantly on. At the centre his contacts were all one-to-one with therapists in relatively quiet settings.

Information processing

Head injury commonly results in reduced speed in processing incoming information, which means there may be long pauses as the meaning is worked out and appropriate responses developed. Hartley and Jenson (1991) found fewer words and slower, less complete units of communication. Information processing problems are often exacerbated further in group settings. Indeed people often deliberately avoid group settings as they are unable to keep up with the flow of conversation. Decreased information processing seems to be a core deficit in all degrees of severity of head injury (for example, Ellmo et al., 1995).

Interpretation of sensory information

If complex visual information is misperceived it may be hard for the client to interpret the feelings and intents of others, which are often reflected non-verbally through facial expression, eye contact and body language. There may be a tendency to invade the personal space of others and even to choose inappropriate social behaviours in a given context because visual clues are missed. More specifically, understanding of spatial terms and the ability to use them may be affected, so that making use of and giving directions becomes difficult.

Memory

Memory is a complex area and may have a multifaceted impact on communication. The most obvious result is seen in the individual who constantly repeats ideas, statements and questions, which can be particularly irritating and difficult for communication partners. There may be problems staying on the topic and purpose of the interaction, so that discourse becomes disorganized and verbose. Understanding will be affected as information is not retained at all or in part and messages are incomplete or mixed up. When communicating, speakers need to be able to take into account how much background information is shared with the listener, in order to avoid either overexplaining or underexplaining. This may be a problem for the head-injured person who has memory impairment.

Learning will be influenced by memory loss, which may extend into the ability to learn from routine social situations and thus to acquire or improve social skills.

Executive function

Ylvisaker and Szekeres (1989) attributed various communication deficits after traumatic brain injury directly to impaired executive functioning. This area is described more fully in Chapter 4, but some of the implications for communication are highlighted in Table 6.1.

Having considered some possible implications of specific cognitive impairments, it is important to note that these rarely happen in isolation. The overall picture of the individual with cognitive-communication disorder is of impairment at the discourse level and in the way language and non-verbal behaviours are used socially. Snow, Douglas and Ponsford (1997) indicate the lack of normative data and huge diversity that makes study of discourse difficult.

Hartley (1995) outlines three patterns of abnormal discourse production – confused (characterized by dysfluencies and inaccuracies); impoverished (reduction in content and amount of output, concreteness and poor cohesion); and inefficient (accurate but long, tangential and rambling output). Snow, Douglas and Ponsford (1998) found no significant improvement in conversational abilities over a period of an average of 2:10 years post injury. There were still marked difficulties with information transfer – meeting the needs of the listener – so that more responsibility rests on the other person in the interaction.

Motor speech disorders

Motor speech disorders may, of course, coexist with language and cognitive impairments, or with other sequelae of a head injury. The term encompasses disorders with the physical production of speech.

Dysarthria

Dysarthria is a disorder of speech due to weakness or paralysis of the muscles of respiration, phonation, resonance and articulation. Dysarthria is 'one of

Table 6.1. Executive functioning and communication.

Self-awareness	Fails to read social clues.
	Egocentric conversation topics.
Goal setting	Flattened affect.
	Does not seek information.
	Does not seek clarification.
	Focus on inessentials not overview.
Inhibition	Makes tactless or rude comments.
	Interrupts others.
	Talks excessively.
	Inappropriate laughter and comments.
	Unpredictable responses.
Initiation	Appears passive and disinterested.
	Does not start or maintain conversation.
	Does not ask for clarification/explanation.
Flexible problem solving	Rigid ideas/views reflected in conversation.
	Unable to see other points of view.
	Concrete interpretation of information.
	Difficulty understanding abstract ideas/language.
Planning and organization	Lack of consistency between saying and doing.
	Illogical, confusing discourse.
	Difficulty sequencing discourse.
	Unable to explain/give directions clearly.
	Fails to appreciate overview.
Self-monitoring	Focus on irrelevant as much as on relevant detail.
	Confabulation.
	Fails to correct.
Creativity	Rigid approach.
	Focus on inessential detail.
	Difficulty making inferences/links.

the most persistent sequelae of severe traumatic brain injury, often beyond resolution of concomitant language disorders' (Sarno and Levin, 1985). Estimates of prevalence vary from 8% to 100% (Rusk, Block and Lowmann, 1969; Dresser et al., 1973; Groher, 1977), but Sarno, Buonaguro and Levita's finding of 34% in 1986 was corroborated by Olver, Ponsford and Curran (1996).

This persistent nature of dysarthric speech after head injury is frequently commented upon. Thomsen (1984), for example, looked at 15 subjects who all still had dysarthria 10 to 15 years after the injury. This would seem to be important in relation to the ability to return to work, study, leisure activities and social life, although Murdoch and Theodorus (1999) point out that little research has been done in this area.

There appears to be wide variability in severity and type of dysarthria, as might be expected given the variability and complexity of damage possible after head injury. The lesion site will largely determine whether signs of spastic, hypokinetic, ataxic, flaccid or mixed dysarthria present. Duffy (1995) suggests spastic dysarthria may occur most frequently but any type may be found after head injury, partly as a result of other injuries sustained at the time. Flaccid dysarthria may be due to neck trauma, for instance.

The dysarthric client may have abnormal articulation, respiration, resonance, prosody and/or phonation. The specific features in any individuals will determine the overall degree of intelligibility that they can achieve, which in turn will affect their ability to interact socially. The implications on everyday functioning or activity limitation of dysarthric impairment may be profound, but may not relate directly to the objective severity of the impairment. A young person whose social life is pub-and-club based may have great difficulty coping in those noisy backgrounds, despite having only mild impairment on objective assessment. Another client whose interests are quieter may manage well despite an apparently more severe disorder.

A 57-year-old man who had fallen from a ladder presented with dysarthria, which made his speech minimally intelligible beyond the use of one-syllable words. If listeners were cued in to the subject and in a quiet environment, those short words were clear. However, the effect of the dysarthria was severe for two main complicating factors. Firstly, his insight was poor and there was no carry-over between rehabilitation and his home environment – unless constantly prompted to limit his speech to short words, he would speed up and become completely unintelligible. The second factor was that his carers, despite lip service to the need to follow up therapy goals, did not reinforce the need to slow down. They were used to him and he had few concrete needs to communicate within his home. The fact was, however, that although his bodily needs were met, he was denied any opportunity for social interaction.

Other motor disorders include a pseudo-foreign accent, when a person post-morbidly speaks with an altered accent, often recognizable to listeners as a regional accent, this is described by Duffy (1995) as rare. When it is found it is usually due to head injury or stroke. This appears to relate to changes in prosody, but is considered separately from dysarthria – although the two may coexist. It often presents with mild or with no effect on intelligibility. In illustration, a 24-year-old man spoke fully intelligibly after a severe head injury, but with a marked north-eastern accent despite having no links with that part of the country. He was initially concerned by the change, but over time became used to this 'new' voice, and chose not to undertake remedial therapy. Others may, of course, continue to be distressed.

Dysphonia is the term used to describe disorders of voice resulting from damage to or weakness of the vocal cords. Voice disorders often coexist with dysarthria in neurological conditions, but may occur in isolation. People may sound hoarse, harsh, strained or have altered pitch, for example. This may be due to weakness or paralysis of the vocal cords due to nerve damage, but the most likely cause after closed head injury with diffuse, rather than focal, damage is as a result of intubation in the acute phase of treatment. It may also be seen as an emotional response to any trauma, according to Duffy (1995). An ENT examination will establish the state of the vocal cords and aid differential diagnosis.

Articulatory and phonatory dyspraxia may also occur after head injury. Articulatory dyspraxia is a disorder of motor programming, where the fine voluntary movement necessary for speech is impaired despite adequate muscle tone and power. It is characterized by increasing difficulty producing sounds and words as their complexity increases. Thus consonants are harder than vowels and consonant clusters harder than single sounds. Speech is produced in a hesitant way, as if 'groping'for the correct sound. Phonatory dyspraxia affects the ability to produce voice at will. Aphasia almost always coexists with this condition as the relevant neuroanatomical areas appear to overlap.

Assessment

General principles

Above all is the need for assessment to have a clear purpose – if it does not contribute to the clinical picture in a way that advises management decisions, it should not be undertaken. Miller, Halper and Cherney (1991) state that assessment should allow an accurate differential diagnosis, identify strengths and weaknesses, establish pre-treatment baseline measures, develop individual goals and plans, determine prognosis and define family counselling plans. However, it is not possible to get all the necessary information at once, and it is important that assessment is not seen as a discrete operation. Whether formal or informal, assessment is part of a continuing process throughout the treatment programme

There are certain difficulties inherent in attempting to assess communication, as a result of the complexity of the process. Most assessment depends on a knowledge of what is normal, to provide a baseline. However, while this may be possible for aspects of the process (such as language and motor performance in speech) communicative behaviour is such a vast subject, with such wide variations between sociocultural groups, that it is impossible effectively to describe 'normal' behaviour. Not only do specific abilities need to be considered but, as was mentioned earlier in the chapter, communication is very much influenced by the context. Decisions as to what is acceptable for each individual must often be subjective. For example, an academic client, who completed *The Times* crossword daily before his accident, may be distressed by difficulty finding words. Another client, with fewer verbal interests, may never even have heard those same words. This means that it is important to cast the assessment net as widely as possible across sources, situations and settings (Body and Parker, 1999).

It is worth reiterating that insight and motivation will be important factors in how to approach the assessment of each individual, as will the existence of other impairments. Severe physical or sensory difficulties, for example, will often create specific problems by affecting the ability to use standardized test materials.

Records

The first step is a review of pertinent records. In the community this may present difficulties as medical notes may be sited elsewhere and access may be difficult. However it is worth pursuing all avenues to establish as much detail as possible about the individual's injury and subsequent progress both in general and in relation specifically to communication.

It has been stated elsewhere in this book that the same information should not be gathered repeatedly if there is good communication between team members, and much of interest to the speech and language therapist can be gathered from other team members' accounts of clients and their history. For example, medications may have side effects on language, speech, communication or cognition, which will have relevance to decisions on management. Similarly information about level of insight and any cognitive difficulties may be apparent from a neuropsychology report. This information should be documented and easily accessible to all team members.

Interview

Specifically in relation to communication, it will be worthwhile interviewing clients and their family/friends or professional carers to establish how communication has changed and to gain a picture of clients' premorbid communication styles and patterns. Often the client, especially if he has difficulty at the level of insight, will present a different picture of current communication skills from that put forward by his family or carers. There are many examples of head-injured clients who firmly believe they have no communication difficulty, despite the family describing marked changes in the way they communicate. It is useful to use this interview to discover both client's and family's expectations and hopes for the future. The individual will have had complex and varied communicative roles, responsibilities and relationships. It is useful to gain an insight into what communicative demands were part of his life pre-morbidly. It may be that some couples' social lives were very much interwoven and it is worth considering the impact upon the carer of the communication impairment and of the possibility of increased social isolation for him or her.

Formal assessment

Formal or standardized assessments are almost always part of the overall assessment process. Not only do they help decision making in relation to diagnosis and management and provide a baseline for change, but they are useful ways of communicating information about the individual to other members of the team and to outside agencies. However, Snow and Ponsford (1995) advise caution with formal assessment, as isolating linguistic skills tends to obscure pragmatic considerations. Testing done in quiet, distraction-free settings and with clear stimulus-response paradigms obviously bears little resemblance to real life.

Ylvisaker and Holland (1985) also cite features of formal assessment in a clinical setting that will threaten the usefulness of results. They point out that attention/concentration and initiation/information-processing deficits may be masked by the orderly environment and stimulus-response patterning of clinical interaction. They state that clinicians' ability to adapt their communication to benefit the interaction may create a halo effect, and that the supportive situation minimizes the consequences of failure and prevents useful risk-taking.

Such issues need to be recognized, but so must the danger of throwing the baby out with the bathwater! Some of the benefits of formal assessments are listed above and, as a by-product, formal one-to-one sessions can also have a role in building rapport, providing boundaries, facilitating self-disclosure and allowing information giving or counselling. Formal testing is the most reliable approach if test results need to be related to normative data, used for pre- and post-treatment measures, or to provide a baseline if progressive disorders are suspected.

Snow and Ponsford (1995) are in favour of exploring all qualitative and quantitative avenues and sources, and stress the value of not adopting a battery approach to assessment. It is not always necessary to use all subtests within a formal assessment – although, of course, it must also be appreciated that norms will no longer be valid. Screening by informal tasks or use of subtests from standard tests can direct where the focus of intervention should fall and which formal assessments will be most useful. Other factors such as severity level, premorbid factors, and goals will also influence test selection. There is also undoubtedly the factor of clinician experience, style and preferences.

Motor speech assessments

There are no motor speech assessments specifically for people with head injuries, and indeed there may be no need to develop such an assessment as the existing ones are generally accepted (for example The Frenchay Dysarthria Assessment – Enderby, 1983). However the concurrent existence of cognitive problems may mean administration needs to be adapted.

Language assessments

Much of the research that has been done on the language skills of head-injured clients has been based upon traditional aphasia tests. These have taken the form of multimodal batteries (such as the Boston Diagnostic Aphasia Test of Goodglass and Kaplan (1972) or the Western Aphasia Battery by Kertesz (1982)) or focused on one mode. The trend in aphasiology to work from a psycholinguistic model, exemplified in the PALPA (Kay, Lesser and Coltheart, 1992), has also been seen in head injury rehabilitation. However, all these tend to be impairment based and as, by definition, they attempt to access specific language skills, they do not pretend to investigate the complex interplay of cognitive, linguistic and other factors that are accepted as affecting communication after diffuse brain injury. They also do not look at the activity limitation that might result from the impairment, and Coelho (1999), for example, points out the ceiling effect of aphasia tests applied to head-injured people.

It would appear from these comments that aphasia batteries make poor tools to use clinically with a head-injured population; however, given the dearth of appropriate assessment materials for this group, they are often still used, as was seen in a survey of specialist SLTs in 1998 (RCSLT Special Interest Group Head Injury, Simpson, 1999). Ellmo, Graser and Calabrese (1994) reported a survey of speech and language pathologists, which indicated a generally low level of satisfaction with traditional aphasia tests in this area, especially in relation to mild head injury. Higher level subtle changes are not detected even when functionally significant (Wertz, 1978). However, Body and Parker (1999) suggest that some standardized tests developed for aphasia, such as those listed above, *may* have a value, despite a lack of specific norms. Head injury often does not cause impairments that fall into neat categories and wider questionnaires and assessments may give useful information. Miller, Halper and Cherney (1991) and Hartley (1995) offer comprehensive lists of tests available for linguistic (and cognitive) processes that may provide useful information.

Discourse analysis

A great deal of interest has focused on formal discourse analysis recently. This technique is being used increasingly as it can detect subtle non-aphasic impairments and allows analysis on a number of levels. Samples of discourse are taken that exemplify different styles (genres), such as descriptive, narrative, procedural and conversational. These samples are transcribed for analysis (for example, Coelho, 1999), which may focus on aspects such as logical story structure, cohesion, semantic/pragmatic coherence, total output (productivity), speaking time, response appropriateness, self-initiated compensatory strategies (Penn and Cleary, 1988), and topic and content (for example, Ehrlich, 1988; Mentis and Prutting, 1991). Some of these studies have included consideration of the ability of the conversational partner to meet the client's needs (Peter, 1995) or on the client's role as partner in an interaction (Parsons et al., 1989).

The methodology of such assessment is difficult in relation to context and sampling techniques, measures and norms, and there are huge implications for the busy clinician in that techniques are time consuming. However, it is important to consider the discourse level rather than isolated linguistic parameters. Most head-injured people have intact linguistic processing at the clause level but it breaks down at discourse level (Togher, Hand and Code, 1999).

Cognitive communication assessment

Cognitive assessments may be very relevant to determining the impact of cognitive impairment on communicative ability, and in planning intervention. Such assessments of attention, perception, memory and executive functioning may be administered by other members of the team but have great significance to communication rehabilitation, and provide useful insights into determining an overall course of action.

Little attention had been given to establishing specific assessments of communication in head-injured people and relevant norms until recently, when increased interest has led to batteries such as the Measure of Cognitive Linguistic Abilities (MCLA) (Ellmo et al., 1995) and the as-yet unpublished Mount Wilga Assessment. Still predominantly adopting an impairment-based approach, these access similar areas to the aphasia tests in that they look at comprehension, expression, reading and writing. However, they stem from the principle that communication and cognition are inextricably linked and that the language changes are not aphasic in nature. High level and subtle deficits in comprehension and expression (such as understanding and using inferences) need to be defined by assessment, as well as more obvious behaviours, such as word finding, in order to allow appropriate intervention strategies. Miller, Halper and Cherney (1991) also suggest academic achievement tests that depend on language and may be useful particularly if considering educational or vocational placements.

This section has focused on formal assessment but clinicians must sometimes have the courage of their convictions even in 'these days of the Reign of Terror of evidence-based practice' (Sheridan, personal communication) to use non-standardized or informal assessments if they will direct possible management. Similarly subtests of standard assessments may be used in a non-standard way. Experience is necessary in order to feel confident about such approaches and the value of support from other specialist therapists is important.

Pragmatic assessment: behavioural observation, rating scales and checklists

As was explained earlier, the study of pragmatics looks at the actual way in which language and general communicative behaviours are used in the 'real' world. Pragmatic assessment is important as it addresses communicative ability from the view of everyday life. However, it is a difficult area to address successfully. If it is attempted in clinic it is artificial in that it ignores real-life settings, but to look at only one real-life context may not be much more informative, as everyone communicates differently in different contexts. Similarly considering only one communication partner will only give part of the picture.

A major difficulty that has already been highlighted is the vast range that constitutes what is considered 'normal' behaviour. Premorbid demographic variables must be separated out from the effects of organic damage, which can be a difficult process, although use of multiple sources in assessment may help, asking others to describe the client's premorbid communicative style. It may also be of interest and value to observe how the client's family and friends interact.

McGann and Werven (1995) point out another danger in that clinicians will have different communicative styles and social and ethnic backgrounds, which means all clinicians will have stereotypes and personal stigmas. These must be reduced as much as possible in creating conditions for objective and non-judgemental assessment. All assessments of social communication need to recognize that in attempting to evaluate the functional implications of cognitive communication impairment it is crucial to recognize and respect the heterogeneity of the population.

Rating scales and checklists

A systematic examination of all aspects of social behaviour is needed, in both terms of perception and use. Behavioural observation is a useful technique if a systematic system of recording observations can be established. This can allow the client's behaviour to be observed in as many different settings as possible and with different communication partners. The problem with this approach is largely practical – it is not usually possible to find the time in a busy practice to observe each individual in numerous settings, and even when it is possible there is the additional factor that the presence of an observer immediately changes the communicative interaction. A multiple source approach (that is, asking others in their social/family circle to complete rating scales) may go some way to meeting this practical need, and will be discussed in more detail later in the chapter.

Assessment via behavioural observation can usefully look at everyday communication skills on both receptive and expressive levels. Listening behaviours, and conversational and speaking skills can all be evaluated in this way. Systematic recording is conducted using checklists and rating scales, which may be based on interviews, unstructured conversation, role play, or in 'natural' settings, specifically selected to be relevant to the individual. Beukelman, Yorkston and Lossing (1984) suggest an environmental needs assessment, to consider differing demands and strategies. For example, a busy office environment will create very different demands from a relatively isolated job; and someone living alone will have different demands from a parent of young children.

What most scales and checklists have in common is that they attempt to record both verbal and non-verbal aspects of communication. Some attempt to look at communication as a whole – the La Trobe Communication Questionnaire (Douglas, O'Flaherty and Snow, 2000) and the Profile of Functional Impairment in Communication (Linscott, Knight and Godfrey, 1996) are two examples. The Pragmatic Profile expands Speech Act Theory (Prutting and Kirschner, 1983) by formulating three broad categories – verbal, paralinguistic and non-verbal. The verbal aspects include speech acts, topic, turn taking, lexical selection and communicative style. Paralinguistic aspects include intelligibility and prosody, for example, and non-verbal include proxemics and kinesics. However little reference is made to sociolinguistic background and most rely entirely on subjective judgements.

Many scales have been devised for communication specialists to complete, but following the principle that multiple sources are useful in evaluating communication, others have been designed for non-specialists. Such scales need to be easy to administer, avoid jargon and have face validity. Different levels of explanation will be needed depending on the abilities and knowledge of the people involved. If this approach is taken, it is important to have agreement from the client. Scales developed for non-specialists include The Family Questionnaire (Ellmo et al., 1995), Conversational Rating Scale (Spitzberg and Hurt, 1987) and the Conversational Rating Scale (Ehrlich and Barry, 1989).

Functionally based rating scales and checklists may also be relevant to how dysarthria leads to activity restriction, although formal motor speech assessments do include sections on intelligibility, which will be relevant to the ability to function. However, as with other specific language and cognitive-communication impairments, it is important to establish measures in different and, where possible, real-life situations. Intelligibility in a quiet assessment room will usually be vastly different from intelligibility in a busy office or at home.

Multiple sources and settings

Body and Parker (1999) discuss the use of multiple informants in the assessment of communication after traumatic brain injury. They suggest three underlying principles – to provide different perspectives on superficially similar areas (for example, written instructions may take many forms and make vastly different demands); to recognize that communication in the widest sense involves everybody; and to ensure account is taken of variations in function under different circumstances. To illustrate its value, they point out how commonly friction can occur in families because traumatic brain-injured people deal with some communicative interactions and not others, which is perceived by the family as obstructive. An example of this is seen in a 45-year-old father, who appeared to be able to concentrate enough to talk to a friend about cricket but whose family complained he did not 'bother' to try to join in conversations at home. It became apparent that his attention deficit meant he was unable to cope with the background noise at home, where children had the television on.

Possible sources that can be tapped in assessment include the head-injured person himself, carers or family members, and other professionals. Snow and Douglas (1999) suggest comparing different sources to identify overlap or discrepancies. Settings will obviously depend on the lifestyle of each person but it is important also to consider the different roles that will be expected of the person. For example, evaluation may focus on a person's role as husband or wife, as parent, as child and as friend. Certain roles may be particularly difficult to resume and cause apparently disproportionate anxiety and disability. It may also be important to establish crucial roles for the present and roles that may occur in the future in order properly to evaluate communicative ability. For example, if a head-injured person plans to return to paid employment the work context will need to be evaluated and consideration given to the communicative demands that will be made.

The vast range of possible settings and sources for each and every individual means it is often the practicalities of the therapist's time and priorities that determine how far this approach can be taken. While accepting the value of using multiple sources and looking at many settings, it is realistic to seek to select the most characteristic or most important to investigate first. However it is worth bearing in mind that the individual's life may be very limited when first discharged from hospital into the community, and the resultant restriction on situations and people with whom communication can occur may falsely suggest the person is communicating adequately. Later, as they perhaps attempt to resume other roles and enter new situations, problems may emerge. This highlights the need to continue the assessment process throughout involvement with a client.

The communication partner

There is increased recognition of the need to consider how the head-injured individual interacts with others. As communication is a two-way process the abilities of regular communication partners may be relevant to the rehabilitation process. Specific factors – such as a partner's deafness – have obvious implications, but there is mounting evidence that some people communicate more effectively with head-injured individuals than others.

Togher, Hand and Code (1999) look at a method of analysing how social roles are affected by head injury (exchange structure analysis). They look at the behaviour of both participants in context, recognizing that the communicative partner can inhibit language and communicative choices by the client. As a result they state – 'If we view the therapy interaction as only one of many contextual configurations that our clients may be faced with, it becomes clear that we need to be spending less time talking with them and more time facilitating their interaction with others.'

Assessment of any individual other than the 'impaired' person is not generally undertaken in any systematic way. However it may be a valuable source of information. Most clinicians will anecdotally recount how clients appear to communicate better with certain people. If presented in an understanding way, with clear explanations as to the value, most families and carers respond well to questions about their own communicative style and skills. This aspect will be considered further in the section on management.

Goal setting

As part of the multidisciplinary team, the communication specialist will be part of the setting of the long-term goal for the client. The intermediate goals towards that long-term aim and the short-term process goals may be specified by the client and the speech and language therapist after discussion, but working to achieve the goal is likely at some point to involve others in the team. Indeed others in the client's world must be part of the process, and at times goals may relate to or involve particular people or groups. Communication has been defined as context dependent and goals may need to be specific to context.

Goals should allow the client to experience success in a communicative situation and must have face validity. This can be difficult in working with dysarthria, where some goals may be thought useful by the therapist who wants to work on isolated parameters, such as respiration, but which the client fails to see as significant. Time spent on explanation may help, but there may well be times when it is more appropriate to begin with goals that are immediately of value to the client – that is, usually, direct work on the spoken word. Later in the therapeutic process, with a more developed relationship, additional goals may be introduced.

The need to be part of the overall working towards a long-term goal is important. For example, if that goal is to enable a client to remain at home without support while a partner or parent is at work, it could be relevant to look at the ability to use the telephone for various purposes. Partners may want to know that clients can call emergency services, telephone a neighbour or friend, or telephone them at work depending on the level of emergency or need.

Functional goals, such as the example above, can be set alongside more impairment-based therapeutic work. However the latter should always have a real-life purpose in sight. Academically interesting goals do not help the client towards independence. Cherney, Halper and Miller (1991) adopt a process-specific approach with suggested goals within cognitive and linguistic areas of functioning. They also highlight the fact that all goals should be kept in mind even when work is being done on other aspects; for instance, eye contact may be one goal and can be encouraged even when not the specific focus of a therapy task. However the team may end up with a lot of simultaneous goals and discussion will then be needed to set priorities.

Management

Snow and Douglas (1999) state 'the overriding aim of both individual and group therapy is to teach traumatically brain-injured speakers communication skills and behaviours they can successfully employ in the real world'. This section will consider individual and group approaches, including discourse level therapy, cognitive therapy, social skills work and compensatory strategies. It will also discuss indirect techniques involving working through families and other carers, and through other members of the team.

Individual therapy

Management must be driven by the goals. Individual work will often be appropriate, either alone or alongside group work. As much as possible the individual work should relate clearly to real life, so from the very beginning consideration must be given to transfer and generalization of skills. This may mean techniques such as role play, bringing in natural reinforcers, or the use of other people who have particular relevance. Overall the goal of communication therapy is to rebuild communicative competence and skilled social behaviour.

It is important to involve the client actively so that roles addressed are relevant and motivating. As the individual therapy progresses and attempts are increasingly made to integrate the abilities that have been the focus of therapy into real-life settings, community teams have a great advantage. The communicative demands of different activities can be analysed within the individual's lifestyle, and worked on sequentially through a hierarchy of difficulty or anxiety. This analysis and follow-through need not be the role of any one member of the team, although this statement does highlight the need for the whole team to have knowledge of communication. Specific targets need to be set, with self-monitoring a crucial part of any programme. This enables self-initiated strategies to be incorporated into interactions. The programme may need to operate within a variety of settings and contexts to effect change in general. Thus a task may be discussed and tried in role play in the clinic and then attempted in a variety of settings. Failure can be an important part of the learning process but is rarely part of clinical practice. It can be crucial to enabling a client to cope with the real world, although it may not be appropriate if there is severe memory loss, for instance, which prevents the individual being able to learn from experience.

IG, a 46-year-old man, illustrates this approach. His communication was severely impaired and he was encouraged to use a mixture of verbal and non-verbal means to get a message across. Thus, he could mix occasional spoken words with written words, which he could show, gesture, and facial expression. He was embarrassed about going out and needed considerable role play in the rehabilitation centre, with a variety of staff, to demonstrate to him that he could go into a shop. Time was spent enabling him to plan ahead and feel prepared for possible questions. He then went out with a rehabilitation assistant. The motivation to go alone came from his desire to buy a present for his wife, as a surprise for her birthday.

Many head-injured people can benefit from an educational approach to adapting their social behaviour – increased knowledge about what social communication involves, what can go wrong and how to cope, can help awareness and motivation to adjust. Videos and audiotapes can be useful techniques to demonstrate differing aspects of communication. These may be created as teaching aids, but equally may be tapes of television soaps, for example, which demonstrate when communication works or does not work. Tapes of the client himself can also provide useful feedback and discussion.

Individual therapy for specific language disorder (aphasia) will not be discussed in this volume. There are a wide variety of references available and, as was stated earlier, even if it is accepted that aphasia can occur after head injury it is not specific to that population. It is worth repeating that work on aphasia may well be complicated by the concurrent existence of cognitive-communication disorder. Similarly, therapy for dysarthria, while an important part of the speech and language therapist's work with head-injured clients, is not specific to this group and is clearly covered elsewhere (for example, Duffy, 1995; Murdoch and Theodorus, 1999). Again work may have to be adapted in relation to co-existing cognitive-communication disorder.

Discourse level therapy

Snow and Douglas (1999) focus on discourse-level intervention. They advise beginning with clear explanation of different types of discourse - conversational, narrative and procedural – and the 'rules' that govern their structure. These rules then become the focus of therapy. As return to work, for example, is affected by the ability to sustain conversation (Brooks, McKinlay and Symington, 1987) this approach may well be valuable. Snow, Douglas and Ponsford (1998) found that conversational disabilities did not spontaneously improve over time and are associated with psychosocial handicap. Douglas (1990, 1992) describes a systematic behavioural approach to identifying and ameliorating discourse changes.

Hartley (1995) also describes specific discourse therapy. Looking at both comprehension and expression, she outlines clearly a progression of tasks. In relation to comprehension she suggests focusing on self-monitoring; identifying what makes a good listener; identifying strategies that help listening (such as restraining oneself from interrupting); training in the different ways in which language is used; obtaining information and following directions; and recognizing factors that interfere with the process. Discourse production therapy focuses on the abnormal patterns of behaviour shown by the client and covers different types (or genres) of discourse. However lack of insight or denial on the part of client or family will have an impact on the usefulness of such approaches. In addition there are large normal variations in such behaviours and this can be very difficult to build into therapy plans.

Cognitive therapy

Chapter 4 considers management of cognitive impairments and these techniques may be fruitful in relation to communication. For example, attention training may help an individual to focus better on auditory or written information, or anger management techniques may be used to stop a person interrupting conversations inappropriately. Similarly, coping with stress strategies, assertiveness training, and problem-solving training may all have value, and this list is by no means comprehensive. It does highlight the need to know the relationship between communication and different cognitive skills. As Snow and Ponsford (1995) point out, repeated practice on cognitive tasks does not automatically improve communication in real life, but a number of cognitive rehabilitation studies do indicate successful intervention (Coelho, DeRuyter and Stein, 1996).

Social skills

It has been widely recognized for some time that, as Marsh (1999) states, 'Chronic social isolation appears to be the defining characteristic of the long term psychosocial consequences of traumatic brain injury.' Bond and Godfrey (1997) concluded in their study that head-injured people have many fewer socially rewarding experiences, and many other studies support these views.

Social skills are the behaviours that allow individuals to build and maintain social relationships. To be socially skilled means having a knowledge of social rules, roles and routines, the ability to perceive and interpret social cues and the ability to regulate behaviour (Ylvisaker, 1995). Approaches to training have followed information processing and cognitive models, but Ylvisaker, Urbanczyk and Feeney (1992) developed a communication model. This area is perhaps the best example of the need to adopt a multidisciplinary approach, as social skills cross a variety of disciplines' traditional areas of expertise. As Snow and Douglas (1999) point out, partitioning a client into discrete disabilities for different professions does not work.

Social skills work is often seen as predominantly a group therapy and indeed for some this may be the approach chosen. However, often individual therapy can focus on specific behaviours that are then practised in the group setting. The focus may be on very specific microlevel behaviours (such as eye contact or turn taking) or on wider social behaviours (perhaps assertiveness or anger control). Cultural and ethnic variations must be considered and the clinician may need to involve family members or relevant local organizations or individuals.

Motivation and opportunity

Individual therapy may need to look at increasing the individual's enjoyment of communication. Social isolation and anxiety may grow as a result of constant apparent failure to communicate effectively – finding a situation in real life, in *their* real life, in which successful, rewarding communication is experienced may open therapeutic avenues in the future by raising motivation. At the extreme it is possible for social phobia to develop, even in cases of apparently mild communicative disorder, and it is obviously worth taking steps to prevent such a possibility.

The earlier example of IG is also applicable here. He had no enjoyment from communicating anywhere but within his home. His embarrassment and fear of looking stupid prevented him from attempting to go out. The experience of succeeding in shopping tasks opened other social opportunities and increased his confidence.

Compensatory techniques

Individual work may involve looking at compensatory techniques – internal or external. Again some techniques developed by other members of the team may be applicable within communication work, but some may stem from the speech and language therapist. External aids may include checklists, diaries or organizers, for example. These may be especially useful if considering the written word, but can have a place in spoken communication. For instance, a checklist of listening skills can be used overtly in an organized group setting with the aim of internalizing the list. Agreed cues can be used – for example, a phrase or subtle visual reminder from a member of the family or a friend can be used to limit excessive talkativeness or interrupting behaviour.

External compensatory strategies would also include environmental manipulation, a concept well known to speech and language therapists. The physical setting can be set up to facilitate communication by such apparently simple procedures as placing chairs appropriately, to encourage face-to-face interaction. Most usefully, perhaps, with this client group is reducing environmental distractors, such as background noise.

It has been stated that it is important not to base judgements on performance in a quiet, distraction-free clinical setting, and this is in recognition of the fact that performance tends to be better than in real-life settings where there are constant distractions. However there may be instances where distractions can be minimized – for example, to facilitate reading if a client with attention problems is attempting to study, it may be possible to establish which room in his home is furthest away from traffic noise and so on. Structuring the day can be used to reduce the communicative demands on an individual – routine can also be used to achieve other cognitive aims.

The social environment can also be manipulated. Working with the family or carers to adapt their communicative style may be one approach. Another would be in considering the number of people to whom the client is exposed at any one time, which may be valuable as group settings are often hardest. Clients may find restrictions to their lifestyle hard to accept, even when appreciating the need. A young woman who enjoyed clubbing, became upset that she could not effectively communicate in the club setting, and indeed became quite stressed by the noise level. However, she could not accept advice to choose environments to suit her ability to cope with noise, because she would not accept that she might not be able to enjoy clubbing again.

Task analysis allows manipulation at the task level – for example, it may be possible to modify or adjust the demands of a task by removing time constraints. Careful evaluation of individual tasks in a work setting may mean such modification (with a supportive employer) can make the difference between remaining in work or not. Such issues will be discussed in Chapter 7.

Another external compensatory strategy would be the use of alternative or assisted communication, which ranges from simple alphabet charts to complex computer technology, or simple amplification. This approach will be of most use with the individual who is severely dysarthric but has the prerequisite language and cognitive skills, and early use is thought to prevent frustration and increase motivation.

Group therapy

It is generally accepted that group approaches offer more natural communicative opportunities in that they provide peer support (and, indeed, criticism) within a social setting. It is important, however, that groups are chosen according to the individual's needs. This is not always practical in a community rehabilitation setting; for example, there may not be the numbers of similar clients to create the ideal group. Compromise may be necessary, but for each group member the group must be part of the process toward achieving his personal long-term goal. On this there should not be compromise.

In relation to head-injured people and communication, groups are often used to develop social communication skills by looking at non-verbal behaviours and the importance of context, as well as listening and conversational skills. Hartley (1995) suggests specific approaches such as group activities, social skills training and applied behavioural techniques, such as those described in Chapter 5.

It has been mentioned that group work is commonly used in social skills training. The format usually includes discussion, rehearsal, feedback, prompting, and sometimes homework assignments (for example, Marsh 1999). Numerous studies have looked at specific programmes (for example, Braunling-McMorrow, Lloyd and Fralish, 1986; Brotherton et al., 1988; Yuen, 1997). McGann, Werven and Douglas (1997) stress the need for the client to be equal in the therapeutic process, so the therapist does not judge success or failure, but merely facilitates the group. Snow and Ponsford (1995) see group therapy as an adjunct rather than a substitute for individual therapy.

Various texts offer practical planning suggestions, covering such factors as the selection of group members, timing and frequency and so on (see, for example, Snow and Douglas, 1999). Evaluation of the group is essential, but less often mentioned is the need to look beyond the group to evaluate whether skills have generalized and are of use to individuals in 'the real world' (Cockburn and Wood, 1995).

Barriers to individual or group work

The very nature of head injury means there will be individuals with whom communication therapy is not possible, even if they have a severe handicap as a direct result of poor communication skills. Non-compliance may be due to a variety of reasons (such as lack of insight, passivity, and depression) and there may be opportunity within the team to analyse the nature of the non-compliance and seek to address the issues. It is common to find individuals (or families) who want to be cured and do not accept that they should play an active part in rehabilitation. A case illustrating this was seen in a young man with cognitive-communication disorder and pseudo-foreign accent syndrome, who unrepentantly and repeatedly stated that it was the therapists' job to make him better and that he should not be expected to undertake home-based activities.

It may be that timing is crucial and that clients need space to adjust to the overwhelming consequences of their head injury before being ready to accept the need for therapy. More specifically, it may be that the person cannot at first accept the need for an alternative communication method but that experience of living with the impairment brings home to him the need.

Reluctance to undertake therapy may also be due to the use of tasks that have little or no face validity for the client. If this is recognized the tasks can be adapted or more detailed explanations provided to increase the client's motivation and involvement in the process. This danger of setting tasks that mean little to the client is perhaps a hangover from the early days of rehabilitation under a medical model, when it was assumed patients would do as they were told by 'the experts'.

In a community service there may be people for whom discharge from hospital creates unexpected problems or suddenly forces them to face the situation. Clients often see going home as marking the end of their 'illness', when in fact it may mark the beginning of living with their disabilities. This means a need for continued involvement, albeit at a distance, in order to be ready to intervene when it is wanted. As insight improves over time, or as problems become apparent in community life, people may become more open to intervention, so it is important not to alienate them initially.

Working with carers and family

Loss of communication skills – whether due to specific speech or language disorder or to cognitive changes – will not just affect the injured person.

There can be wide-ranging social implications for family and friends. At times the social ramifications may even be greater for the carer, whose ability to communicate with his or her partner is restricted and whose opportunity to communicate with others is also affected by the role of carer. This may be most obviously true for the carer whose relative lacks insight or is passive about the changes to his social life.

Carers whose relatives have communication difficulties, whether specific or due to cognitive changes, will face very particular burdens. Communicating with family, friends and others is central to life. Suddenly these carers may find themselves having to take responsibility for all interactions and no longer be able to communicate easily and naturally. This may extend to their own interactions with others if the head-injured person is present. The carer role combined with communicative failure often eventually leads to social isolation for the carer no less than the client.

Andrews and Andrews (1991) state that 'family members will be capable of being effective participants in therapy when they feel confident and capable, when they know that their views and ideas are respected, and when their contributions are positively regarded by professionals.' It is important to identify who to involve and how those involved interact with each other. Not all will view the client or, indeed, the rehabilitation process and goals in the same way, and consideration needs to be given to ensuring a consistent approach by discussion and negotiated compromise.

In relation to communication there are three main roles for the speech and language therapist in working with carers' education in general (teaching about communication and what has happened to their relative or friend); education in a more specific sense (looking at how to adapt in order to improve communicative interactions with the individual and, in some cases, how to assist with homework exercises); and offering support by recognizing the carer's life has also been affected and that the carer will have his or her own needs.

General education

The first two educative roles for the communication specialist with families and other carers will overlap to some extent. Educating people as to the nature of communication and the nature of the difficulties that their relative might face is not as straightforward as it seems. The danger for the speech and language therapist is to assume knowledge about normal communication. Most people never question their ability to communicate or consider the many different aspects and abilities involved. Providing a framework not only helps to describe the client's difficulties and thus understand what has gone wrong but, perhaps even more importantly, it provides a basis for relatives to adapt their own behaviour. To be told, out of the blue, to make conversation literal as the client cannot appreciate abstract language any more, will mean little, if anything, to most people. Setting it in the context of what normal communication entails may well enable informed adjustment of their own skills. This assumes clear and appropriate explanations at the right level for each family and avoiding jargon.

In relation to teaching about the actual difficulties the client faces, written advice sheets can be valuable if individualized. However they will have greater meaning for the carer if behaviours are described in terms of how they affect everyday life and even more so if the carer can *see* the behaviour. For example, if a client has difficulty with non-literal language, it might be useful to ask him to explain some common abstract phrases (such as proverbs) which will demonstrate the tendency to take the literal meaning rather than the implied – although, in the latter case, timing is important as it may be someone is not ready to face the full ramifications of the disability. This may be apparent in a desire to explain away difficulties, perhaps as due to lack of use or practice.

Adapting the communication skills of others

Togher, Hand and Code (1997) found that communication partners do interact differently with traumatically brain-injured people – they give less information, ask for less information and use fewer checks. Thus they concluded partners may disempower by their contributions to the interaction. However, Bond and Godfrey (1997) found partners got much less enjoyment from communication as a result of the increased burden they have to shoulder. This indicates the need to be realistic in what is expected from carers, and to value them as individuals even when retaining the primary responsibility to the client. The way carers react may be a healthy adaptation to cope with the situation. Whether one should work with partners must depend on individual circumstances.

Booth and Swabey (1999) describe a programme for group training of communication skills for carers of adults with aphasia. Such an approach may well have relevance to the carers of head-injured adults, although as they found there can be problems with the generalized advice needed in groups. Wilkinson et al (1998), also working with aphasic people and their partners, describe a three-way analysis of communication. This means the client and carer themselves recognize and identify issues, rather than the therapist prescriptively telling them what to do, and see language as 'a vehicle through which communication, relationships and self are connected'. Ylvisaker (1998) did focus on head-injured people and looked at training partners in relation to their own communication style, by using video to analyse discourse. Again the need for the partner to analyse and discuss actively is stressed, rather than the therapist adopting a prescriptive approach.

In addition to enabling carers to adapt their communication skills, some may respond well to being involved in therapy procedures. Andrews and Andrews (1991) suggest three types of assignment that may be appropriate – noticing, intervention and assessment/monitoring. Noticing would be paying attention to what circumstances lead to a particular behaviour – for example, does the client's language become more difficult to understand when there is background noise? Intervention might involve asking the family to respond in a certain way to specific behaviours – if the client makes eye contact, reward him with your full attention. An assessment and monitoring role might include recording whether he is more intelligible when pacing himself, by tapping his foot, for example. This also helps to increase the family's awareness of progress. The more involved a family feels in rehabilitation, the more likely it is to accept such roles. However this is not right for every family and it is not appropriate to exert pressure on those who feel unable to be involved. Premorbid abilities, styles, coping behaviour and the nature of the existing relationship will all affect their level of involvement.

The supportive role

The supportive role is important. It is clear the communicative partner may well have very negative views about the effects of communication impairment (O'Flaherty and Douglas, 1997). It may be relevant to involve other professionals who can have a direct responsibility to support the carer. This is discussed more fully in Chapter 9.

Different members of the family or other carers will have differing needs based not only on their individual character, but also on the role they have in the head-injured person's life. For example, although writing about stroke, Jordan and Kaiser (1996) make the valuable point that children can end up 'losing' both parents – one to the disability and one to the carer role. Whatever the nature of the relationship – parent, child, spouse, friend – communication difficulty places very specific strains on that relationship.

It is important to consider family needs throughout the process of rehabilitation. At the end of rehabilitation, which may be difficult for both client and carers, links to future support mechanisms must be made. In the case of communication impairment, problems can re-emerge later as a result of a crisis or a change in circumstance and it may well be appropriate to reassure people that they can contact the speech and language therapist at any time.

Working through other professionals

Throughout this volume runs the central philosophy that a team approach is critical and that boundaries between professions should be blurred. However there remain the core knowledge bases of the different specialisms, which should be a resource for the whole team.

As in the work with carers, there may be both general and specific educative roles. Glenwright, Davison and Hilton (1999) describe a case study of an aphasic client whereby the client's ability to understand was significantly improved as a result of a training session enabling staff to modify their language appropriately. This would seem a potentially valuable role for the speech and language therapist working with head-injured clients.

Good communication between team members should also enable communication goals to be considered in all interactions, regardless of discipline. Similarly, of course, the speech and language therapist should follow through other disciplines' programmes whenever possible.

Evaluation and outcomes

Despite evidence of some degree of spontaneous recovery, communication disorders are often a long-term problem for the head-injured client. Levin et al. (1981) suggest full language recovery is likely after mild head injury, but that anomia may persist for six months. After more severe head injury persistent, often subtle, language impairment is likely. Other work has been quoted in this chapter highlighting the persistent nature of dysarthria after head injury and of social communicative disability.

It is difficult to distinguish the effect of therapy from spontaneous recovery, but it is still important to try to make this distinction by taking baseline measures and systematic data collection. Evaluation is even more complicated when attempting to affect behaviour in the community, rather than addressing specific impairments in a clinical setting.

Enderby (1997) has suggested outcome scales for dysarthria, dysphasia and dysphonia, and a core scale that may be adapted to cover head injury. However the scales are only intended to provide general outcome data and are not sensitive enough to establish whether recovery or therapeutic intervention has led to a change in the measures. There is also considerable variability between therapists using the scales (Enderby and John, 1999) reflecting the complexity of factors involved. More specific measures have been used, most notably via single case studies, to provide evidence that speech and language therapy is effective for language disorders following stroke or head injury, if targeted to specific deficits and needs and if intensive. However, if general, non-specific or low intensity there is little or no evidence of efficacy (Wertz, 1987; Enderby and Emerson, 1996). However, what is not known is whether a team approach, where communication goals are worked on by all team members, means that less intensive specific speech and language therapy is a valid approach.

In relation to cognitive-communication disorder little objective effort has been made to assess the value of therapeutic intervention, although there have been evaluations of social skills groups and cognitive therapy (Coelho, deRuyter and Stein, 1996). They point out that few studies have looked specifically at communication and that techniques used are generally not sensitive enough.

Body and Campbell (1995) did attempt to devise a system whereby clinical and research needs could be met. They stress the importance of considering available resources and the feasibility of data collection. Evaluation may be a matter of relating back to the goals set for individual clients and recording whether they were achieved; however this approach presupposes appropriate goal setting and is complicated by the fact that goals will often need to be revised and updated, even as therapy continues.

Overall it is imperative that a valid and reliable method of evaluating communication therapy with this client group is devised. At present much therapy is based on clinical judgement and anecdotal evidence of value, and this is not always adequate justification for intervention.

Conclusions

After head injury, communication is commonly impaired either in specific ways or in relation to social communication generally. However, historically most intervention has been employed as a result of extrapolating from work with people who have focal neurological damage. Research is developing understanding of how diffuse closed head injury can affect language, speech, and social communication skills. Recent developments have recognized the need to look at all aspects of intervention – assessment, individual therapy, group work, work with families – in terms of their value specifically with head-injured people.

There are increasing numbers of studies looking to create assessment materials and therapy programmes, although evaluative studies are greatly needed to back up this work. As in many areas of rehabilitation the clinician needs to seek to evaluate individual casework, since it may well be that this channel is most productive, as has been seen in aphasia research. However, it is early days and many questions remain to be addressed.

The overriding importance of communication for every individual must drive clinicians and researchers to continue to develop and extend work in the field, seeking to reduce the social handicap that all too often results from head injury.

References

Andrews MA, Andrews JR (1991) Family based treatment: a systematic model for involving families. In Halper AS, Cherney LR, Miller TK (eds) Clinical Management of Communication Problems in Adults with Traumatic Brain Injury. Gaitnersburg MD: Aspen, pp. 147–58

Beukelman DR, Yorkston KM, Lossing CA (1984) Functional communication assessment of adults with neurogenic disorders. In Halper AS, Cherney LR, Miller TK (eds) Clinical Management of Communication Problems in Adults with Traumatic Brain Injury. Baltimore: Aspen, pp. 101–15.

Body R, Campbell M (1995) Choosing outcome measures in Chamberlaine MA, Neumann V, Tennant A (eds) Traumatic Brain Injury Rehabilitation – Services, Treatments and Outcomes. London: Chapman & Hall, pp. 245–58.

Body R, Parker M (1999) The use of multiple informants in assessment of communication after traumatic brain injury. In McDonald S, Togher L, Code C (eds) Communication Disorders Following Traumatic Brain Injury. Hove: Psychology Press, pp. 147–74.

Body R, Perkins M, McDonald S (1999) Pragmatics, cognition and communication in traumatic brain injury. In McDonald S, Togher L, Code C (eds) Communication Disorders Following Traumatic Brain Injury. Hove: Psychology Press, pp. 81–112.

Bond F, Godfrey HPD (1997) Conversation with traumatically brain injured individuals: a controlled study of behavioural changes and their impact. Brain Injury 11(5): 319–29.

Booth S, Swabey D (1999) Group training in communication skills for carers of adults with aphasia. International Journal of Language and Communication Disorders 34(3): 219–309.

Braunling-McMorrow D, Lloyd K, Fralish K (1986) Teaching social skills to head injured adults. Journal of Rehabilitation 52(1): 39–44.

Brooks DN, McKinlay W, Symington C (1987) Return to work within the first seven years of severe head injury. Brain Injury 1: 5–19.

Brotherton FA, Thomas LL, Wisotzek IE, Milan MA (1988) Social skills training in the rehabilitation of patients with traumatic closed head injury. Archives of Physical Medicine and Rehabilitation 69: 827–32.

Cherney LR, Miller TK (1991) A classification system for cognitive, linguistic, speech and swallowing disorders in the traumatically brain injured adult. In Halper AS, Cherney LR, Miller TK (eds) Clinical Management of Communication Problems in Adults with Traumatic Brain Injury. Gaitnersburg MD: Aspen, pp. 9–18.

Cherney LR, Halper AS, Miller TK (1991) Treatment of Communication Problems. In Halper AS, Cherney LR, Miller TK (eds) Clinical Management of Communication Problems in Adults with Traumatic Brain Injury. Gaitnersburg MD: Aspen, pp. 57–101

Cockburn J, Wood J (1995) Developing communication skills: a group therapy approach. In Chamberlaine MA, Neumann V, Tennant A (eds) Traumatic brain injury rehabilitation – services, treatments and outcomes. London: Chapman & Hall.

Coelho CA (1999) Discourse analysis in traumatic brain injury. In McDonald S, Togher L, Code C (eds) Communication disorders following traumatic brain injury. Hove: Psychology Press, pp. 55–80.

Coelho CA, DeRuyter F, Stein M (1996) Treatment efficacy: cognitive-communication disorders resulting from traumatic brain injury in adults. Journal of Speech and Hearing Disorders 39: S5–S17.

Davis GA, Holland AL (1981) Age in understanding and treating aphasis. In Beasley DS, Davis GA (eds) Aging: Communication Processes and Disorders. New York: Grune & Stratton, pp. 106–32.

Douglas JM (1990) Traumatic Brain Injury: Language and Communication Deficits. Paper given at New Zealand Speech-Language Therapists' Association biennial conference, Christchurch, New Zealand.

Douglas JM (1992) Communication Awareness Training following Traumatic Brain Injury. Paper given at North Australian Association Speech and Hearing Conference, Melbourne.

Douglas J, O'Flaherty C, Snow P (2000) Measuring Perception of Communicative Ability: The Development and Evaluation of the La Trobe Communication Questionnaire Aphasiology. Aphasiology 14(3): 251–68.

Dresser AC, Meirowsky AM, Weiss GH, McNeel ML, Simon GA, Caveness WF (1973) Gainful employment following head injury: prognostic factors. Archives of Neurology 29: 111–16.

Duffy JR (1995) Motor Speech Disorders – Substrates, Differential Diagnosis and Management. St Louis: Mosby.

Ehrlich JS (1988) Selective characteristics of narrative discourse in head injured and normal adults. Journal of Communication Disorders 21: 1–9.

Ehrlich JS, Barry P (1989) Rating communicative behaviour in the head injured adult. Brain Injury 3(2): 193–8.

Ellmo WJ, Graser JM, Calabrese DB (1994) Methods of Assessment Utilized by Speech and Language Pathologists Working with Brain Injured Adults: A National Survey. Edison NJ: JFK Johnson Institute.

Ellmo WJ, Graser JM, Krchnavek EA, Calabrese DB, Hauck K (1995) Measure of Cognitive-Linguistic Abilities. Vero Beach FL: The Speech Bin.

Enderby PM (1983) Frenchay Dysarthria Assessment. San Diego CA: College Hill Press.

Enderby PM (1997) Therapy Outcome Measures. London: Singular.

Enderby PM, Emerson J (1996) Speech and language therapy – does it work? British Medical Journal 312; June 29, pp. 1655–8.

Enderby PM, John A (1999) Therapy outcome measures in speech and language therapy – comparing performance between different providers. International Journal of Language and Communication Disorders 34(4): 417–29.

Glenwright S, Davison A, Hilton R (1999) Communication training and aphasia: a case study. British Journal of Therapy and Rehabilitation 6(9): 430–5.

Goodglass H, Kaplan E (1972) The Assessment of Aphasia and Related Disorders. Philadelphia: Lea & Fabinger.

Groher M (1977) Language and memory disorders following closed head trauma. Journal of Speech and Hearing Research 20: 212–23.

Hagan C (1984) Language disorders in head trauma. In Holland A (ed.) Language Disorders in Adults. San Diego CA: College Hill Press, pp. 245–81.

Hartley LL (1995) Cognitive-communication Abilities Following Brain Injury: A Functional Approach. San Diego CA: Singular.

Hartley LL, Jensen PJ (1991) Narrative and procedural discourse after closed head injury. Brain Injury 5(3): 267–85.

Holland AL (1982) When is aphasia aphasia? The problem of closed head injury. In Brookshire RL (ed.) Clinical Aphasiology Conference Proceedings. Minneapolis MN: BRK Publishers, pp. 345-9.

Jordan L, Kaiser W (1996) Aphasia: A Social Approach. London: Chapman & Hall.

Kay J, Lesser R, Coltheart M (1992) Psycholinguistic Assessments of Language Processes in Aphasia. Hove: Psychological Press.

Kertesz A (1982) Western Aphasia Battery. New York: The Psychological Corporation.

Levin HS, Grossman RG, Sarwar M, Meyers CA (1981) Linguistic recovery after closed head injury. Brain and Language 12: 360-74.

Linscott RJ, Knight RG, Godfrey HPD (1996) The profile of functional impairment in communication (PFIC): a measure of communication for clinical use. Brain Injury 10: 397-412.

Marsh NV (1999) Social skills deficits following traumatic brain injury: assessment and treatment. In McDonald S, Togher L, Code C (eds) Communication Disorders Following Traumatic Brain Injury. Hove: Psychology Press, pp 175-210.

McDonald S, Togher L, Code C (1999) The nature of traumatic brain injury: basic features with neuropsychological consequences. In McDonald S, Togher L, Code C (eds) Communication Disorders Following Traumatic Brain Injury. Hove: Psychology Press, pp. 19-54.

McGann W, Werven G (1995) New management concept – social competence and head injury: a new emphasis Brain Injury 9(1): 93-1102.

McGann W, Werven G, Douglas MM (1997) Social competence and head injury: a practical approach. Brain Injury 11(9): 621-8.

Mentis M, Prutting CA (1991) Analysis of topic as illustrated in a head injured and a normal adult. Journal of Speech and Hearing Research 34: 583-95.

Miller TK, Halper AS, Cherney LR (1991) Evaluation of comunication problems in the traumatically brain injured adult. In Halper AS, Cherney LR, Miller TK (eds) Clinical Management of Communication Problems in Adults with Traumatic Brain Injury. Gaitnersburg MD: Aspen, pp. 27-56.

Murdoch BE, Theodorus DG (1999) Dysarthria following traumatic brain injury. In McDonald S, Togher L, Code C (eds) Communication Disorders Following Traumatic Brain Injury. Hove: Psychology Press, pp. 211-34.

O'Flaherty C, Douglas MJ (1997) Living with cognitive-communication difficulty following traumatic brain injury: using a model of interpersonal communication to characterise the subjective experience. Aphasiology 11(9): 889-911.

Olver JH, Ponsford JL, Curran CA (1996) Outcome following traumatic brain injury: a comparison between 2 and 5 years after injury. Brain Injury 10(11): 841-8.

Parsons CL, Snow P, Couch D, Mooney L (1989) Conversational skills in closed head injury: Part 1. Australian Journal of Human Communication Disorders 17: 37-45.

Penn C, Cleary J (1988) Compensatory strategies in the language of closed head injured patients. Brain Injury 2(1): 3-17.

Peter C (1995) Conversations avec une patiente souffrant de lésions traumatiques bifrontales: ajustements mutuels. Revue de Neuropsychologie 5: 53-85.

Prutting CA, Kirschner DM (1983) Applied pragmatics. In Gallagher TM, Prutting CA (eds) Pragmatic Assessment and Intervention Issues in Language. San Diego CA: College Hill Press, pp. 29-64.

Rusk H, Block J, Lowmann E (1969) Rehabilitation of the brain injured patient: a report of 157 cases with long term follow up of 118. In Walker E, Caveness W, Critchley M (eds) The Late Effects of Head Injury. Springfield MA: Charles C Thomas, pp. 327–32.

Samuel C, Louis-Dreyfus A, Couillet J, Roubeau B, Bakchine S, Bussel B, Azouvi P (1998) Dysprosody after severe closed head injury: an acoustic analysis. Journal of Neurology, Neurosurgery, Psychiatry 64: 482–5.

Sarno MT, Levin HS (1985) Speech and language disorders after closed head injury. In Darby JK (ed.) Speech and Language Evaluation in Neurology: Adult Disorders. New York: Grune & Stratton, pp. 323–39.

Sarno MT, Buonaguro A, Levita E (1986) Characteristics of verbal impairment in closed head injury patients Archives of Physical Medicine and Rehabilitation 67: 400–5.

Simpson S (1999) Results of the Head Injury Specific Interest Group 'Surveyette'. Head Injury Specific Interest Group Newsletter (April): 4–6.

Snow P, Douglas J (1999) Discourse rehabilitation following traumatic brain injury. In McDonald S, Togher L, Code C (eds) Communication Disorders Following Traumatic Brain Injury. Hove: Psychology Press, pp. 271–320.

Snow P, Ponsford J (1995) Assessing and managing changes in communication and inter-personal skills following traumaic brain injury. In Ponsford J, Sloan S, Snow P (eds) Traumatic Brain Injury: Rehabilitation for Everyday Adaptive Living. New York: Erlbaum.

Snow P, Douglas J, Ponsford J (1997) Conversational assessment following traumatic brain injury: a comparison across two control groups. Brain Injury 11(6): 409–29.

Snow P, Douglas J, Ponsford J (1998) Conversational discourse abilities following severe traumatic brain injury: a follow up study. Brain Injury 12(11): 911–35.

Spitzberg BH, Hurt HT (1987) The measurement of interpersonal skills in instructional contexts. Communication Education 36: 28–45.

Thomsen IV (1984) Late outcome of very severe blunt head trauma: a 10-15 year second follow up. Journal of Neurology, Neurosurgery and Psychiatry 47: 260–8.

Togher L, Hand L, Code C (1997) Analysing discourse in the traumatically brain injured population: telephone interactions with different communication partners. Brain injury 11(3): 169–89.

Togher L, Hand L, Code C (1999) Exchanges of information in the talk of people with traumatic brain injury. In McDonald S, Togher L, Code C (eds) Communication disorders following traumatic brain injury. Hove: Psychology Press, pp. 113–46.

Varley R (1995) Lexical-semantic deficits following right hemisphere damage: evidence from verbal fluency tasks European Journal of Disorders of Communication 30: 362–71.

Wertz RT (1978) Neuropathologies of speech and language: an introduction to patient management. In Johns DF (ed.) Clinical Management of Neurogenic Communication Disorders. Boston: Little, Brown.

Wertz RT (1987) Language therapy for aphasics is efficacious but for whom? Topics of Language Disorder 8: 1–10.

Wilkinson R, Bryan K, Lock S, Bayley K, Maxim J, Bruce C, Edmundson A, Moir D (1998) Therapy using conversational analysis: helping couples adapt to aphasia in conversation. International Journal Language and Communication Disorders 33: 144–50.

Ylvisaker M (1995) personal communication. In Coelho CA, DeRuyter F, Stein M (1996) Treatment efficacy: cognitive-communication disorders resulting from traumatic brain injury in adults. Journal of Speech and Hearing Disorders 39: S5–S17.

Ylvisaker M (1998) Socially co-constructed narratives: competencies associated with an elaborative/collaborative style. In Ylvisaker M (ed.) Traumatic Brain Injury Rehabilitation: Children and Adolescents. Newton MA: Butterworth-Heinemann.

Ylvisaker M, Holland A (1985) Coaching, self-coaching and rehabilitation in head injury. In Johns DF (ed.) Clinical Management of Neurogenic Communication Disorders. Boston: Little, Brown, pp. 243-57.

Ylvisaker M, Szekeres SF (1989) Metacognitive and executive impairments in head injured children and adults. Topics in Language Disorders 9: 34-42.

Ylvisaker M, Urbanczyk B, Feeney TJ (1992) Social skills following traumatic brain injury. Seminars in Speech and Language 13: 308-22.

Yuen HK (1997) Case report: positive talk training in an adult with traumatic brain injury. American Journal of Occupational Therapy 15(9): 780-3.

CHAPTER 7

Vocational rehabilitation

DAVID MCLEOD, ROGER JOHNSON, SAMANTHA JONES

Introduction

One of the most important social roles in our society is that of wage earner. A return to competitive employment after brain injury is generally considered a major goal and the ultimate challenge for rehabilitation professionals: 'Vocational rehabilitation should be made available to all categories of disabled persons and should promote employment opportunities to disabled persons in the open labour market' (International Labour Organization, 1983).

According to O'Neill et al. (1998) successful employment is associated with good social integration and improved home and leisure activities. Return to work provides emotional satisfaction and an opportunity for socially acceptable behaviour (Lloyd and Samra, 2000). Employment gives a sense of identity and improves self-esteem, as well as giving opportunities for social development (Low, 1994). Garner (1995) pointed out that return to work is highly valued by family, friends and the wider community, as well as by disabled people themselves.

Work plays a central part in enabling an individual with brain injury to maximize their potential. It helps them to achieve a sense of worth and to feel that they are making a contribution to society. Employment can also be a medium through which rehabilitation goals can be continued. For example, where an individual is experiencing deficits in higher level cognitive functions, work can provide the challenge necessary to test out abilities and to facilitate further recovery.

Return to work after head injury must take account of many factors in addition to fitness to work or the impact of disability. These include the timing of a return to work, the employer's attitude to the employee's return, aspects of employment law, occupational health assessment and safety issues, sick pay, benefits, insurance and other financial implications.

The role of vocational rehabilitation (VR) is to manage and advise on such issues as well as to promote fitness to work. The aims include the following:

- to facilitate a gradual return to work or education through work experience, voluntary work, supported placement, pre-vocational or vocational training, further education and sheltered workshops;
- to assist individuals to retain and maintain their existing employment where appropriate, or to obtain new employment;
- to support the individual in adjusting to change related to employment;
- to support and advise the individual in matters relating to Tribunals under the Disability Discrimination Act 1995 and other relevant legislation;
- to offer advice and support to employers;
- to help individuals explore opportunities for other forms of occupation within the community if formal employment is not a realistic option.

Vocational rehabilitation is one strand of the overall rehabilitation process. The pathway individuals follow in their efforts to return to work will often rely upon other aspects of their rehabilitation programme. What differentiates VR from other interventions is not only its focus upon vocation and related issues, but also the perspective from which the individual is viewed within the rehabilitation process, the work environment and wider society. Anthony and Blanch (1987) view VR within a social model of disability. This view of disability focuses upon the barriers to successful employment and enables the VR worker to adopt a stance that is distinct from the medical model of disability associated with medical services.

The consequences of brain injury represent a particular challenge to vocational rehabilitation. Neuropsychological disabilities are much more difficult to perceive or understand than physical ones, yet their pervasive effects on function can represent a severe handicap and one that may be difficult or impossible to accommodate in the workplace. Those with observable difficulties will often be accepted more readily by their work colleagues, and some allowances made for any unusual behaviour or reduced performance. Many people with an acquired brain injury exhibit subtle or fluctuating deficits that other people find hard to recognize and therefore they do not accommodate them. For example, a person with impaired memory and attention may be perceived as 'normal' by work colleagues and no special allowances will be made, yet a person with a minor weakness in an upper limb may be viewed as 'disabled' and treated in a more supportive way. In practice, impaired memory may be more disabling than a mild physical complaint. An employer may see a person with executive dysfunction and poor initiation, due to frontal lobe damage, as lazy or unmotivated. Such lack of understanding on the part of others will be further compounded if clients lack insight into their own difficulties. This may make them appear uncaring to others. Ross (1982) recognized that an individual's motivation to overcome his difficulties is a key factor in returning to work successfully. Lack of insight may allow individuals to maintain unrealistic expectations or to present themselves as more competent than they are in practice. People with acquired brain injury often maintain the aspirations that they held prior to their injury (Thomas and Menz, 1990).

Employment outcome after head injury

The incidence for successful return to work after severe head injury is difficult to establish. Figures from outcome studies vary widely because investigators have looked at groups of patients with differing levels of severity of injury and different employment histories. There has been no consensus about how soon after injury outcome should be assessed and few have attempted to look at stability of employment after head injury over a lengthy period of time. Moreover, different research studies have used different criteria to define what constitutes a return to work (Humphrey and Oddy, 1980; Wehman et al., 1995).

For some, the level of employment they can manage after head injury will decline. Some people also appear to change their jobs more frequently than they did beforehand (Oddy et al., 1985; Brooks et al., 1987; Wehman et al., 1993). Few studies have looked at longer term outcomes, several years after head injury. Those that have done so suggest that rather little change in work status occurs once two years or so have elapsed after the injury. Thus, Thomsen (1984) looked at a series of patients 10 to 15 years after their injuries and found little change in occupational outcome compared to two to three years post injury. A study by Johnson (1998) suggested considerable stability in employment status between about three years and about 10 years post injury. Those who had settled back into work within two years of injury were mostly still in stable employment 10 years after the event. Those who failed at their first attempt to work tended to develop an unstable pattern of work, with short-lived jobs and frequent changes. A third group made little or no attempt to work following their injuries and nearly all these people were still unemployed at 10 years post injury.

Estimates of the likelihood of a successful return to formal work vary widely. An overview of outcome studies suggests that only about 30% of those with severe head injury will return (Greenwood and McMillan, 1993), but for those who do settle back into work, including those who are assisted by vocational rehabilitation programmes, the long-term prospects for remaining in employment are good (Johnson, 1998).

Many factors interact in determining employment outcome after brain injury and there is no single factor that can be used as a predictor of work outcome (Crepeau and Sherzer, 1993; Dikmen et al., 1994). These authors drew attention to some association between successful return to work and stable pre-injury employment, together with the importance of access to resources for vocational rehabilitation. The principal issues that have been suggested as predictors of work outcome are as follows:

Previous level of employment

A study by Brooks et al. (1987) found that 50% of those with severe head injury, previously employed in managerial and similar level jobs, returned to work, whereas only 21% of unskilled workers did so. A reason for this difference may be that in skilled and professional workplaces there are better resources to accommodate disabilities. Support from work colleagues is perhaps more likely. Nevertheless, Johnson (1987) showed that schemes for support in the workplace, for clients with disabilities due to head injury, could be just as well set up for those in unskilled jobs as in other kinds of work. However, there may be a greater need for these employers to have access to advice and support from a vocational rehabilitation service about how best to do this.

Age and severity of injury

Age at the time of injury, and severity of injury, have been suggested as predictors of work outcome (Brooks et al., 1987; Ponsford et al., 1995; Wehman et al., 1995). Neither is reliable in practice but they show some predictive value at the extremes. Thus, older people may be less likely to work again after severe head injury, and may opt for early retirement (Brooks et al., 1987; Crepeau and Sherzer, 1993). Minor head injury (post-traumatic amnesia of less than 24 hours) rarely leads to significant employment difficulties (Wrightson and Gronwall, 1981), whereas those with very severe head injuries and multiple handicaps are unlikely to attempt to work again (Johnson, 1987).

Nevertheless, some older people, and some who sustain very severe injuries and considerable neuropsychological disability, do return to work successfully (Oddy, Humphrey and Uttley, 1978; Newcombe, 1982). Thus, neither age nor severity of injury should be used to exclude people from vocational rehabilitation opportunities.

Disabilities

The implications for employment of physical or sensory disabilities may be fairly easy to recognize. However, employment outcome after head injury will inevitably be affected by cognitive disabilities and by problems with communication or changes in behaviour. Some of these deficits may be difficult to detect or to anticipate before a return to work is made. For example, mild problems with sustained attention, or changes in speed of work, may only become evident once the person is back in a work environment. The specific cognitive skills required for the job must be adequate, and social skills must be reasonably good (Gronwall, Wrightson and wadell, 1990).

It has been stated that the number and severity of neuropsychological symptoms will predict work outcome (Godfrey et al., 1993; Wehman et al., 1995), although there is some controversy about this relationship, There is better consensus that behavioural disabilities are particularly likely to disrupt work (Sale et al., 1991; Wehman et al., 1993; Groswasser et al., 1999). The importance of good social interactions within the workplace has also been recognized for clients with mental health problems (Anthony and Jansen, 1984). Small changes in irritability or other features of disinhibition will disrupt relationships with work colleagues. Even mild problems with impulsiveness or motivation, for example, can lead to unreliability. These factors are likely to lead to early breakdown of employment unless they are tackled at the outset.

Support at work

Special support when a return to work is first attempted after head injury, and rehabilitation interventions that extend into the workplace, appear to increase the chances of a successful return. Moreover, success is more likely where support and training within the workplace continue for at least several months (Johnson, 1987; McMillan and Greenwood, 1993). The importance of continued job support has also been recognized in the rehabilitation of people with mental health problems (Cook, 1992). Return to previous employment tends to be more successful than starting new work. This is probably because the opportunities for support are better in the former case and because re-establishing old skills is easier for someone with a brain injury than learning new ones. A high rate of successful return to work (73%) was reported for a series of patients with very severe head injuries who went back to their previous employment (Johnson, 1987). A high overall return rate of 42% in this study appeared to be due to the benefits of continuing rehabilitation into the workplace.

In practice, a wide range of factors need to be taken into account when planning a vocational rehabilitation programme. The principal ones are summarized in Table 7.1.

Table 7.1. Barriers to employment following acquired brain injury

Cognitive deficits	Executive dysfunction; attention; memory; perceptual deficits
Communication difficulties	Expressive and receptive language problems, reduced literacy skills
Physical disabilities	Mobility, dexterity, fatigue
Sensory loss	Vision, hearing, sense of smell
Emotional disturbance	Depression, anxiety, anger; frustration, loss of confidence, post-traumatic stress disorder
Behavioural issues	Disinhibition, aggression, loss of concern, inertia
Social problems	Separation from partner, housing problems, care of children
Welfare rights	Benefits, financial constraints
Unrealistic expectations	Lack of insight
Legal issues	Liability for injury, compensation claims; criminal proceedings

Assessment

According to Lloyd and Samra (2000):

> work assessment is the first stage in work-related rehabilitation. It not only evaluates the occupational skills of the person but also takes into account other factors such as self-care, mental state, motivation and social relationships that are essential for a competent work performance.

Botterbusch (1989) claims that vocational evaluation can be split into two major sections: clinical and psychometric. Psychometric testing, as used in occupational work, was developed through military and personnel psychology. Standardized tests were developed to measure aptitudes, interests, temperament, personality traits, and academic levels. Results were validated against job requirements. When working with clients with traumatic brain injury, tests of cognitive function, designed to identify neuropsychological deficits, may prove of equal or greater importance. Moreover, some cognitive deficits can interfere with the ability to complete vocational measures, such as questionnaires about interests or personality. For example, responses from clients with executive dysfunction may be unreliable because of poor decision making or impulsiveness.

Clinical methods of assessment are more subjective and rely on the intuitive skills of the evaluator. The client may be observed in real or simulated work conditions. Techniques include behavioural observation and analysis techniques, or establishing how the client reacts in specific situations or under certain conditions.

The clinical and psychometric approaches can be used together to good advantage, complementing and supporting each other. Psychometric tests allow objective measurement, which can be compared to appropriate normative data, whereas 'clinical' observation will not allow the evaluator to identify covert traits and symptoms. On the other hand, psychometric test performance can be adversely affected by negative attitudes to this kind of assessment on the part of the client – perhaps because he is unable to see the relationship between the tests and real work. Moreover, test performance is not always a reliable predictor of performance in practice and in this respect clinical observation can prove more reliable.

Activities that closely resemble actual operations carried out in industry or other vocational settings ('work samples') provide a useful tool for the evaluator. They can be used to test practical abilities, including intellectual and physical aptitudes. They may also measure motivation to work, interpersonal relationships, stamina, initiative, and other variables that cannot be tackled by psychometric measures. Clients will generally show good co-operation on assessments of this kind as they can be seen to be relevant to establishing work capabilities. Moreover, cultural, social and language limitations inherent in many psychometric tests can be circumvented by practical evaluation of performance in work-like settings.

Performance on work samples can be measured against normative data for industrial standards. Work samples can also be used to train clients until their performance matches that of the standard required in the workplace.

Job-site evaluation is a further measurement tool. This enables all parties to assess performance in the setting of the client's workplace and without the protection and security of work sampling. It allows a realistic assessment of the client's ability to cope with the normal psychological and social pressures of employment, such as stress of work demands, time constraints, and criticism. The evaluator can observe factors such as productivity, sustained concentration, fatigue, or behaviour with colleagues, for example. Job-site evaluation provides the client with good feedback about his readiness for work. It enables him to make direct comparison of his performance with that of his colleagues, and with his own previous standards. This can be particularly beneficial where the client is showing difficulties with insight.

Job-site evaluation is cost effective. Many employers are able to offer time-limited work experience placements as goodwill gestures and will frequently assist in evaluating performance and behaviour during the period of the placement. It is a particularly useful strategy for brain-injured clients where accurate assessment of readiness for work may be very difficult by any other means. Moreover, it provides a first step towards a return to work and forms a basis on which to educate and inform employers and work colleagues about the nature of the disabilities that need to be accommodated.

A further advantage of using job-site evaluation, rather than formal re-employment, is that if the work placement proves unsuitable, or it is evident that a return to work is premature, then the plan can be relatively easily revised or modified. On occasion, a further period of rehabilitation may be indicated.

In summary, the tools and techniques available for vocational assessment all have their particular advantages and disadvantages – no single tool is likely to be effective if it is used in isolation. Langman (2000) identified a range of psychological and educational tests designed to measure personality, intelligence, aptitudes and vocational interests, for diagnostic purposes (Table 7.2).

For clients with brain injury, specific tests of neuropsychological function are particularly important too. Above all else, practical evaluation within the workplace, or in work-like settings, is likely to prove essential for those recovering from head injury. It is often the case that the subtle neuropsychological symptoms these people have, or the impact of these problems, can only be identified clearly by *in vivo* assessment.

Table 7.2. Psychological and educational tests frequently used in vocational rehabilitation

Personality	Minnesota Multiphasic Personality Inventory, Sixteen Personality Factor Questionnaire
Intelligence	Wechsler Adult Intelligence Scale III
Achievement	Wide Range Achievement Test – revised
Vocational aptitudes	General Aptitude Test battery, Non-Reading Aptitude Test Battery, Differential Aptitude Test, Crawford Small Parts Dexterity Test
Vocational interests	General Occupational Interest Inventory

The timing of vocational rehabilitation

Many factors can determine the timing and nature of VR input in relation to the overall rehabilitation process. Any of the 'barriers to employment' (Table 7.1) could result in an unsuccessful return to work or other undesired outcome. Gronwall, Wrightson and Wadell (1990) recognized that members of the rehabilitation team are together likely to hold the information that will answer the question: 'When should this person begin the return to work process?'

Time needed for recovery

The longer the period of time a person is off work, the more difficult their return and subsequent re-integration is likely to be (Niemeyer et al., 1994). If they are off work for too long, loss of confidence will be aggravated and their vulnerability to depression increases (McMillan and Greenwood, 1993). Moreover, an early return to work can aid further recovery and adaptation. The point has already been made that if employment has not been re-established within two years of severe head injury then return to work becomes very unlikely. The reasons for this are unclear. The long-term unemployed in the normal population show a deterioration in mental health and it may be that effects of this sort, when combined with the disadvantages of head injury, make it extremely difficult for the client to achieve a return to work.

On the other hand, there are considerable dangers in attempting to return to work too soon after head injury. This is a common problem because many people who have sustained a brain injury are determined to get back to work as soon as possible but are not well able to judge their ability to cope with it. They may be physically fit and easily convince themselves that, once back at work, difficulties with memory or concentration will resolve. Others may lack insight and appear to be unaware that they have any problems. From the employer's point of view, the disabilities may not be immediately evident. They are likely to be impressed by the client's motivation and eagerness to work, and unwittingly collude with them in arranging a premature return.

Head injury problems may be greatly aggravated if a client returns to work and fails. This event is very often followed by a pattern of unstable employment (Johnson, 1998). Failure at the first attempt to work after head injury seems to seriously reduce the chances of the person settling back into employment in the longer term. In Johnson's series of patients, all of whom had sustained very severe head injuries, none who eventually returned to work successfully made an initial return before five or six months post injury. Ideally, rehabilitation should continue to a point where the best possible level of recovery has been achieved before work is attempted. As the majority of the recovery following brain injury will take place in the first six months, this may be the minimum period off work for those with severe head injury.

Thus, a rough guide, following a severe head injury, is that a return to work should not be attempted earlier than about six months, and not later than 18 months after the injury. If two years have elapsed since injury, without a return to work, then sheltered work or other alternative occupation should be considered.

Insight

Lack of insight can be a significant factor in determining a person's readiness to start the return to work process. If clients are not aware of their difficulties, or the effect that their actions or behaviour may have on others, much damage to working relationships can be done. Under such circumstances the individual is likely to fail, not only because of a poor level of performance but also due to breakdowns in working and personal relationships with colleagues. Demotion, redundancy, resignation, or dismissal are likely to follow (Gronwall et al., 1990).

It may be helpful or necessary when working with clients who have impaired insight to provide them with 'evidence' of their limitations. Such evidence may be obtained through work-like tasks. Sometimes, it may be necessary to allow a premature return to previous employment before a client who is adamant that he is fit to do so is able to accept the implications of cognitive or behavioural disability. For some clients, this can be the only way forward despite the effect that too early a return may have on their relationships with colleagues and on the prospects of their job remaining open to them. In these circumstances particular care is needed about the way a work trial is set up and to ensure that the outcome can be used positively.

Financial considerations

Financial constraints may affect decisions about when to return to work. It is usually best for the vocational rehabilitation worker to establish a good understanding of these issues as early as possible. For many people there are financial pressures to return sooner rather than later and most employers will expect the employee to return to work within a specified time frame. Others may be more flexible as to when the employee returns and be happy to take the advice of the rehabilitation team into account. The policies of the employing organization about sick pay or insurance against ill health may also influence decisions about work. Sometimes, alternative outcomes need to be considered, such as the possible benefits of retirement on medical grounds or a redundancy deal.

Many employees have little or no contact with their employers during the initial stages of rehabilitation, and this can lead to misunderstandings later. The VR worker can facilitate communication between the employee and the employer; act as an advocate on the employee's behalf, and advise employers as to their responsibilities under current legislation. Issues relating to benefits and the implications of the Disability Discrimination Act are dealt with later in this chapter.

In this last respect, early involvement of the vocational rehabilitation worker is clearly important - perhaps soon after the injury. As far as the client making a return to work is concerned, there is a balance to be struck between the hazards of doing this too soon and of leaving it too late. In the early months following injury, the client must be encouraged to focus on therapy and on efforts to maximize recovery and insight. Six to 12 months after injury the emphasis must shift to looking at how a return to work might be achieved. If plans about work are put off for too long then the client's motivation, confidence and mood may start to deteriorate.

Goal setting

Employment prospects will be best served by establishing a work rehabilitation programme that reflects the goals held by the client (Lloyd and Samra, 2000). Park, Duran and Fisher (1997) stated that goals should reflect what the client needs or wants to be able to do and the level of performance that the client needs to achieve. A particular problem when working with those affected by head injury is that clients may have unrealistic goals due to lack of insight and difficulties in judging their disabilities and circumstances.

Any intervention should be based upon collaboration between the client and the rehabilitation specialist. This is of fundamental importance, especially if the VR practitioner is to take on the role of advocate. If the goals of the individual and the practitioner conflict, then neither is likely to be satisfied with the outcome (Neistadt, 1995). Thus, even where there is a lack of insight, it is important to try to identify goals that can form a compromise between those of the client and those of the VR worker, but which can be agreed by both.

Providing this principle is followed then the importance of an assessment to establish appropriate plans for work is clear to both the client and the VR worker. A baseline of performance is established and, if this is clearly documented, it provides 'an objective basis to determine the appropriateness, effectiveness, and necessity of intervention' (American Occupational Therapy Association, 1995). It also gives a measure by which the outcome of a vocational rehabilitation programme can be judged.

Goals may reflect an individual's subjective experiences (for example, increased confidence or self-esteem), providing these factors can be 'operationalized' (Anton, 1978). This is achieved by identifying observable ('objective') behaviours that the client would expect to change in relation to subjective criteria (Spreadbury in Creek, 1998). For example, a reduction in the frequency of support sought from an employer by clients who have returned to the workplace may be an indicator of their increased confidence. However, it is important to identify other factors that might also contribute to such changes (for example, structure provided in the workplace; use of cognitive strategies). By documenting such observable changes it is possible to use this information to demonstrate progress to the client, to their relatives, and to an employer. Such changes, however small, may hold great significance for the individual and significantly influence the outcome of VR intervention.

Evaluation and outcome measures

The method of documentation and type of 'tool' used to measure outcomes will depend upon the expected or desired change. The outcome of vocational rehabilitation can be rated according to the level of vocational activity achieved (Table 7.3).

Table 7.3 does not represent a complete list but gives an indication of the range of outcomes. A change in the level of support that a client needs can be an index of the progress made during a VR programme and therefore a measure of the effectiveness of the intervention.

Specialist vocational outcome measures are currently used by some services. For example, the Community Head Injury Service in Aylesbury has developed a vocational assessment incorporating interviews, formal tests of cognitive function and observation of work attitude, performance and behaviour (Tyerman, 1999).

Table 7.3. Levels of vocational outcome

Open employment, full-time (previous work or new work)

Open employment, part-time

Supported employment

Vocational training

Education course

Voluntary work

Sheltered employment

Day centre activities

Management

Occupational therapy and vocational rehabilitation

Some brain-injury rehabilitation teams include a VR worker but many do not. Other professionals, and particularly occupational therapists, therefore often involve themselves in vocational rehabilitation programmes. In our experience there are many cases where the role of the OT and VR worker overlap. For example, the development and practice of memory and attention strategies to compensate for deficits may enable the individual to return to work activities that would otherwise be too challenging for them. Many aspects of

VR for those with brain injury necessarily draw upon, if not depend upon, the skills or knowledge of other multidisciplinary team members.

Vocational rehabilitation for those with head injury must accommodate a range of different needs. A majority of people will have been employed at the time of their injury and their best, and usually preferred, option is to return to their previous work. For those who were unemployed or in education at the time of the injury, or seeking new jobs for other reasons, rather different strategies are necessary. Some clients may seek help from a community rehabilitation team only after they have attempted to return to their jobs but failed to cope. A further group of clients are those who have disabilities that preclude work. For these people VR needs to address the alternatives to open employment that may be available to them.

Liaison with other agencies

Specialist provision will vary depending on local brain injury services and available expertise: where such provision is health based it will be necessary to add placement expertise; where it is employment based it will be necessary to add brain injury expertise; where it is social services based it will be necessary to include both brain injury rehabilitation and placement expertise (Tyerman, 1999). It is therefore vital that links are formed with agencies that can provide the employment expertise and support to the community rehabilitation service. Some of the agencies and schemes with whom the community rehabilitation team may work in partnership to provide a comprehensive VR service are shown in the appendix to this chapter.

In practice, relatively few people with head injury return to employment via employment service schemes or other agencies. This is probably due to a combination of factors. Many schemes are more suited to the needs of those with physical disability than to dealing with the neuropsychological impairments that follow head injury. The majority of head-injured people have little or no physical disability and their priority is to return to their previous work and their previous employer. This means that the most useful vocational rehabilitation strategies to help clients with head injury are those that aim to work directly with employers and to exploit the workplace as the environment in which much of the vocational rehabilitation takes place. Nevertheless, close collaboration between the brain injury rehabilitation service and the employment service will enable individuals to access other resources where appropriate, and help establish links with local providers of education, training and work experience placements. Such joint working will enhance the support provided to clients seeking employment, returning to previous work or undertaking vocational training. Contact with the Employment Service can be made through the local Disability Employment Adviser (DEA).

In vivo rehabilitation strategies

Return to previous employment, and establishing good strategies for support in the workplace, is particularly beneficial to those recovering from head injury for several reasons. It provides an opportunity to test work skills out and on this basis to adapt the previous job to accommodate the worker's altered abilities. Alternatively the client may be tried out in different jobs within the organization to identify the level of work best suited to him. To begin with, it is always wise for the brain-injured client to start back at work on a part-time basis – with both shorter hours and a limited number of days per week. Fatigue is one of the commonest problems after head injury but a cautious start also makes sense simply on the grounds that it is easy to increase demands but much more difficult to reduce them if the initial plan proves too ambitious. Usually, a gradual increase in hours and in demand is necessary over a period of months.

The workplace can be used for continued skills retraining, perhaps in conjunction with further therapy sessions at the community rehabilitation centre. Training at work can be particularly effective. The client is likely to be well motivated and better able to judge his own performance in a familiar work setting compared to what he can achieve in a therapy session. Skills are acquired within the context where they must be applied and therefore there are no problems of transferring skills learnt in one setting to their application in another. It is important to set targets for the work the person is doing, and to monitor performance or errors that may arise due to poor memory or other impairments. Work colleagues can sometimes be involved in maintaining a record of performance.

Introducing these measures depends on a good level of understanding on the part of the employer and on a preparedness to accommodate their disabled employee. Thus, negotiation and education via the VR worker is of particular importance. This can be time consuming but in this way successful re-employment can be achieved, with relatively low levels of professional input, and low cost, compared to many other models of employment rehabilitation.

The length of time for which support or training may be needed in the workplace is easily underestimated. To be effective, an average period of about eight months is probably needed for those recovering from severe head injury. This is based on the findings of the study by Johnson (1987) for people returning to their previous work and on the report by Wehman et al. (1990) on the duration of support in their job coaching schemes for clients entering new employment after head injury. A long period of time for training to be effective is probably necessary because the process of learning and the acquisition of compensatory strategies are particularly slow after head injury.

For those returning to work after head injury but starting new jobs, the opportunities for continued training or therapy in the workplace are much more limited. Some schemes through the employment services can provide a degree of support but their limitations are that they are really designed to accommodate permanent, physical disability. There is little provision for training cognitive skills or the possibility of change.

There has been a much greater interest in training people within new work settings in the US. Kreutzer et al. (1991) and Wehman et al. (1990) have described vocational rehabilitation strategies and job coaching schemes there and they have published a series of subsequent papers. There is little scope or provision for vocational rehabilitation along these lines within the UK – perhaps because this approach is expensive with a need for training specialists to work with each client for lengthy periods of time.

Provision from the employment services, such as the job introduction scheme, lasts for too short a time to be of benefit to most head-injured people. The job introduction scheme is in any case designed to assess the suitability of a job rather than provide training. The supported placement scheme also offers little in the way of training and is more akin to sheltered work. It can continue indefinitely and therefore offers some scope for support to brain-injured clients with permanent disability.

The work preparation scheme does offer time-limited training but the benefit for head-injured clients will vary according to the resources of local providers and the suitability of the training they can offer. Residential courses may suit some clients but for many people with head injury they are inappropriate. This may be because they are unable to offer suitable training or because the disabilities many of these clients have mean that it is difficult for them to live away from their usual sources of support or care. Others may feel unable to live away from home and from family commitments for training, which can last for as much as nine months.

For those seeking new work after head injury the best strategy may be to identify alternatives to work that will allow a period of *in vivo* training before formal work is attempted. These strategies can also be a useful stage in helping a client return to his previous work but they are particularly important where support in the workplace is unlikely to be available.

The principal options here are voluntary work or informal arrangements to help in businesses run by family or friends. These settings allow the client's abilities to be observed and they require work activities to be carried out according to the demands set by the requirements of the job. At the same time, there can be a degree of support and some flexibility about hours and about the level of demand made on the client. As far as possible, the work should be matched to the client's skills or interests in order to enhance motivation. Sometimes, specific skills or knowledge that a client has can be applied in a voluntary work setting.

The use of strategies whereby a client makes an indirect return to work after head injury is extremely common. Johnson (1998), in his series of patients, noted that 87% went back to work on a trial basis, to an easier job for an initial period, or via alternative activities, such as voluntary work, study courses or training. Returning to work after head injury without an intermediate stage of this kind carries a high risk of failure.

Once the indications are that the client may be ready to move on to formal work, the level of job the client should seek will need careful evaluation. Part-time work may be best at first and work will probably need to be at a lower or easier level than before their injury. All too often clients are too ambitious when applying for new jobs after head injury and expect to be able to work at their previous level. If the work is now too difficult, even if only slightly so, then occasional mistakes, mild slowness or other minor problems, can quickly lead to the job being lost. This is particularly likely if clients, and perhaps their history, are not known to new employers and a normal performance is expected.

Alternatives to formal work

If open employment is not an option, alternative forms of work can provide an opportunity to develop confidence, engage in purposeful activities and enable the individual to rebuild his self-esteem. Many people still feel the need to make a contribution to society or their local community through a work-related activity.

The three main models of alternative employment in rehabilitation work are:

- supported employment or sheltered work;
- clubhouse model;
- social firms.

Supported employment schemes, including sheltered work, are the most widely used strategies for helping those with brain injury to return to work. The clubhouse model and social firms are used within the mental health and learning disability services, and may be unavailable or difficult to access for those with brain injury.

Supported employment

Supported placement schemes (SPS) are designed to encourage employers to provide opportunities for disabled people, working alongside non-disabled colleagues. Placements need to be individualized, focusing on the person's strengths and abilities (Lloyd and Samra, 2000). A sponsor (for example, a voluntary employment agency or local authority) assists the host company (employer) with provision of suitable work for the disabled employee, and also provides tools and any training required. The sponsor helps to set up the placement and can assess health and safety risks, clarify issues such as day-to-day supervision and provide support to the company and the employee. An agreed amount is paid to the employer to cover costs (of special support needed, losses in production or other expenses), and the sponsor will usually monitor the placement at regular intervals .The sponsor can in some cases also be the employer. The SPS is shortly to be replaced by 'work step schemes'. It is believed these will be structured differently to SPS but will have a similar aim of providing supported work opportunities.

Supported placement schemes can be of benefit to clients with head injury although they are defined in terms more suited to those with physical and permanent disability. After brain injury the need is commonly one of accommodating the more cryptic disabilities of cognitive or behavioural impairments and with a need for training aimed at moderating these symptoms.

Sheltered workshops are another form of supported employment that can form a stepping-stone to open employment or provide a viable alternative in the long term. Resources will vary in different localities.

The advantages of sheltered workshops are that they can provide a secure base for building confidence, a choice of training opportunities and specialist support. This offers an invaluable environment for people who need to develop or practise skills but who lack confidence and motivation, or who require supervision.

The disadvantages are that sheltered work can fail to provide incentives for a person to move on. Difficulties may arise due to the commercial requirements of the workshop if they depend upon the productivity of those attending to generate their revenue. Moreover, head-injured clients, particularly those with behavioural difficulties, often do not fit in well to facilities of this sort. Some younger people, particularly those with little or no physical disability, can prove antagonistic to a working environment that they perceive as principally for physically handicapped people. They may also be opposed to doing work that is usually of a very straightforward and routine nature.

Clubhouse model

Clubhouses are member-run facilities offering a restorative environment where individuals can regain confidence, develop personal and work skills and overcome isolation (Pozner et al., 1996). These are user-led schemes where members contribute to the planning and running of activities, and to education and transitional employment programmes. They have paid facilitators who work alongside the members. Clubhouses have been piloted and associated with mental health projects. Each clubhouse provides options for support, leisure and daytime activity as well as assistance in developing work skills. They focus upon transitional employment that is waged and time limited. This provides the opportunity for members to experience paid work in ordinary competitive employment (Pozner et al., 1996). To achieve this, the whole clubhouse applies for a job, which then 'belongs' to the clubhouse. All appropriate members are trained to do the work, and each individual then does the job for a set period of time before it is handed to another member of the clubhouse. By working through a series of such placements each member can gain experience, develop work skills and build up a history of work experience.

The advantages of this model are that it provides realistic work experience, the individuals are paid, and they can be well supported. The disadvantages are that placements can be hard to find and sustain, and employers may be concerned about the changes in staff and consistency of the work done. The application of this model in head-injury rehabilitation is likely to involve additional difficulties. The variation between individuals in the nature and severity of disabilities would make it hard to establish a group of individuals fit to carry out the same series of jobs. Nevertheless, a project based on this model has been implemented for people with traumatic brain injury in the US. Four out of nine clubhouse programmes are reported to have been successful (Jones, 2001).

Social firms

Social firms, also known as 'social enterprise' or 'cooperatives', are set up with the aim of providing opportunities for disabled people to work. They are small- to medium-sized enterprises that provide paid employment for individuals who have been unable to sustain open employment but who can function productively if they are accommodated in a supported and flexible work environment (Pozner et al., 1996).

Advantages of social firms are their small team approach, participatory and cooperative structure and non-stigmatizing ethos. Disadvantages can be that they require deft commercial skills and they can have expensive set-up costs. Historically, they have been targeted at individuals with learning difficulties or enduring mental health problems. Currently there is no list of social firms available but as far as we are aware there are none in the UK specifically set up for those with brain injury.

Welfare rights

Welfare rights form an important part of the initial stages of the vocational rehabilitation process. An informal check that clients are receiving the benefits that they are entitled to should be made at the outset. Changes in clients' financial situation can affect many areas of their lives and can influence decisions made about when to return to work. Satisfactory benefits arrangements provide a 'buffer' of time and security during which the client can consider the advice of the rehabilitation team and their own feelings before making a decision about work. Benefits such as income support, disabled person's tax credit, incapacity benefit or severe disablement allowance can enable a person to begin a programme of graded work experience whilst maintaining some degree of financial security.

If an informal return to the workplace is to be made this may affect the company sick pay scheme or eligibility for statutory benefits. However, if work is commenced on an unpaid basis in the first instance, or if it can be described as a part of a rehabilitation programme, then benefits can continue and a small amount can be earned under the 'therapeutic earnings rule'. Eligibility for this needs to be established and agreed with the local social security office before work starts. Clients who are in receipt of incapacity benefit, severe disability allowance or other incapacity related benefit are allowed to do voluntary work without this affecting their benefit, although work for close relatives is excluded (Disability Rights Handbook, 2000–1).

Health and safety and insurance issues must also be assessed. Company insurers will need to be informed that an employee with some degree of disability is attending work. Certain aspects of the client's work may not be possible if their disabilities mean there might be a safety hazard. The most common problem of this sort after head injury arises if there is a risk of fits. Physical or sensory handicaps more often lead to safety concerns – in the use machinery, for example – than neuropsychological impairments. However, the safety implications of cognitive deficits, and more particularly any impairment in behavioural control, must be carefully evaluated. If the client is self-employed it is particularly easy for safety hazards and insurance issues to be overlooked.

Useful references about Welfare rights are the Disability Rights Handbook (2000) and the Welfare Benefits Handbook (George et al., 2000). It is advisable to seek advice about up-to-date legislation from the Joint Commissioning Team Welfare Rights Unit, or their helpline, or other informed sources. Training courses in welfare rights can equip a VR worker with the basic tools and knowledge necessary for giving advice and assistance where necessary. Much time may be needed when working with head-injured clients helping them to complete benefits forms, acting as an advocate for them, or representing them in negotiations or disputes such as an appeal tribunal.

Employment law and the Disability Discrimination Act 1995

Part 1 (section 1) of the Disability Discrimination Act 1995 (DDA) defines disability as a physical or mental impairment which has, or has had, a substantial and long-term adverse effect on an individual's ability to carry out normal day-to-day activities. Part 2 makes it unlawful for an employer who has 15 or more employees to discriminate against a disabled employee or job applicant in relation to employment by 'treating that person less favourably, for a reason which relates to his or her disability, than [the employer] treats or would treat others to whom that reason does not or would not apply'. The DDA also places a duty upon employers to make reasonable adjustments to working practices or the working environment where these would otherwise act as a barrier to the disabled employee or place them at a disadvantage.

The 'reasonable adjustments' referred to in the Act can include reallocation of certain duties to others; transferring the person to an existing, alternative vacancy; making adaptations to the premises; providing support or equipment; altering working hours; or allowing absence from work for the purposes of rehabilitation, assessment or treatment. The employer is responsible for making the necessary adjustments to the workplace or the conditions of employment (Thurgood, 1999).

Employees are not obliged to disclose their disability. However, not doing so could leave employees at a disadvantage if at a later stage they take sick leave that is related to an undeclared disability or if work conditions, which could have been adjusted, are the cause of difficulties in coping with the job (Thurgood, 1999).

There is evidence that disabled people face prejudice and direct discrimination when applying for jobs. Educating employing organizations and exposing some of the myths regarding disabled workers would improve the employment opportunities available to all disabled people. For example, a misconception held by some employers is that their field of occupation is unsuitable for disabled people; or that adaptations to the workplace would be too difficult. Most people disabled by head injury need little or no alteration to the workplace. Physical or sensory handicaps are relatively easy to recognize and adaptations in the workplace in accordance with the DDA may be quite clear. The cognitive or behavioural changes that can follow head injury are more difficult to accommodate. Nevertheless the Act does specify that adaptations should be made where appropriate in the workload, or the number of hours worked. These provisions can prove particularly useful to those with neuropsychological impairments.

Awareness of the support and special funding available to clients is essential, as this could greatly increase their chances of a successful return to work.

Funding for travel costs, equipment, adaptations or the provision of support could come via the employment service (for example, under the Access to Work Scheme), from the individual (for example, private funding from a compensation settlement), or from voluntary organizations.

Conclusions

Failure to achieve employment following severe head injury can often be due to a lack of appropriate support and training rather than because these people are incapable of work (Johnson, 1987). Re-employment after head injury may be achieved even where there are quite significant neuropsychological disabilities.

Employment rehabilitation, which makes use of the previous workplace, or similar *in vivo* training strategies, appears to be particularly important for those with brain injury. This is because it accommodates their particular vulnerabilities. The amount of new learning is minimized and support from employers and colleagues can be enlisted. Another important element in vocational rehabilitation for those with head injury is the need for support and training to continue over a long period of time. This is probably because the development of compensatory strategies for neuropsychological deficits, and establishing new habits, is a very slow learning process.

In a study on a specialist vocational assessment and rehabilitation for persons with severe traumatic brain injury, Tyerman (1999) concluded that 'without specialist vocational provision many persons with severe Traumatic Brain Injury fail in their efforts to return to employment'. The study highlighted the value of observations and ratings of work attitude, behaviour and performance on simulated work activities in the community, alongside vocational interviews and assessments by neuropsychologists, occupational therapists, speech and language therapists and by physiotherapists. Tyerman emphasized the importance of a service framework within which it is possible to integrate core elements of brain injury rehabilitation with graded vocational rehabilitation activities.

Appendix: Agencies and Schemes for Vocational Rehabilitation

Charitable organizations specializing in vocational and employment issues

Accessed directly or by referral from other services (for example employment service; social services; rehabilitation centre). *Funded* by statutory authorities, grants, charitable organizations or privately.

- *Shaw Trust.* Supports the recruitment and training of disabled and disadvantaged people; supports existing employees to keep working; supports organizations to make 'reasonable adjustments' under the DDA 1995.
- *Rehab UK.* Brain injury vocational centres: assessment and planning; work preparation and job training; job placement and follow-up support.
- *The Papworth Trust.* Vocational assessment and rehabilitation programmes; community placements.

The employment service – disability employment adviser (DEA)

Accessed via the Job Centre: provides advice, support and access to funding and other schemes (for example, Work Preparation; Access to Work; Work Step Scheme). Occupational psychologist – for work-focused assessment.

Benefits agency; social services; welfare rights helpline

Access by telephone or in person at local centre. Access to benefits and advice.

Sheltered workshops

Access by contact according to local resources or via the job centre.

Training and enterprise councils (TECs)

Access via the job centre. Identify and provide support for specialized learning; programmes are targeted at specific client groups; work-based training.

Educational resources

Access via local schools, colleges, universities or training centres.

Addresses

National Vocational Rehabilitation Association
The Membership Secretary
Old Rectory Cottage
Old Bolingbroke
Lincs. PE23 4HB
E-mail: jill.price@crawford-thg.com

The Papworth Trust
Papworth Everard
Cambridge
CB3 8RG
Tel: 01480 830341
Fax: 01480 830781

Rehab UK
12 Gough Square,
London EC4 3DE

Brain Injury Vocational Centres:
Glasgow: telephone 0141 354 0200
Aberdeen: telephone 01224 625580
Fife: telephone 01592 643444
Tyne and Wear: telephone 0191 232 0234
London: telephone 020 7378 0505

Shaw Trust
Shaw House
Epsom Square
White Horse Business Park
Trowbridge
Wiltshire
BA14 0ZZ

Telephone: 01225 716350
Fax: 01225 716334
Minicom: 0345 697288
E-mail: stir@shaw-trust.org.uk

References

American Occupational Therapy Association (1995) Elements of clinical documentation (revision). American Journal of Occupational Therapy 49: 1032-5.

Anthony W, Blanch A (1987) Supported employment for persons who are psychiatrically disabled: an historical and conceptual perspective. Psychosocial Rehabilitation Journal 11: 5-23.

Anthony W, Jansen M (1984) Predicting the vocational capacity of the chronically mentally ill. American Psychologist 39: 537-44.

Anton J (1978) Studying individual change. In Goldman L (ed.). Research methods for counselors: practical approaches in a field setting. Wiley, New York. Cited in Creek J (ed.) (1998) Occupational Therapy: New Perspectives. London: Whurr.

Botterbusch KF (1989) Fourth National Forum on Issues in Vocational Assessment. Menomonie: University of Washington.

Brooks N, McKinley W, Symington C, Beattie A, Campsie L (1987) Return to work within the first seven years of severe head injury. Brain Injury 1: 5-19.

Cook J (1992) Job ending among youth and adults with severe mental illness. Journal of Mental Health Administration 19: 158-69.

Creek J (1998) (ed.) Occupational Therapy: New Perspectives. London: Whurr.

Crepeau F, Sherzer P (1993) Predictors and indicators of work status after traumatic brain injury: a meta-analysis. Neuropsychological Rehabilitation 3: 5-35.

Dikmen SS, Temkin NR, Machamer JE, Holubkon AL, Fraser RT, Win RH (1994) Employment following traumatic head injuries. Archives of Neurology 51: 177-86.

Disability Rights Handbook, April 2000-April 2001. London: Disability Alliance Educational and Research Association.

Garner J (1995) Prevocational training within a secure environment: a programme designed to enable the forensic patient to prepare for mainstream opportunities. British Journal of Occupational Therapy 58: 2-6.

George C, Allirajah D, Donnelly C, Fitzpatrick P, Frobisher F, Hynes B, Mitchell S, Robinson S, Simmons D, Stagg P, Tait G, Thurley D, Turville P (2000) Welfare Benefits Handbook 2000/2001. 2 edn. London: Child Poverty Action Group.

Godfrey H, Bishara SN, Partridge FM, Knight RG (1993) Neuropsychological impairment and return to work following severe closed head injury: implications for clinical management. New Zealand Medical Journal 106: 301-3.

Greenwood RJ, McMillan TM (1993) Models of rehabilitation programmes for the brain injured adult. I: Current provision, efficacy and good practice. Clinical Rehabilitation 7: 248-55.

Gronwall D, Wrightson P, Wadell P (1990) Head Injury: The Facts. A Guide for Families and Care-givers. Oxford: Oxford University Press.

Groswasser Z, Melamed S, Agranov E, Keren O (1999) Return to work as an integrative outcome measure following traumatic brain injury. Neuropsychological Rehabilitation 9: 493-504.

Humphrey M, Oddy M (1980) Return to work after head injury: a review of post war studies. Injury 12: 107-14.

International Labour Organization (1983) Employment and Disability. Geneva: ILO.

Johnson RP (1987) Return to work after severe head injury. International Disability Studies 9: 49-54.

Johnson RP (1998) How do people get back to work after severe head injury? A 10 year follow-up study. Neuropsychological Rehabilitation 8: 61–79.

Jones M (2001) A return to productive activity utilizing the clubhouse model with people with traumatic brain injury. Conference presentation: Towards a Productive Life after TBI, the European Platform for Vocational Rehabilitation and Rehabilitation. UK, February 2001.

Kreutzer JS, Wehman P, Norton MV, Stonnington HH (1991) Supported employment and compensatory strategies for enhancing vocational outcome following traumatic brain injury. International Disability Studies 13: 162–71.

Langman C (2000) Employment Issues After Brain Injury. Conference presentation. September 2000.

Lloyd C, Samra P (2000) Occupational therapy and work-related programmes for people with a mental illness. British Journal of Therapy and Rehabilitation 7: 254–61.

Low C (1994) After the rhetoric – equal opportunities policy in the 1990s. Rehabilitation Network 4: 14–19.

McMillan TM, Greenwood RJ (1993). Models of rehabilitation programmes for the brain injured adult. II: model services and suggestions for change in the UK. Clinical Rehabilitation 7: 346–55.

Neistadt ME (1995) Assessing clients' priorities: whose goals are they? Occupational Therapy Practice 11: 37–9.

Newcombe F (1982) The psychological consequences of closed head injury: assessment and rehabilitation. Injury 14: 111–36.

Niemeyer L, Jacobs K, Reynolds-Lynch K, Bettencourt C, Lang S (1994) Work hardening: past, present and future – the work programmes special interest section national work-hardening outcomes study. American Journal of Occupational Therapy 48: 327–36.

Oddy M, Humphrey M, Uttley D (1978) Subjective impairment and social recovery after closed head injury. Journal of Neurology Neurosurgery and Psychiatry 41: 611–16.

Oddy M, Coughlan T, Tyerman A, Jenkins D (1985) Social adjustment after closed head injury: a further follow up 7 years after injury. Journal of Neurology Neurosurgery and Psychiatry 48: 564–8.

O'Neill J, Hibbard MR, Brown M, Jaffe M, Vandergoot D, Weiss MJ (1998) The effect of employment on quality of life and community integration after traumatic brain injury. Journal of Head Trauma Rehabilitation 13: 68–79.

Park S, Duran L, Fisher AG (1997) Evaluation and intervention planning: enhancing ADL performance. In Fisher AG (ed.) Assessment of Motor and Processing Skills. 2 edn. Fort Collins: Three Star Press, pp. 87–117.

Ponsford JL, Olver JH, Curran C, Ng M (1995) Prediction of employment status 2 years after traumatic brain injury. Brain Injury 9: 11–20.

Pozner A, Ng M, Hammond J, Shepherd G (1996) Working it Out. Brighton: Pavilion Publishing.

Ross PJ (1982) Basic work assessment and rehabilitation procedures. British Journal of Occupational Therapy 45: 270–2.

Sale P, West M, Sherron P, Wehman PH (1991) Exploratory analysis of job separation from supported employment of persons with traumatic brain injury. Journal of Head Injury Rehabilitation 6: 1–11.

Thomas DF, Menz FE (1990) Conclusions of a national think tank on issues relevant to community based employment for survivors of traumatic brain injury. American Rehabilitation 33: 20-4.

Thomsen IV (1984) Late outcome of very severe blunt head trauma: a 10–15 year second follow up. Journal of Neurology Neurosurgery and Psychiatry 47: 260-8.

Thurgood J (1999) The employment implications of the Disability Discrimination Act 1995 and a suggested format for developing reasonable adjustments. British Journal Occupational Therapy 62: 290-4.

Tyerman AD (1999) Working out: a joint DOH/ES traumatic brain injury vocational rehabilitation project. Abridged report. Aylesbury: Aylesbury Vale Community Healthcare NHS Trust.

Wehman PH, Kreutzer JS, West MD, Sherron PD, Zasler PD, Groath CH, Stonnington HH, Burns CT, Sale PR (1990) Return to work for people with traumatic brain injury: a supported approach. Archives of Physical Medicine and Rehabilitation 71: 1047-52.

Wehman PH, Kregel J, Sherron PD, Nguyen S, Kreutzer JS, Fry R, Zazler ND (1993) Critical factors associated with the successful supported employment placement of patients with severe traumatic brain injury. Brain Injury 7: 31-44.

Wehman PH, West MD, Kregel J, Sherron PD, Kreutzer JS (1995) Return to work for persons with severe traumatic brain injury: a data based approach to programme development. Journal of Head Trauma Rehabilitation 10: 27-39.

Wrightson P, Gronwall D (1981) Time off work and symptoms after minor head injury. Injury 12: 445-54.

CHAPTER 8
Psychosocial issues

ROSEMARY GRAVELL

The term psychosocial encompasses 'notions such as adjustment to disability, ability to pursue a normal life, ability to play a variety of social roles, ability to maintain social relationships, quality of life, satisfaction with life . . . and the ability to cope with the demands of life' (Oddy, 1997). In some ways all the chapters in this book that consider specific aspects of rehabilitation are therefore related to psychosocial issues. Physical, cognitive, communicative and behavioural aspects may all affect an individual's psychosocial state – for example, a physical disability may limit the social roles he can take on and a communication disorder will inevitably affect social relationships. However, the psychosocial consequences of head injury are worthy of consideration in their own right, not least because they are often cited as the most persistent of all the disabilities. They have rarely been given the attention they deserve in rehabilitation settings, perhaps because they are difficult to identify, measure and treat.

Psychosocial issues involve external factors, which can be objectively assessed, such as the ability to perform certain social and work tasks, and internal factors, which are subjective and personal, such as the sense of wellbeing and self-esteem (Prigatano, 1986). Commonly, consideration of personality falls into this area.

This book is concerned with reintegration into the community. The persistent nature of psychosocial problems, such as decreased social contact, loneliness and depression, suggests that they may be the greatest challenge to successful reintegration. After severe brain injury, Tate et al. (1989) indicate that between 40% and 75% may still have psychosocial problems, six to eight years post-injury. Hellawell, Taylor and Pentland (1999) looked at moderate traumatic brain injury and found deterioration in psychosocial outcomes between 12 and 24 months after injury. Mathias and Coats (1999) studied people who, after mild head injury, were diagnosed with post-concussional syndrome, and also found increased emotional problems over time.

270

Kinsella, Packer and Oliver (1991) postulate that cognitive impairment acts as a 'protective buffer' limiting the development of emotional distress consequent to social isolation. While this may be true for some, there is evidence that psychosocial problems are the greatest concern for many clients (for example, Klonoff, Snow and Costa, 1986) and, indeed, for their families (for example, Lezak, 1978). This chapter will consider what psychosocial effects may result from head injury and which clients may be most at risk. Current assessment approaches and possible management options will then be outlined.

This chapter draws on various research findings and it is worth noting, at this stage, the enormous methodological difficulties faced by researchers in this field. Often broad areas, such as personality, are broken into a variety of factors for study purposes but results will not necessarily extend to other factors within that broad area. Finding matched control groups can be difficult. Often studies cannot be directly compared because of methodological differences.

Interpretation of results can also be potentially misleading. It is important to remember that the head-injured population is not representative of the general population. More of those with head injury will have pre-existing psychosocial problems. Thus, comparisons between, for example, rates of depression in the former and the latter will not necessarily indicate the effects of head injury *per se*. It may reflect characteristics of the group of people who are more at risk of head injury.

The development of psychosocial problems

Psychosocial problems seem to develop gradually, with evidence suggesting clients will face different issues at different times after the initial injury. Individual aspects of psychosocial problems will be discussed but it will become apparent that these aspects overlap with each other and interact in various ways. Discussing each area helps to focus on particular issues but most clients will present a more complicated picture. The study of head injury is never that simple! To illustrate the gradual development of psychosocial problems and the mixture of issues that arise over time it may be helpful to consider an individual case history.

When he was 25 years old, JD was in a car accident. He was admitted to a specialist unit and received acute care and initial rehabilitation as an inpatient. He presented with executive dysfunction, marked attention problems, mild cognitive-communication disorder and left-sided weakness. He did not initially cooperate with rehabilitation efforts, as he expressed the belief that he would soon be better. He used the evidence of rapid initial recovery of some physical function to support this belief. At this stage he was in the relatively protected hospital environment and therefore few demands were put on his executive and cognitive skills. His wife and parents and a variety of friends and colleagues visited him.

After eight weeks, he was discharged home and was referred to a specialist day rehabilitation centre. He began to express anger at what had happened and his family reported that they felt his personality had changed, although they noted his friends seemed less aware of this, in their shorter interactions.

Six months after the accident JD began to raise issues about his relationship with his wife. He had established a rapport with one member of the team, and in individual sessions he expressed an inability to understand why his wife did not want to resume sexual relations. She, in discussion with another team member, described feeling as if he was not the same person and that they had lost their former level of communication. At the same time, she expressed guilt about this as other people did not appear to see him as so altered. She also noted the fact that his friends no longer visited as much and he seemed unmotivated to try to maintain former friendships.

JD was cooperating in rehabilitation to a reasonable degree but still made comments suggesting that he believed that he would recover fully. It became apparent that he did not want to join in any social situation involving more than two or three people. He was anxious about how people would judge his physical appearance, and in team meetings several members expressed concern over his self-esteem and mood.

One year after his accident he was becoming more insightful about his difficulties and less optimistic about his recovery. His mood was very low and he talked of feeling isolated. His wife began to discuss her own future and the possibility of separation. His only regular social contact by this stage, apart from her, was his parents. Despite expressing a lack of satisfaction with his social life, he did not appear motivated to engage in previously enjoyed or new leisure pursuits, despite having the physical ability to do so. He was referred for treatment of his depression.

Five years after the accident, he was divorced and lived alone, with support from his parents and a social services carer. He continued to feel lonely and isolated. He had not been able to return to employment. The comment he most regularly heard from those who knew him at the time of the accident was how well he had done!

This offers only a broad outline of the problems experienced by one individual but it does illustrate the persistent nature of psychosocial problems and how they change and develop over time. It also suggests how the problems are directly related to the individual's environment and the people around him. Particular issues will now be discussed, but it is important to bear in mind this overall context.

Adjustment to disability

Adjustment to disability is the ability of an individual to come to terms with the fact that certain elements of his disability are permanent. This is obviously not an issue restricted to head-injured clients. However, it is an important aspect within the rehabilitation process and there may be specific factors affecting those with head injury. As people do adjust it will become apparent in their readiness to adapt their lifestyle to their impairment and to make realistic future plans. It is normal for mood to be depressed, as clients go through a grieving process, mourning what has been lost. If this depression is prolonged or extreme, intervention may be needed. Even after mild to moderate injury clients often face reduced confidence and a need to revise their sense of self. Additional physical and cognitive impairments may compound the difficulties of this adjustment process and the ability of the person to cope with decreased independence and competence. Reduced insight will also be a factor. Tyerman and Humphrey (1984) note that head-injured people may perceive themselves as less able than they were pre-injury, but at the same time tend to see themselves as better than other 'typical' head-injured clients.

Adjustment will take differing courses and periods of time depending on the individual person and his needs. Not all clients will be able to adjust fully to their disability, and as a consequence will never reach their potential in terms of functional ability. One such client, BE, a young man who had been injured in a traffic accident, repeatedly refused to attempt suggested tasks in the belief he would 'get better anyway'. He had severe physical, perceptual and cognitive problems and, in the opinion of the rehabilitation team, would never be able to live independently. He continued to believe he would resume his former lifestyle.

As well as the impairment level and degree of insight, other factors may be implicated in the adjustment process. For example, the way individuals perceive the incident in which they were injured can be relevant. Bulman and Wortman (1977) found self-blame in accident victims (not just those with head injury) to be associated with good coping, whereas those who blamed others or fate coped less well. Another example, is described by Roueche and Fordyce (1983) who suggested that adjustment is more likely if the patient, family and staff all view the situation from a similar realistic perspective.

Personality

After head injury, changes in personality are often cited by clients, and relatives, as a major cause of stress. 'Personality' is a somewhat nebulous, hard-to-define term and yet is consistently heard within discussion about head injury. Prigatano, Pepping and Klonoff (1986) define it as 'patterns of emotional and motivational responses that develop during our life-time; these are highly influenced by early life experiences, are modifiable although with difficulty, and greatly influence (and are influenced by) cognitive processes'. No clear distinction can be made between personality and behaviour changes, and many clinicians prefer the latter term. This is because it is easier to define and therefore plan management in terms of behaviour (that is, what is observed) than the more abstract characteristics of personality. Behaviour change is discussed in Chapter 5.

Reported personality changes may include changes in concern and emotional responsiveness, in attitudes and the way they are expressed, in level of interest in former pursuits, and in sense of humour. Relatives may describe inertia, egocentricity, childishness, inflexibility, passivity, irritability and aggression. Clinicians in the field will often hear the words 'he is not the same person', even after what may seem to outsiders to be relatively mild changes. Subtle differences in 'personality' can have lasting and profound effects on relationships. Certain traits may appear to be exaggerated versions of the former personality but, equally, former traits may be less apparent – for example, individuals described previously as rather chauvinist might become more extreme and outspoken in their views after head injury, whereas others may become more liberal in their attitude.

Personality changes are associated with marital break-up, social isolation and unemployment (for example, Zencius et al., 1990) and it is notable that they have the greatest impact on psychosocial skills and outcome (Brooks, 1984). Often there seems to be an increase in severity of psychosocial issues over time (Brooks and McKinlay, 1983).

It has been generally accepted that pre-trauma personality is important to psychosocial functioning, but there is little empirical evidence of this. Tate (1998) looked at pre-morbid psychosocial factors and their influence on rehabilitation outcomes, to evaluate the assumptions that pre-morbid adjustment and personality are relevant. He felt that early studies might have used outmoded measures of pre-morbid social maladjustment (such as illegitimacy) and that their conclusions were therefore value judgements. In severe head injury, Tate did not find these factors to be correlated to outcome. Malia, Powell and Torode (1995) looked at four aspects of personality – locus of control, humour, optimism and easy-going disposition – and did not find that pre-trauma personality made a significant difference. Easy-going disposition and the use of humour *post-trauma* did make a difference. However, it may be that only certain personality factors are relevant to psychosocial functioning or that all personality variables are relevant, but operate via other mediating influences. Further research is needed to investigate more fully. What Malia et al. did find was that time post injury affected the changes in personality that were reported.

Social issues and family relationships

Chapter 9 looks at issues from the perspective of the carer and many of the same studies are relevant here. Carers have, by definition, a pre-existing relationship with the injured person, but for the individual with brain damage it is often the ability to maintain or to make new relationships outside the family that causes most concern. The more severely head injured may well have little contact outside the family – Thomsen (1984) found two-thirds of her sample had no outside social contacts. Others have also found this, with head-injured people more likely to have their primary attachment to a parent. Oddy et al. (1985) found that 60% of their sample had no boyfriend or girlfriend, and that this was perceived as the major problem – both by the client and the family. Often head injury affects young people, predominantly men, when they are at the early stages of forming relationships but the injury forces a renewed dependency on the family (Oddy, Humphrey and Uttley, 1978). The years between 20 and 40 are the crucial period for the development of both friendship and romantic relationships (Erikson, 1959).

It appears that between six months and two years post-injury, social support networks decrease and pre-injury friendships dissolve (Oddy and Humphrey, 1980). This will not be helped by long periods away from social contact in hospital or rehabilitation centres. This results in a lack of peer support – which, Altman and Taylor (1973) postulate, may also affect the opportunity to relearn social skills. Increased dependency on the family limits the opportunity to make new friends. Oddy et al. (1985) found loneliness to be the greatest difficulty in their long-term follow-up study. Employment helped to reduce social isolation. Thomsen (1984) found the two main problems cited by head-injured subjects 10–15 years after the injury were memory and social isolation. Head-injured clients may find their only contact is with family or paid support workers.

There may be a variety of reasons for decreased social contact, but the main reason is change in behaviour or personality. Head injury may cause specific impairments that make the client less acceptable to his social group – perhaps physically or behaviourally. Particularly in a younger age group, friends may not know how to handle the situation. Physical impairment may also restrict the ability to get to community social activities. Emotionally, low self-esteem can develop and clients may not be prepared to enter social situations. Cognitively, people may be apathetic or passive, or not able to initiate communication. Cognitive-communication disorder and more specific, focal speech and language disorders were discussed in Chapter 6 and have obvious social implications. Certain social settings make the resultant handicap worse – for example, noisy environments or groups will accentuate the effects of a communication difficulty or attentional deficits. Often, of course, a combination of factors will be involved, complicating the picture further. For example, a person may use a physical difficulty, which could actually be circumvented, as an excuse if there are self-esteem and confidence issues causing anxiety about social situations.

AD was a 40-year-old man who sustained a head injury at work. He coped reasonably within his very supportive family, but when he and his wife attempted to go out with friends, as they had done previously, he became quite anxious and withdrawn. Their usual outing was to a local pub and the combination of noise and being in a group of people made him unable to cope. He described himself as feeling 'stupid' and 'isolated'. Eventually they stopped these outings, which reduced his anxiety but also reduced both his and his wife's social opportunities. In turn, the loss of contact with friends caused both to feel isolated and depressed.

Perhaps rehabilitation efforts in general do not recognize enough that social contact and meaningful friendships are critical to the quality of life. However, this may reflect the very great difficulty in helping people deal with psychosocial changes rather than a lack of awareness of the issue. People with severe head injury are at high risk of loneliness and social isolation – potentially for the rest of their lives.

Sexual problems

Sexual problems are common after head injury. Kosteljanetz, Jensen and Norgard (1981) cite 58% of people with post-concussional syndrome have sexual problems, while O'Carroll, Woodrow and Maroun (1991) found 50% of their neurologically impaired subjects to be sexually dysfunctional. Problems may be physical or psychological, and may affect partners not just the head-injured client. Direct physical effects may include specific neurological damage and non-specific effects of fatigue, pain and so on. Psychological effects may develop after a head injury. The individual may feel anxious, unattractive, guilty, angry, or fearful. Partners may feel they are no longer attracted to the person, perhaps because they feel they are not 'the same person', or because they might be frightened of hurting the client. Problems might also be relationship based as roles change and different dependencies are established.

Banks (1998) suggests a classification of problems into dysfunction, difficulties and dissatisfaction. The dysfunction category would include changes in desire/drive, arousal, and orgasm. Sexual difficulties would encompass relationship factors, such as the ability to relax, to indulge in foreplay, or a sense of revulsion. Dissatisfaction appears to relate more to difficulties than to dysfunction, which fuels further anxieties about attractiveness and self-image problems.

There has been little research into the effect of head injury on sexuality, with the studies that do exist often suffering from cultural and gender bias, which will affect the relevance and generalizability of the results. Problems that have been noted include erectile dysfunction, and hypo- or hypersexuality (such as excessive masturbation). While most discussion clinically seems to be concerned with those who are disinhibited, either physically or verbally, in fact the opposite problem is much more likely to occur. Kreutzer and Zasler (1989) found hyposexuality to be common in men after brain injury as a result of decreased self-confidence, perceived sexual appearance, and depression. Garden, Bontke and Hoffman (1990) cite 75% of women and 55% of men as having decreased post-injury sexual activity. The reason clinical discussion focuses so often on disinhibition and hypersexuality, is that these cause more obvious problems in relation to community reintegration. Management of disinhibited behaviour is addressed in the chapter on behavioural issues.

Rosenbaum and Najenson (1976) state that 'sexual difficulties are seldom dealt with in detail in the literature despite the fact that they arise in clinical practice and range from minor (performance anxiety) impotence in the injured patient to severe relationship disturbances and feelings of frank distaste on the part of an injured patient's spouse'. They go on to say that sexual disturbance is more likely the more a person has changed in personality and behaviour.

Coughlan (1998) referred to the need to develop and to maintain relationships. Starting or developing relationships will depend on self-esteem, opportunity, the reactions of others, sexual experience and knowledge, and the ability to modify behaviour. Maintaining a sexual relationship after a head injury, may depend on the pre-injury state of the relationship, the partner's personality, enjoyment of sex and reaction to the injured person, concern over children, the ability of the head-injured person to be aware and to modify behaviour and the willingness of both to adjust.

To illustrate problems that arise in rehabilitation work, it may be of interest to consider three case histories. BB was a 35-year-old man who had been married for two years, but in the same relationship for 10 years. Having made a good physical recovery he was keen to resume a sexual relationship with his wife, but did have language and cognitive problems albeit at a mild level. His wife, however, found that even these relatively mild changes had subtly affected his personality and she could no longer feel sexually attracted to him. She still expressed her love for him but, after some months, decided that separation was the best option. BB could not understand why she did not want to have a sexual relationship, having limited insight into his changed character and therefore being unable to modify his behaviour. Subsequently BB did develop a sexual relationship with someone else, who did not know him prior to the injury.

GR was a 40-year-old woman who was severely physically, linguistically and cognitively affected after her injury. She lived at home with her husband and it became apparent to rehabilitation staff that she was in a highly vulnerable position when she managed to communicate that her husband was making sexual demands that she did not want but was not able to reject.

The final illustration is of a young head-injured woman, in her late teens, who experienced very low self-esteem based upon her altered physical appearance and mobility difficulties. She would not attempt to resume her former active social life because she felt unable to risk rejection, having convinced herself that no one could possibly find her attractive. Interestingly, her view was based on her knowledge of how she would have viewed others in her position before she was injured.

These cases are not isolated examples and, clinically, it is likely such cases are the tip of the iceberg. It may be that individual clients do not feel able to discuss such issues or that rehabilitation staff do not feel able to address them. Often it appears that, when sexual concerns are discussed, it is with the member of the team, regardless of profession, with whom the client has time to build a rapport. Team members, however, need to be aware of the possibility of such issues and to respond appropriately to hints from the client.

Vocational and leisure activities

Vocational issues are dealt with in Chapter 7, and as such will not be considered in detail in this chapter. However, it is worth noting that both work and leisure pursuits are relevant to discussion of psychosocial problems. Oddy (1997) notes that, in severe head injury, after 12 and 24 months, people had 50% fewer leisure activities than pre-injury, not attributable to physical limitation. Interestingly, however, relatives did not rate them as being more bored and it may be that cognitive issues mean some clients are content to be restricted. Rehabilitation must obviously address leisure time, perhaps particularly for those unlikely to return to employment. It may be, as Oddy (1997) suggests, that one goal of such intervention may be to help relatives.

Chronic unemployment can add to depression and feelings of low self-esteem (Wehman and Kreutzer, 1990). Occupation or goal related activities do seem to be important to the individual's feelings of self-worth.

Psychiatric conditions

House (1997) categorizes the most common presenting problems seen by psychiatric services in neurological rehabilitation settings as disorders of mood (including depression, anxiety and irritability), negative syndromes (such as apathy and passivity), poor compliance, relationship problems and provoked mental illness (when the stress of a neurological disorder appears to provoke a severe mental illness). However, most clients with head injury, as well as other neurological conditions, will probably never see a psychiatrist. It is likely to be only the obviously severely affected individuals who are referred, while others are managed by the rehabilitation team. The differential diagnosis between organic and reactive disorders may not be easy but when the problems are perceived as due to the organic brain damage it can be difficult to gain access to psychiatric services. There may also be a difference in relation to the length of time since the injury – those with acute symptoms who are in an inpatient situation may have easier access to such services. This volume is concerned predominantly with community services, however, and it is important that all rehabilitation staff are aware of the possible psychiatric sequelae of head injury. It is also important that the brain injury and psychiatric services work together.

The overlap between psychiatric symptomatology and possible cognitive or behavioural consequences of head injury is considerable. Members of the team may need to refer outside the team, for example to a community mental health team or to a neuropsychiatrist. The most likely psychiatric conditions in a community-based head-injured population are the mood disorders – depression, mania and/or anxiety.

Mood disorders

Depression and anxiety have been found to be common after severe head injury. For example, Tyerman and Humphrey (1984) looked at subjects between two and 15 months after the incident and found 60% to have clinical symptoms of depression. Different studies suggest vastly different levels of anxiety after head injury, ranging from 11% to 70% (Klonoff, 1971; Lewis, 1942). In fact, estimates of the frequency of depression and anxiety after brain injury vary widely (McCleary, 1998). Even after minor head injury there is evidence of significant depressive symptoms – Rutherford, Merrett and McDonald (1977) found 6% to be severely depressed. Bowen et al. (1998) looked at newly injured patients to evaluate how many would have significant mood disorder six months after injury. Of their sample of 99, 38% had anxiety and/or depression and they found those people who were unoccupied before the injury were three times more likely to have a mood disorder. Others have also noted that symptoms may not start until six months or more after the injury (Varney, Martzke and Roberts, 1987). This may be due to individuals only recognizing the reality of their situation as they attempt to resume their former lifestyle and activities.

Fedoroff et al. (1992) compared acute and delayed onset depression. Of their small sample group of 66, 26% had major and 3% minor depressive symptoms, associated with premorbid vulnerability and, at the acute stage, specific lesion location. However at follow-up the lesion site did not correlate, while poor social functioning was significantly associated throughout. In a second study (1993) they looked at 41 subjects who were not initially depressed and found 27% diagnosed with major depression and 9% with minor depression.

Jorge, Robinson and Arndt's 1993 paper suggests only personal psychiatric history significantly differentiated those with acute depression from the non-depressed group. Those with acute depression did appear to show a link to left dorsolateral frontal and basal ganglia lesions. The people who developed delayed onset depressive symptoms had significantly poorer social functioning, but tended to have less severe depression and less impairment of daily living skills than the acute group. The authors suggested that there are different etiological mechanisms between acute (neurophysiological changes) and delayed (poor social functioning) onset. That is, that the nature of the depression changes over time towards more psychological symptoms.

Jorge, Robinson and Arndt (1993) looked at whether there are symptoms that are specific for depressed mood in patients with traumatic brain injury. They compared autonomic (for example, lack of energy) and psychological (for example, hopelessness, self-esteem) symptoms in clients who described themselves as depressed and those who did not. They found that the 'depressed' did have more symptoms, but that symptoms that discriminated between the depressed and the non-depressed varied over time. Psychological impairment in excess of the apparent severity of the injury and poor cooperation are strong indicators of persistent depression, as is premorbid psychiatric history (Kraus, 1999). Apathy is commonly seen with depression (Kant, Duffy and Pivovarnik, 1988).

Mania has also been found to be more common than in the general population – Jorge, Robinson and Arndt (1993) suggest an incidence of 9%, and link it to right limbic lesions, family history or pre-existing sub-cortical atrophy. Again, the incidence comparison is somewhat misleading because of the nature of the head-injured population.

There are methodological issues in many of the studies of the incidence of depression. Many focus on a certain demographic group – young, white males of lower social-economic background, often with a history of drug abuse. Some control for conditions that may complicate the argument, but in fact are relevant to consideration of depression after brain injury. For example, Ridsdale et al. (1996) note a higher incidence of depression and suicide in those with epilepsy. Harrison (2000) also draws attention to the fact that some medications have side effects that can mimic psychiatric symptoms.

The high incidence of anxiety and depression is often noted but the relationship to social support systems has not been studied to a great extent. Relatives report anxiety and depression (McKinlay et al., 1981) and the reports do not diminish over time (Brooks, Campsie and Symington, 1987). From the perspective of the client, Tyerman and Humphrey (1984) found 64%

of their small sample of 25, had significant psychiatric disturbance. Kinsella, Moran and Ford (1988) noted that the availability of a confidant was an important predictor of depression. Various researchers do suggest a link with social interactions (for example, Elsass and Kinsella, 1987; Ranseen, 1990).

After a significant head injury it is normal to suffer psychological reactions and face problems adjusting to the changes caused by the injury. It is when the reaction is prolonged or particularly severe that specific management concerns arise. However, for all those suffering head injury, rehabilitation staff need to acknowledge and address psychological needs as well as physical and cognitive, in order for rehabilitation to be at its most effective. As Morton and Wehman (1995) point out, mood may affect long-term rehabilitation outcome, so untreated emotional problems can waste resources.

Assessment

Much of the research mentioned suggests high levels of psychosocial problems persisting over a long period and severely affecting individuals' ability to cope and to lead fulfilling lives. However, clinicians will know that not all clients fit this pattern and some appear to cope remarkably well. Indeed more research now is focusing on discovering which factors do put people at risk of long-term handicap. Those at risk in general or in specific areas need to be identified so that intervention can be targeted.

Many factors may be implicated, including cause, severity, lesion site, neurological impairments, time since injury, age, education, socioeconomic, and premorbid factors (such as substance abuse, relationship status and psychiatric history). Lishman (1973) made a distinction between direct neurological factors and indirect influences on psychosocial adjustment. The latter may include responses to the environment, litigation and so on. Similarly, Kendall and Terry (1996) suggest a range of antecedent variables may be implicated but, if so, some may be more important than others. For example, Vilkki et al. (1994) found executive abilities more predictive than intelligence or memory. Tate and Broe (1999) studied a variety of biographical, injury, impairment and psychological measures (such as self-esteem). They found in severe brain injury the main determinants of psychosocial function were initial severity and consequent neuropsychological impairments (particularly behavioural), and time since injury. Other studies were mentioned earlier that did not find premorbid personality to be relevant to outcome.

Overall, focus has been on only a few variables and much more research is needed to establish who is at risk of persistent psychosocial difficulty. Factors such as financial state, environmental resources, coping strategies and so on may be equally important. There is no proven method of predicting outcome and thus establishing a proactive programme to support community reintegration. However, Morton and Wehman (1995) state that 'Clinicians will need to diagnose and treat these problems much earlier in the community re-entry process in order to have effective rehabilitation for clients with traumatic brain injury'.

It is important that behavioural deficiencies and social maladjustment pre-injury are not mistaken for the effects of head injury, but it is equally, if not more, important that impairment is recognized when it does exist. Weinstein and Wells (1981) note one case where four admissions to psychiatric hospital were made before an organic cause was discovered. Rehabilitation teams must be aware of and sensitive to the psychosocial situation and the changing needs of the individual.

Assessments of psychosocial functioning include scales to be filled out by professional rehabilitation staff, carers' report forms and self-report scales. Self-report scales have been viewed with some doubt because of the high incidence of problems with insight and awareness after head injury. However, several studies have found that brain-injured people can accurately perceive and rate themselves. Malia, Powell and Torode (1995) found their subjects were more in tune with relatives' ratings than were the control group. Others, too, have indicated that self-reporting is valid after head injury (for example, Tyerman and Humphrey, 1984; Kinsella, Moran and Ford, 1988). Even if clients do report a different perspective from carers, such reports can indicate where there is a need for educational programmes.

Indeed, there are problems with all these approaches – for example, clinicians are limited by a lack of knowledge about the person pre-injury, which makes it difficult to interpret findings as the result of injury, rather than pre-existing characteristics. They also cannot assess in the various situations a client will face in daily life and clinical situations will often lack the emotional overlay that may elicit the problem. Self-report, although validated by studies like the above, may need caution especially in very severe head injury, when insight is likely to be affected. Carers' forms will be subjective and potentially emotionally biased.

There are, however, advantages in each case. Clinicians can assess from a knowledge base and experience. Carers will often see the situations in which the client's problems emerge and that the clinician is not able to experience. The client's evaluation is important for obvious reasons - particularly when considering psychosocial aspects.

There is a lack of assessments of psychosocial function created specifically for head-injured clients, despite the need for a satisfactory standardized assessment of social, personality and emotional sequelae. Such an assessment would have both clinical and medico-legal value. Some general scales have been used and others have been adapted for this population, and a few do exist which were developed specifically to apply to head-injured clients.

Scales developed for other populations include the Minnesota Multiphasic Personality Inventory, which has been analysed in relation to brain-injured clients (Alfano et al., 1991). The Neuropsychological Behaviour and Affect Profile (Nelson, Satz and D'Elia, 1994), which has subscales for indifference, inappropriateness, depression, mania and pragnosia (which refers to pragmatic aspects of communication), and the Neurobehavioural Rating Scale (Levin et al., 1987) were devised for traumatic brain injury. Jackson et al. (1992) modified the Katz Adjustment Scale, which was developed for psychiatric clients, to use in traumatic brain injury and spinal injury. Earlier use had found inconsistent results as to which factors were affected by brain injury, but their study established clinically relevant syndromes, in the areas emotional/psychosocial, physical/intellectual, and psychiatric.

The Headley Court Psychosocial Rating Scale was specifically designed for use with head-injured clients (Malia, Powell and Torode, 1995). Watts and Perlesz (1999) attempted to develop a psychosocial outcome risk indicator (PORI), on the principle that the broad context is needed rather than individual factors, in a clinical situation. They used this screening instrument in a study that suggests some value in predicting individuals and carers at risk of poor psychosocial outcome after 12 months, although a larger study is needed to back this pilot study. The screening consisted of the self-rated PORI scale, the Community Reintegration Questionnaire (Willer, Rosenthal and Kreutzer, 1993), the General Functioning Subscale from Epstein, Baldwin and Bishop's (1983) Family Assessment Device, the Problem Checklist (Kay, Cavallo and Ezrachi, 1995), and a general health questionnaire.

Specialist assessment will be needed for specific issues and referral outside the team may be required. Where such a service exists, specialist neuropsychiatry is preferable. Psychiatric assessment will seek to assess the stresses arising from any impairment and other areas of the person's life, to identify coping strategies and to explain the current mental state (House, 1997). Assessment will be through interview, if possible of the family as well, and behavioural observation. Similarly sexual difficulties will often need specialist assessment, looking at the individual's history and preferences, physical examination and clinical diagnostic investigations. The environment may need to be considered as inappropriate behaviours may be being inadvertently reinforced.

Management

At the beginning of the chapter, Prigatano's (1986) distinction between external and personal issues was mentioned. This distinction is useful in relation to management planning. The external issues relate to the objective ability to do social and work 'tasks', and management would often be through a functional approach, seeking to enable an individual to do those tasks. Most chapters in this volume discuss management techniques that would be appropriate to this element of psychosocial functioning. There are some specific issues, such as psychiatric or sexual problems, which have not been covered elsewhere, which will be briefly outlined below. The personal issues are more subjective and harder to address, and it is these that encompass aspects such as self-esteem and confidence, and general psychosocial functioning. In relation to the personal, subjective issues, intervention may include counselling or psychotherapy, environmental management, or the provision of education/information, to increase understanding and insight.

A proactive role might be appropriate in dealing with those considered to be at risk of psychosocial dysfunction, if such people can be identified. An annual review system going on for perhaps five to 10 years, may identify some affected clients as their circumstances change over time, but non-attendance may reflect those who have slipped through the net.

The timing of intervention is crucial. If it occurs too soon, when a client is not fully aware of the nature of the difficulties, little will be achieved. However, if intervention comes too late, it may not be possible to alter clients' beliefs about themselves or change behaviours, and social support networks may already have broken down. This means constant reviewing of the individual's needs and abilities, and good team communication.

Another principle would be to recognize, and respond appropriately to, normal reactions of depression and anxiety, as well as picking up on when those reactions develop into more specific psychological conditions. A balance is needed between realistic hope and telling the 'full story'. It is of course possible for clinicians to be too pessimistic, but false hope can also be damaging to the process of adjustment. Attention does need to be given to clients' confidence and self-esteem, as these are factors in people's ability and motivation to be socially active.

Society as a barrier to adjustment

This section of the chapter will consider general approaches and, briefly, some specific management techniques. It is worth mentioning one fundamental influence on rehabilitation of psychosocial problems, which is that social life does not happen in a vacuum and, therefore, the way in which society in general reacts to people with disabilities will always be a factor. This is not specific to people with head injury and there is not scope in this volume to address the issue, but it is a central factor that all rehabilitation workers need to bear in mind. To illustrate the point, consider HW, an 18-year-old whose physical rehabilitation was at a stage where he could attempt walking in a local town, if accompanied. His first excursion was marked by shoppers actually stopping to stare at him. Rehabilitation staff are so used to the world of disability that they can easily forget the way other people react. The importance of environmental support to enable maximal functioning is highlighted elsewhere in this volume and must not be underestimated.

Counselling/psychotherapy

Oddy (1997) claims that psychological therapy is 'an essential ingredient for any comprehensive rehabilitation service'. Prigatano (1986) supports this and feels it can help clients to consider the implications of what has happened and to foster a sense of realistic hope. The unconditional and non-judgemental nature of psychological therapies may help to raise self-esteem and acknowledge emotions that may be hard to discuss in other settings. However, cognitive issues can make this approach difficult. Alderman and Burgess (1990) described some of the limitations to using formal cognitive behavioural therapy with clients who have severe brain injury. Prigatano (1986) indicates how important it will be to structure interactions in line with the client's cognitive skills. For example, in working with a young man with marked memory problems it may help to limit the issues covered per session and to provide brief written summaries.

Environmental

A supportive social environment outside the rehabilitation setting is important to facilitate progress (Prigatano, Fordyce and Zeiner, 1984). It is, however, critical that relationships have meaning for clients and are not just artificially thrust upon them. This is easier said than done. Rehabilitation staff may be able to find appropriate community-based facilities offering a variety of social and work-related support – for example, the centres run by the charity Headway can be an invaluable resource. For some clients these centres, by bringing together people who have had similar experiences, enable friendships to develop, which do have meaning for the individuals. For others, friendships do not develop, and unfortunately rehabilitation clinicians cannot create friendships for their clients. These centres can have other roles as well, not least being able to offer respite to the families.

Education/information

Education and information have been addressed many times in this volume and they are no less relevant to psychosocial functioning, particularly when an individual's insight into these issues is reduced. Raising awareness can be the first step towards dealing with the issues. As is the case with more specific areas of functioning, education may be provided individually or with particular carers, or in group settings. The goals of each will differ from specific, individual points and advice, to general information. A group setting may be especially valid as it can provide opportunity for clients to meet others in a supportive setting and to talk with people who face similar issues.

Specific approaches

Psychiatric intervention

Psychiatric intervention will follow the general principles of psychiatric practice with other groups of clients, although some of the difficulties of differential diagnosis may be particularly pronounced in this group.

Knowledge of brain injury may help in distinguishing between cognitive impairment or behavioural anomalies and psychological conditions. House (1997) suggests the two routes of individual counselling and medication. The former is constrained when there are severe memory problems or a severe communication disorder. Tate and Broe (1999) point out that counselling may well be of benefit if depression is a dynamic process, changing over time from neurophysiological routes to psychological.

Sex therapy

Again, detailed discussion of specific therapies is outside the scope of this book. Actual physical sexual difficulties, such as erectile dysfunction, will need specialist therapies. In the case of erectile dysfunction, for example, this may include vacuum, injection, medication or implants – obviously not part of the repertoire of the average head injury rehabilitation team! Referral to specialists is essential. The psychological reasons for sexual problems, within the individual or the relationship, may well also benefit from specialist counselling, beyond the expertise of a rehabilitation team. However, it is important that rehabilitation staff are open to the possibility of this as a problem and able to respond appropriately if the subject is introduced.

Aylott et al. (2000), although written for nurses, does highlight generally applicable issues for staff. These include poor training/information, lack of professional experience of such problems, religious or personal views that may intrude, the need for the centre to have the right culture, and risk of embarrassment or lack of confidence to respond. All members of the team need to know how to handle such matters and what to do if issues are beyond their ability or difficult for them within their personal opinions.

Conclusion

Within the rehabilitation team it is important to be aware of the limitations of both individual and combined expertise. Care must be taken to ensure up-to-date knowledge within the service of the specialist help that can be accessed. However, every member of the team must be open to the possibility of psychosocial problems. Not all clients will be able to raise issues in a direct way because of continued misconceptions and stigma in society about problems such as depression or sexual difficulties. Many clients feel that psychosocial aspects are signs of weakness or inadequacy, or that they are somehow less relevant than the specific issues traditionally dealt with by the separate rehabilitation disciplines. It is clear that a physical problem can be mentioned to a physiotherapist, but there is no clear person with whom social problems can be discussed. It is not putting it too strongly to say that it is the team's duty to ensure clients, and families, can address these problems openly and in a non-judgemental setting.

References

Alderman N, Burgess PW (1990) Integrating cognition and behaviour: a pragmatic approach to brain injury rehabilitation. In Wood RL, Fussy I (eds) Cognitive Rehabilitation in Perspective. London: Taylor & Francis, pp. 204–28.

Alfano DP, Finlayson MA, Stearns GM, MacLennan RM (1991) Dimensions of neurobehavioural dysfunction. Neuropsychology 5: 35–41.

Altman I, Taylor DA (1973) Social Penetration: the Development of Interpersonal Relationships. New York: Irvington.

Aylott J, Beavan P, Blackburn M, Caulfield H, Davies S, Dennis S, Encabo B, Heath H, Stagg J, Thorpe L, White I (2000) Sexuality and Sexual Health in Nursing Practice. London: RCN.

Banks R (1998) The impact of illness and injury on sexuality. Paper presented at Sexuality after Head Injury – Perspectives on Assessment and Treatment conference, Sheffield.

Bowen A, Neumann V, Conner M, Tennant A, Chamberlain MA (1998) Mood disorders following traumatic brain injury: identifying the extent of the problem and the people at risk. Brain Injury 12(3): 177–90.

Brooks DN (1984) Head Injury and the Family. In Brooks DN (ed.) Closed Head Injury: Psychological, Social and Family Consequences. Oxford: Oxford University Press, pp. 123–47.

Brooks DN, McKinlay W (1983) Personality and behavioural change after severe blunt head injury. Journal of Neurology, Neurosurgery and Psychiatry 46: 336–44.

Brooks DN, Campsie L, Symington C (1987) The effects of severe head injury on patient and relative within seven years of injury. Journal Head Trauma Rehabilitation 2: 1–13.

Bulman RJ, Wortman CB (1977) Attributions of blame and coping in the real world. Journal of Personality and Social Psychology 35: 351–63.

Coughlan A (1998) Sexual relationships following head injury. Paper presented at Sexuality after Head Injury – Perspectives on Assessment and Treatment conference, Sheffield.

Elsass L, Kinsella G (1987) Social interaction following severe closed head injury. Psychological Medicine 17: 67–78.

Epstein NB, Baldwin LM, Bishop DS (1983) The McMaster Family Assessment Device. Journal of Marital and Family Therapy 9: 171–80.

Erikson E (1959) Identity and the life cycle. Psychological Issues 1: 5-9.

Federoff JP, Starkstein SE, Forrester AW, Jorge RE (1992) Depression in acute traumatic brain injury. American Journal of Psychiatry 149: 918-23.

Garden FH, Bontke CF, Hoffman M (1990) Sexual functioning and marital adjustment after traumatic brain injury. Journal of Head Trauma Rehabilitation 5(2): 52-9.

Harrison A (2000) Psychological problems in the neurology setting. Professional Nurse August 15(11): 706-9.

Hellawell DJ, Taylor R, Pentland B (1999) Cognitive and psychosocial outcome following moderate or severe traumatic brain injury. Brain Injury 13(7): 489-504.

House A (1997) Psychiatry in neurological rehabilitation. In Greenwood R, Barnes MP, McMillan TM, Ward CD (eds) Neurological Rehabilitation. Hove: Psychology Press, pp. 403-12.

Jackson HF, Hopewell CA, Glass CA, Warburg R, Dewey M, Ghadiali E (1992) The Katz Adjustment Scale: modification for use with victims of traumatic brain and spinal injury. Brain Injury 6(2): 109-27.

Jorge RE, Robinson RG, Arndt S (1993) Are there symptoms that are specific for depressed mood in patients with traumatic brain injury? Journal of Nervous and Mental Disease 181(2): 91-9.

Kant R, Duffy JD, Pivovarnik A (1988) The Prevalence of apathy following head injury. Brain Injury 12: 87-92.

Kay T, Cavallo M, Ezrachi O (1995) Head Injury Family Interview: a clinical and research tool Journal of Head Trauma Rehabilitation 10: 12-31.

Kendall E, Terry DJ (1996) Psychosocial adjustment following closed head injury. A model for understanding individual differences and predicting outcome. Neuropsychological Rehabilitation 6: 101-32.

Kinsella G, Moran C, Ford B (1988) Emotional Disorder and its assessment within the severe head injured population. Psychological Medicine 18: 57-63.

Kinsella G, Packer S, Oliver J (1991) Maternal reporting of behaviour following very severe blunt head injury. Journal of Neurology, Neurosurgery and Psychiatry 54: 422-6.

Klonoff H (1971) Head Injuries in children: predisposing factors, accident proneness and sequelae. American Journal of Public Health 61: 2405-17.

Klonoff PS, Snow WG, Costa LD (1986) Quality of life in patients 2 to 4 years after closed head injury. Neurosurgery 19: 735-43.

Kosteljanetz M, Jensen T, Norgard B (1981) Sexual and hypothamic dysfunction in the post-concussional syndrome. Acta Neurologica Scandinavica 63: 169-80.

Kraus MF (1999) Neuropsychiatric sequelae: assessment and pharmocologic intervention. In Marion DW (ed.) Traumatic Brain Injury 14. New York: Thieme, pp. 173-85.

Kreutzer JS, Zasler ND (1989) Psychosexual consequences of traumatic brain injury: methodology and preliminary findings. Brain Injury 3: 177-86.

Levin HS, High WM, Goethe KE, Sisson RA, Overall JE, Rhoades HM, Eisenberg HM, Kalisky Z, Gary HE (1987) The neurobehavioural rating scale: assessment of the behavioural sequelae of head injury by the clinician. Journal of Neurology, Neurosurgery and Psychiatry 50: 182-93.

Lewis A (1942) Discusssion on differential diagnosis and treatment of post-concussional states. Proceedings of the Royal Society of Medicine 35: 607-14.

Lezak MD (1978) Living with the characterologically altered brain injured patient. Journal of Clinical Psychiatry 39: 592-8.

Lishman WA (1973) The Psychiatric Sequelae of head injury: a review. Psychological Medicine 3: 304–18.

Malia K, Powell G, Torode S (1995) Personality and psychosocial function after brain injury. Brain Injury 9(7): 697–12.

Mathias JL, Coats JL (1999) Emotional and cognitive sequelae to mild traumatic brain injury. Journal of Clinical and Experimental Neuropsychology 21(2): 200–15

McCleary C, Satz P, Forney D, Light R, Zaucha K, Asarnow R, Namerow N (1998) Depression after traumatic brain injury as a function of the Glasgow Outcome Score. Journal of Clinical and Experimental Psychology 20: 270–9.

McKinlay WW, Brooks DN, Bond MR, Martinage DP, Marshall MM (1981) The short term outcome of severe blunt head injury as reported by the relatives of the head injured person. Journal of Neurology, Neurosurgery and Psychiatry 44: 527–33.

Morton MV, Wehman P (1995) Psychosocial and emotional sequelae of individuals with traumatic brain injury: a literature review and recommendations. Brain Injury 9(1): 81–92.

Nelson L, Satz P, D'Elia L (1994) The Neurobehavioural Behaviour and Affect Profile. Palo Alto CA: Mind Garden Press.

O'Carroll RE, Woodrow J, Maroun F (1991) Pschosexual and psychosocial sequelae of closed head injury. Brain Injury 5: 303–13.

Oddy M (1997) Psychosocial consequences of brain injury. In Greenwood R, Barnes MP, McMillan TM, Ward CD (eds) Neurological Rehabilitation. Hove: Psychology Press, pp. 423–33.

Oddy M, Humphrey M (1980) Social recovery during the year following severe head injury. Journal of Neurology, Neurosurgery and Psychiatry 43: 798–802.

Oddy M, Humphrey M, Uttley D (1978) Subjective impairment and social recovery after closed head injury. Journal of Neurology, Neurosurgery and Psychiatry 41: 611–16.

Oddy M, Coughlan T, Tyerman A, Jenkins D (1985) Social adjustment after closed head injury: a further follow-up seven years after injury. Journal of Neurology, Neurosurgery and Psychiatry 48: 564–8.

Prigatano GP (1986) Psychotherapy after brain injury. In Prigatano GP, Fordyce DJ, Zeiner H (eds) Neuropsychological Rehabilitation after Brain Injury. London: John Hopkins Press.

Prigatano GP, Fordyce DJ, Zeiner HK (1984) Neuropsychological rehabilitation after closed head injury in young adults. Journal of Neurology, Neurosurgery and Psychiatry 47: 505–13.

Prigatano GP, Pepping M, Klonoff P (1986) Cognitive, personality and psychosocial factors in the neuropsychological assessment of brain injured patients. In Uzzell BP, Gross Y (eds) Clinical Neuropsychology of Intervention. Boston: Martinus Nijhoff, pp. 136–6.

Ranseen J (1990) Positive personality change following traumatic head injury : four case studies. Cognitive Rehabilitation 8: 8–12.

Ridsdale L, Robins D, Fitzgerald A (1996) Epilepsy in general practice: patient's psychiatric symptoms and their perceptions of stigma. British Journal of General Practice 46(407): 365–66.

Rosenbaum M, Najenson T (1976) Changes in life patterns and symptoms of low mood as reported by wives of severely brain-injured soldiers. Journal of Consulting and Clinical Psychology 44: 881–8.

Roueche JR, Fordyce DJ (1983) Perceptions of deficits following brain injury and their impact on psychosocial adjustment. Cognitive Rehabilitation 1: 4–7.

Rutherford WH, Merrett JD, McDonald JR (1977) Sequelae of concussion caused by minor head injuries. Lancet 1: 104.

Tate RL (1998) 'It is not only the kind of injury that matters, but the kind of head': the contribution of pre-morbid psychosocial factors to rehabilitation outcomes after severe traumatic brain injury. Neuropsychological Rehabilitation 8(1): 1–18.

Tate RL, Broe GA (1999) Psychosocial adjustment after traumatic brain injury: what are the important variables? Psychological Medicine 29: 713–25.

Tate RL, Lulham JM, Broe GA, Strettles B, Pfaff A (1989) Psychosocial outcome for the survivors of severe blunt head injury. Journal Neurology Neurosurgery and Psychiatry 52: 1128–34.

Thomsen IV (1984) Late outcome of very severe blunt head trauma: 10–15 year second follow-up. Journal Neurology, Neurosurgery and Psychiatry 47: 260–8.

Tyerman A, Humphrey M (1984) Changes in self-concept following severe head injury. International Journal of Rehabilitation Research 7: 11–23.

Varney NR, Martzke JS, Roberts RJ (1987) Major depression in patients with closed head injury. Neuropsychology 1: 7–9.

Vilkki J, Ahola K, Holst P, Ohman J, Servo A, Heiskanen O (1994) Prediction of psychosocial recovery after head injury with cognitive tests and neurobehavioural ratings. Journal Clinical and Experimental Neuropsychology 16: 325–38.

Watts R, Perlesz A (1999) Psychosocial outcome risk indicator: predicting psychosocial outcome following traumatic brain injury. Brain Injury 13(2): 113–24.

Wehman P, Kreutzer J (1990) Vocational rehabilitation for persons with traumatic brain injury. Baltimore: Aspen.

Weinstein GS, Wells CE (1981) Case studies in neuropsychiatry: post traumatic psychiatric dysfunction diagnosis and treatment. Journal of Clinical Psychiatry 42: 120–2.

Willer B, Rosenthal M, Kreutzer JS (1993) Assessment of community integration following rehabilitation for traumatic brain injury. Journal of Head Trauma Rehabilitation 8: 75–87.

Zencius A, Wesolowiski MD, Burke WH, Hough S (1990) Managing hypersexual disorders in brain injured clients. Brain Injury 4: 175–81.

CHAPTER 9

Families and carers

CAROL PRATT, KEVIN BALDRY

Introduction: what is a carer?

The practical, social and emotional problems of the survivors of traumatic head injury have long been recognized. However, how best to support their families and friends whilst recovery is taking place and through the rehabilitation process remains a critical question. This chapter will offer an outline of some of the problems that may arise for those families and will discuss the way in which rehabilitation specialists and other professionals can address these issues.

It is usual, at the acute stage of care, to identify the client's next of kin. That person is usually, but not always, a close family member, and as such will usually be very anxious at this time. Most are more than willing to be involved and want to be with their loved one through the traumatic stages of intensive care and hospitalization. After severe head injury families tend to be grateful to staff for keeping their relative alive, and as a result give full cooperation with the medical regime. However, there is a transition once the client leaves intensive care and goes onto the hospital ward. The families begin to take up the threads of their own lives, and have time to reflect upon the care their relative is receiving. Some will become critical. Having been accustomed to one-to-one nursing in intensive care, a staff reduction may be perceived as a reduction in the quality of care. Families who cooperated fully may start to question or doubt medical opinion.

It is during this journey from intensive care to a rehabilitation unit or ward that a metamorphosis occurs – relatives become 'carers'. As such, certain expectations are made and roles placed upon them by professional staff and by others in their environment. Carers, meanwhile, will have had little time to adjust to this new role and will perceive themselves in their pre-injury condition.

The term 'carer' is used extensively in policy documents and research literature as well as in practical and clinical settings. Governmental and health service policies recognize the vital role carers play in the life of anyone with disability, both in practical and in economic terms. It is estimated that full-time carers save the government £34 billion every year (Warner and Wexler, 1998). Indeed this is recognized in recent policy initiatives, such as the launch of the National Health Service National Plan (Department of Health, 2000).

Rehabilitation professionals, as has been seen throughout this volume, recognize that for rehabilitation to be effective, whenever possible, carers must be involved as full members of the multidisciplinary team from the earliest stages. Ward and McIntosh (1987) stated that 'channelling of rehabilitation effort towards the carer is legitimate provided it benefits the patient at least indirectly'.

Some clinicians will have definite ideas about how carers can be part of the rehabilitation programme for a particular client. However, those who find themselves in this new role should be allowed to make choices. It must be remembered that a carer is not a therapist and it should not be assumed that an individual will take on therapeutic tasks. Indeed, there may be both practical and emotional reasons why this is not appropriate and rehabilitation centres must ensure a philosophy and practice that does not judge those who feel unable to be actively involved in rehabilitation tasks, or who feel they must set boundaries. Therapists should be aware of other family and lifestyle commitments. If therapists do not accept people's decisions, it is the rehabilitation programme and ultimately the client who will suffer. The one person who can undermine the best-planned rehabilitation, albeit passively by not doing what has been asked, is the carer. An environment in which the carer feels able to refuse is essential, so that staff can make informed judgements about the programme.

There are numerous examples of people who resist becoming the 'carer'. Practical reasons are well illustrated by the daughter of an elderly person whose physical condition was deteriorating. The daughter lived several miles away, and she was only able to visit occasionally. The staff reacted judgementally towards her, but she noticed a change in them as soon as she explained she was already a full-time carer of a disabled husband. He was an amputee who had suffered a severe stroke, was unsafe to leave alone, and she found it too physically and emotionally draining to drive with him as a passenger.

The emotional aspects of those trying to resist the label of 'carer' are illustrated by the young partner of a severely communicatively and cognitively impaired man who felt unable to change her role from equal partner to carer. They had both been in previous relationships where they felt they had been exploited. They had gone to great lengths to work out the boundaries of their relationship before making a commitment to each other, but the injury and the consequences were beyond anything they had envisaged. It came as a shock to her that she had to change from equal partner to 'carer', and she resisted this role vigorously.

This chapter will use the term 'carer' as defined in the 'Charter for Carers in Suffolk' (Suffolk Carers Charter Group, 1999): 'A "carer" is someone of any age whose life is restricted because they are looking after a friend, relative, partner or other person who cannot manage without help, because of illness, age or a disability of any kind.' Like most labels, the word 'carer' tends to be overused and to belittle or otherwise distort what it signifies. This is not a negative definition, nor does it devalue the person who cares for the client or the client who is cared for. It is a factual comment that no matter how motivated someone is to care, how dependent the client is or is not, the carer's lifestyle will change and be restricted.

The impact of head injury on the carer

Carers will face a variety of issues over time. These may be broadly described as practical, relationship based and emotional, although it should be remembered that these categories overlap in complex ways.

Practical concerns for carers may include their own and their families' financial security, although the Quality Standards for Local Carer Support Services consultation paper (King's Fund, 1999) states that the key issue for carers is primarily about the 'adequacy' of income. Housing is often an issue as financial pressures mean that paying mortgages, loans and so on becomes increasingly difficult. There may also be a need to decide whether to adapt a home for a client with disabilities or whether to move home or take up a place in a residential setting (Barnes, 1997; Great Britain, 2000).

These practical issues will inevitably cause a carer stress as they find themselves having to take the decisions and also having to implement them. It may be a complete role change – one that they have not chosen and do not want.

Relationships will usually be altered and affected by severe head injury in a family member or friend (Brooks and McKinlay, 1983). Even mild or moderate injury may affect relationships, both in the short and long term. Role changes may be forced upon the carer in practical and emotional ways. In the former, it may be that one partner has to take on control of family finances for the first time, or has to become responsible for housework or childcare. Emotionally, it may be that the relationship was based on one strong partner who was the decision maker, who is no longer able to take on this role because of cognitive or communication problems. The client may not be aware of such changes, if insight has been affected, and if he still attempts to take on his former responsibilities it will create further difficulties for the carer. There may be sexual problems as a result of the injury and these have been discussed more fully in Chapter 8. The degree of extra stress on relatives has been researched and documented by, among others, Romano (1974) and Oddy, Humphrey and Uttley (1978).

The emotional impact of head injury on carers is often profound. Many will feel guilty if they try to get on with their own lives, and will feel obliged to give up work and involvement in community life and hobbies or interests. This often results in isolation, as friends and colleagues gradually stop visiting. Reasons for this include embarrassment, inability to cope and lack of understanding. An illustration of the difficulty people have in maintaining friendships can be seen in a young woman caring for her head-injured husband who presented with behavioural problems. She at first expressed the feeling that, although others no longer visited, at least they had each other. However, she went on to discuss the issue in greater depth and admitted that she no longer liked her husband, so could not expect others to put up with him.

Carers may therefore be isolated and may have suffered great loss in terms of their lifestyle but they may also feel that they have lost their relative who is 'no longer the person they knew and loved'. This reaction is particularly common when there is cognitive impairment and/or behavioural issues. Research suggests that carers adjust better and stay in a relationship if the damage caused by injury is only physical (Rosenbaum and Najenson, 1976) and that marital relationships tended to be less stable than parent/child relationships (Panting and Merry, 1972; Thomsen, 1984).

Carers and other family members will go through the same grieving process that any person does after a bereavement. Initial joy and relief that the client has not died will be replaced by sadness and grief over what has been lost. The grieving process is well documented (for example Kübler-Ross 1969) but the individuals concerned may not recognize what is happening to them. It is important that therapists are aware of likely stages in the cycle of grieving. These are classically defined as anger, guilt, blame and denial. Therapists need to be able to recognize these in order to help the client, and be able to refer on to specialist counsellors if necessary.

Factors affecting carers' needs and reactions

A number of factors are involved in determining how an individual will react to being placed in the role of carer. The nature of the impairments and problems faced by the head-injured individual will be one factor. After cognitive changes many carers state, often in highly emotive terms, that the emotional intimacy, companionship and warmth has been lost. Research by

McKinlay et al. (1981) indicates that the amount of stress was related to the incidence of mental and behavioural changes in the patient. Even if the couple or family are able to continue their lifestyle or hobbies superficially, the sense of intellectual sharing may have gone. It is this aspect that seems hardest for carers. It may be that this change is too subtle for the head-injured person to be fully aware but he can, in turn, sense an alteration in his carer's feelings. For example, a young head-injured man asked his wife how he could make things better between them. She reported the interaction to a member of the team with the words: 'How can I tell him when it is so subtle I can't even describe it myself?'

An additional feature of a carer's ability to cope with cognitive changes is the fact that they are often 'hidden' handicaps. Head injury has been frequently described as a 'hidden disability' (see, for example, Social Services Inspectorate, 1996). Others around may find it very hard to appreciate the very real impact on family life if the individual looks as he always did and, at first, seems unchanged. If there is an obvious physical disability people are perhaps more ready and able both to appreciate the needs and offer help and support to the carer. The impact of some injuries can be very dramatic, with profound physical and cognitive impairment, and there may have to be a decision made about specialist long-term care.

Common difficulties reported by carers include aggression, unpre-dictability, role changes, dependency, impoverished communication, restricted leisure and social life, reduced sexual relations, reduced emotional intimacy and lack of awareness in the client of the impact of his behaviour on the family. These issues are discussed and referenced elsewhere in this book.

Timing is another factor (Romano, 1974; McKinlay et al., 1981; Frosch et al., 1997). At the acute and early stages the immediate needs are often practical. The need for reassessment of finances is often identified and, at this time, most employers are helpful and supportive. Employers have by law (Disabled Persons Employment Act 1944) a duty to staff who are ill or have a disability. Practical issues to do with accommodation may be central to discussions about discharge into the community. The difficulties of transition into the community and specialist housing alternatives are discussed in various documents and articles (Geddes, Claydon and Chamberlain, 1989; Barnes, 1997). Once practical considerations are addressed carers will begin to realize the enormity of the task they face after a severe head injury. As time goes on some carers may continue to hope for further recovery despite explanations to the contrary and even if they accept a slowing of progress. Emotional reactions to the situation vary enormously between individuals, as gradually people appreciate the fact that changes will be lifelong. Long-term adjustment is an area with which all rehabilitation teams must be concerned, in relation to client and carer.

Carers' needs will vary depending upon their own situation in relation to the client. Different generations and ages may have different value bases underlying their decisions, and as a result will have different needs. The relationship will also be a factor. Head injury often occurs in young adults and there may well be young children within the home environment who will have particular needs. Similarly in this age group there may be those without partners whose nearest relative is one or both parents (King's Fund 1999).

There is considerable documented evidence of stress on the carers of disabled people (Kinsella and Duffy, 1979). This may be alleviated by periods of respite, or as described in the County of Suffolk 'care breaks'. Ideally, these breaks should be planned, to avoid crises or relationships break down (Barnes, 1997). Eligibility and funding guidelines are laid down in the Community Care Act 1990.

The needs of friends are sadly often neglected, but friends are often crucial to reintegration into the community. As was discussed in Chapter 8, isolation is a real problem for head-injured adults and more consideration should perhaps be given to their pre-existing circle of friends, in order to help friends remain as part of clients' lives when they return to the community. In offering information and education to carers and families, it may be appropriate to widen the audience to include friends and colleagues.

The personality of the potential carer will also influence the ability to cope. Individual coping strategies and expectations will shape the carer role in each case, but whatever carers have to offer, they should have recognition in their own right (Suffolk Carers Charter Group, 1999).

Assessment

In many rehabilitation centres dealing with traumatic brain injury the injured person is invited for screening and assessment. It is often a deliberate policy – as at the Icanho centre in Suffolk and the Sheffield Head Injury Project – to talk to the client and carer separately at the initial screening. These interviews aim to give the team as full an account as possible of the impact of the injury on the carer and family. This first meeting can identify early indications of the stress, distress and adaptation of family members. If there is a specific concern about the carer, a completely separate assessment of the impact of the traumatic brain injury on the family can be undertaken. The carer is also entitled to their own assessment by social services (Community Care Act 1990). This should identify the need for resources, respite, or practical help at home. Many local authorities provide a home care scheme; health authorities have community nurses, and both can facilitate access to schemes within the voluntary sector such as Crossroads Care and the Cheshire Family Support Scheme.

The assessments used by rehabilitation teams will vary with the preferences held by the therapist, but some of the most commonly used are the Family Assessment Device (Epstein, Baldwin and Bishop, 1983), Head Injury Family Semantic Differential II (adapted from Tyerman, 1997) and the Golombok Rust Inventory of Marital State (Rust et al., 1988). If concern is identified about financial issues, a referral can be made to one of the voluntary agencies that specialize in disabilities or debt, if there is no trained welfare rights worker within the team. Practical problems identified can, again, be referred on to specialist agencies if the needs cannot be met within the team.

It must be remembered that in any assessment, carers should be dealt with as individuals, and their culture, race, gender, age, disability or illness must be recognized.

Working with carers

Carers may interact with all members of the team, depending upon the problems their relative faces. However, it may be useful to ensure that one person has responsibility for interactions that do not specifically relate to the individual disciplines. This person may be anyone with whom that carer has a rapport, as long as that clinician has the time and feels comfortable in that role. Some teams have a designated person to assume the role, which enables that individual to acquire the skills and resources to be most effective – it is not uncommon for this role to be taken by a social worker.

The person who assumes responsibility for the carer in this way can act as a facilitator to other team members or act as a bridge/communicator between therapists and the family/home. For example, there are occasions when therapists ask carers to undertake 'homework' activities with the client. The carer may feel unable to express concern over the role – either in general, because it places their relationship on a different footing (as teacher and pupil) or specifically because that task is seen as the latest thing on a long list of demands. A good relationship with at least one member of the team can allow them to air their concerns in a non-judgemental setting, and these concerns can be taken into account when therapy tasks are planned in future.

Factors involved in deciding the most appropriate intervention include the nature of difficulty faced, time since the injury and the carer's approach to her role. Intervention with carers may be practical, educational/informative or emotionally supportive. Each of these areas will be considered in greater detail.

Practical issues

At the acute stage a thorough benefits check by a trained welfare rights worker should be undertaken as soon as possible, to ensure that the client and carer do not lose benefit or entitlement to benefit. Disability brings additional costs (Martin and White, 1998). Often relevant forms are left with clients in hospital with insufficient explanation and there is a failure to make allowances for cognitive impairments. It may be that the family will face real financial hardship before the situation is recognized. Such a delay in administration can lead to short-term problems and even loss of benefit over the longer term. Most social services departments in the UK have county welfare rights units that can be accessed. The voluntary sector has useful resources such as the citizen's advice bureau and the disability advice bureau, which will offer expert advice. Financial checks must be made periodically as the employer's financial responsibility decreases over time. Long-term financial advice may also be necessary, including advice regarding the implications of the injury for pensions.

Families are often embarrassed or inhibited about discussing their financial plight, fearing they will be judged as not coping or seem ungrateful for the advice offered earlier. While the long-term goal must be for families to take on responsibility for their own negotiations, at the acute and early rehabilitation stages they may feel unable to cope. Some clients report that talking to banks, credit card companies and others can cause them to relive the event and experience great distress. Others may be taking on the family finances for the first time and, with yet another new role to assume, will need considerable support and encouragement. For nearly all carers, issues to do with disability benefits will be a totally new area.

It is usually at the screening or assessment stage of rehabilitation that it becomes evident that the client or family is having difficulty managing the practical issues. These issues vary tremendously, with a kaleidoscope of problems coming to light. These could range from debts requiring immediate attention, incurred by non-payment of hire purchase or credit cards, to long-term inability to pay rent or a mortgage. Permission to gather information about finances and the debts incurred must be obtained with sensitivity and in confidence. A signed consent form to enable workers to negotiate on a client/carer's behalf is necessary, and a detailed financial statement, such as that in Table 9.1, can then be taken (George 2000).

What happens next depends on the experience and ability of the worker. Those with debt-counselling skills and welfare rights training who are able to advocate on the client/carer's behalf, will take appropriate action. Others will need to refer to specialist advisors.

Housing issues often have the greatest long-term implications, as clients and their families could lose their homes. Early negotiation with landlords, councils, housing associations or building societies is important. Although none of these agencies encourage debt, they do have designated staff to help people through difficulties.

Table 9.1. Financial statement

A. INCOME	Income weekly/ monthly	B.EXPENDITURE (Do not include debt repayments)	Outgoings weekly/ monthly
Wages/salary		Mortgage	
Wages/salary (partner)		Mortgage endowment policy	
Jobseekers' allowance		Second mortgage	
Income support		Rent	
Family credit		Council tax	
Retirement pension/works pension		Water rates	
Child benefit		Ground rent/service charge	
Incapacity/sickness benefit		Buildings/contents insurance	
Maintenance		Life insurance/pension	
Non-dependants contribution		Gas	
Other		Electricity	
		Other fuel	
TOTAL INCOME	£	Housekeeping/food etc	
		TV rental/licence	
		Magistrates' court fines	
		Maintenance payments	
		Travelling expenses	
		Prescriptions	
		Childminding	
		Other	
		1	
C. TOTAL INCOME	£	2	
Take away TOTAL OUTGOINGS		3	
		4	
First money for creditors figures	£	TOTAL OUTGOINGS	£

D. DEBTS		Priority debts Weekly/monthly	
	Balance owed		Weekly/ monthly offer of repayment
Mortgage arrears			
Second mortgage arrears			
Rent arrears			
Council tax/community charge arrears			
Water/sewage charge arrears			
Fuel debts: gas			
electricity			
other			
Magistrates' court arrears			
Maintenance arrears			
Other			
1			
2			
3			
Total priority debts repayment	£		£

(contd)

Table 9.1. (contd)

E.

	£
First money for creditors figure (from C)	£
Take away from total priority debts Repayment (from D)	£
Second money for creditors figure	£

F.	Credit debts		
Creditor	Balance owed		Monthly offer of repayment
1			
2			
3			
4			
5			
6			
7			
8			
9			
10			
Total owed	£		
Total monthly repayment	£		

The support worker may therefore take initial responsibility, with full permission from the carer, for contacting people in relation to finances. Carers can be encouraged to resume full responsibility when they feel able. Often, when the first shock and anxiety have passed, carers want to feel back in control. It must be remembered that this can be a stressful time for clients. They may be aware that it was their responsibility pre-injury, to manage the finances within the family/relationship and they may be able to appreciate that this aspect of their life is no longer something with which they are able to deal. This can add to their feelings of loss of self-worth, and diminished self-esteem. Careful guidance and support to both parties will be needed at this stage.

Information/education

Practical support will usually be offered on a one-to-one basis, but the crucial role of information provider may be through either one-to-one or group approaches. Those who come into daily contact with the client, especially carers, may have their own requirements for information and advice (Stewart,

1985). Often carers may be given information about the injury at the acute stage and not be able to assimilate it. People may not feel the need to take in too much information as they hope at this time for a full recovery. This means it is not uncommon for carers to have their relative at home, and enter a community-based rehabilitation programme, without knowing exactly what has happened to the client. They may not appreciate what the long-term consequences may be physically, cognitively or behaviourally. The rehabilitation stage is therefore an important point at which to clarify their understanding of what has happened and to provide other necessary information.

On a one-to-one basis, information about the rehabilitation programme is vital if the therapists want to include and work alongside the carer. If medical, psychological or therapy-linked information is required the carer should have the opportunity to see the relevant professional. There will usually be informal contact, but it should be clear that they can make formal times for discussion. This also allows the therapist to be prepared. Some carers report that they find such meetings intimidating, particularly when under stress as a result of their relative's injury, and it may help to suggest they are accompanied by a friend or relative, or another professional with whom they have an established relationship. Staff must be aware of the danger of professional jargon and ensure full understanding and opportunity for questioning at every point. Misunderstandings or misconceptions can be clarified in this way, although it is recognized that people under stress often hear 'selectively' what they would like to hear rather than what is actually said. It is well recognized that often a good deal of the content of consultations involving bad news is frequently not recalled. (Edelstein, 1989). Written information can help to support and explain what has been said.

Groups can be a valuable way of giving information, whether formally or informally structured. Group settings serve several purposes as they bring together those with a common interest or experience. Formal meetings may have a speaker (perhaps a therapist or outside agency) addressing a clearly defined subject, which also makes good use of therapists' time as they have the opportunity to see many carers at once. Carers may feel less inhibited in a group or be helped by hearing questions others are confident enough to ask. There are also disadvantages. There are those people who will not feel comfortable in a group setting, and just as some find comfort in sharing anxieties and experiences, others may find this 'sharing' to be anxiety-provoking or depressing. They may not be able to relate to what they hear, or they might be at a stage where they cannot accept what they hear. This is discussed in more detail by Oddy (1997).

As with information provided on a one-to-one basis, it is important to pitch group education at the right level. Therapists are skilled in their own field but many have little or no training in getting information across to others. Risks include making language too technical or too simple, which may seem patronizing. Visual aids and interactive exercises can be useful to aid understanding and to relax members of a group. It is important to consider how people learn (Preston-Shoot, 1987).

Different relatives and different generations may have quite different needs in terms of information. Primary carers may need a lot of practical as well as emotional support; partners or parents may have defined views on what they should do and find a conflict between duty and their own lives; children may have little understanding of why a parent's behaviour has changed; and friends may have a desire to be involved but not feel able to intrude upon the family. Obviously, at the extreme, all will have unique needs, but in relation to group work it may be helpful to focus on the needs of certain people. This increases the likelihood of shared experience and peer support, and allows staff to plan material appropriately.

In general all groups will depend on the client group, centre, staff and topic. All will use basic group work boundaries and rules, which are discussed in various texts (Preston-Shoot, 1987). Members must feel safe to express views in confidence, must respect other members' contributions, and must feel comfortable if they choose not to speak. Practical issues must also be addressed – for example carers should be offered transport and respite for the client if necessary; otherwise, apart from making it difficult for the carer to attend, it will also convey the message that staff are not really aware of the day-to-day difficulties they face.

There are organizations outside the rehabilitation centre that offer 'support groups', where carers can benefit from mutual support. The Headway Association is specifically designed for people with a head injury; the Carers National Association and the Stroke Association also offer support and social activities to families and carers. The addresses for local groups can be found in telephone directories or through local advice centres. The appendix to this chapter offers a few useful national addresses that may be particularly relevant to carers and to the issues touched on in this chapter.

Children must not be ignored when it comes to education about what has happened. The implications for the young children of someone suffering a head injury are significant (Urbach, 1989). Often they are aware of changes but have been unable to understand explanations or been left to work things out for themselves. It is difficult for adults to understand the possible ramifications of brain damage, particularly if there is no obvious physical handicap, so children will need very careful handling. There is little research into the impact on children who have a parent with a brain injury, and the reasons for this are discussed by Oddy (1997).

Groups for younger children can be run in such a way that they are fun as well as instructive. For example, at the Icanho Centre in Suffolk visual aids and interactive games include an anatomically correct jelly mould of the brain and a game that involves drawing silhouettes of their own heads with the aid of an overhead projector in order to make a simple 'map' of the brain. These activities provide a supportive environment in which children can open up about their own feelings and fears. In extreme cases this may involve child-abuse issues. One child, described how his grandfather, who had had a stroke, would hit out with his walking stick when he lost his temper. At times such as this it is crucial that staff have a clear understanding of their own boundaries and appropriate courses of action should such matters arise. Staff involved must include those with experience of child work and wider child-protection issues.

Any children who are actively involved in the caring role should also be introduced to the services aimed specifically for them. In the UK The Princess Royal Trust Carers' Centre Network offers advice and appropriate contact numbers for 'young carers'.

Table 9.2 and Figure 9.1 offer sample programmes for support groups. Other groups, not simply education or information based, can be established at rehabilitation centres or in the community, to meet the needs of carers. It has been stated that if group members share a common goal (for example, to gain confidence or for support) this will provide a reason for members to invest and interact in the group, thus increasing the sense of unity (Heap, 1977). The groups could be discussion, social action, self-directed, self-help or social in purpose. Membership can be drawn from the whole range of those affected by the head injury, whether it be partners, siblings or other members of the family.

Table 9.2. Sample programme card for carers' information group

PROGRAMME CARD	
Four weekly sessions have been arranged to give carers and relatives a greater understanding of some of the problems relating to brain injury. The sessions will be structured, with a speaker, followed by the opportunity for discussion and questions over coffee.	1. 19.1.00 Speaker : Psychologist Emotional and Behavioural Problems – causes and treatment. 2. 26.1.00 Speaker : Physiotherapist/ Occupational Therapist The Recovery Process
The sessions will be held at Icanho, starting at 4.30 pm and finishing by 6.00 pm. Please let us know if you are able to attend by phoning.	3. 2.2.00 Speaker : Occupational Therapist. Memory Problems and Coping Strategies 4. 9.2.00 Speaker : Solicitor Legal issues in Brain Injury

Table 9.3. Sample programme card for carers' support group

PROGRAMME FOR 2000
January to June

13th January	Let's unpack Christmas: anecdotes, anxieties and the amusing things that happened.
10th February	Aromatherapy and relaxation.
10th March	Informal Meeting.
14th April	A visit from the DIAL Service and your questions answered about benefits and services for people with disabilities.
12th May	Holiday advice, including insurance.
9th June	Informal meeting.

There will be a break in July and August. Later in the year we will distribute the programme for the second half of the year.

Emotional support

Emotional support can be offered in both the group setting or on a one-to-one level. If offering one-to-one support, consideration must be given to the time and place of the meetings. If not, the care regime may be interrupted or the carer may not be able to relax enough to benefit from the contact. Carers will need constant reassurance in their new role and to be helped to recognize the value of maintaining involvement in former activities. Many carers would benefit from staying in employment and maintaining social contacts, as they will provide a major source of support later. Case studies in the National Traumatic Brain Injury Study (Hawley et al., 2000) showed that many good outcomes were associated with the maintenance and reinforcement of family relationships and networks of friends and colleagues.

No therapist can make friends for people, but a carer's position can sometimes be ameliorated by the substitution of other communities and relationships. The professional involved can introduce them to local activities and groups, can provide contact numbers for respite care, social services and local or national organizations working in the area of head injury (such as Headway). The contacts may be for practical or emotional support. Often rehabilitation centres will provide 'in-house' support groups but carers should also be made aware of outside opportunities. Carers will have differing needs and it will depend upon their personality and situation as to which avenues suit them best.

Some carers may benefit from formal counselling, whereas others will respond to more informal approaches. Therapists can listen and absorb stress within sessions with a client and/or carer, and can monitor the need for more specialist intervention, while remaining aware of their own professional and personal boundaries. Therapists need to be confident about facilitating the exploration of carer's feelings or at least recognizing and validating those feelings, while opening other avenues for support. If a carer makes a comment and finds it rejected, brushed over or made light of, they may not open up again. It will also potentially spoil the rapport with that therapist in relation to the ongoing rehabilitation programme.

In summary, rehabilitation staff need to adopt strategies in all their dealings with carers which create a safe environment and encourage openness. These strategies include empathy and understanding, listening and absorbing, informing and explaining, assessing and monitoring, supportive problem solving, providing opportunity for reflection, offering long-term support and facilitating adaptation (Booth, 1998).

A time when considerable emotional support may be needed will be towards the end of the rehabilitation programme. Carers may find it difficult to accept that the situation has reached a plateau and that their relative will not progress further (Walker, 1972; Lezak, 1978). There should be a strategy for the transition from active rehabilitation to long-term support, not just for the client but also for the carer.

Some carers at this stage will face the decision of whether to remain in the relationship or not. There is evidence that there is a particularly high risk of relationship breakdown two years post injury (Oddy et al., 1985; Tate et al., 1989). It is the team's role to remain non-judgemental and supportive, however difficult it may be in certain cases not to feel sympathy for the head-injured client. The carer needs space and information in order to make the decision and the team should maintain contact to ensure the decision is based on clear and appropriate information. It may be necessary to amend or develop new rehabilitation plans around the client's new circumstances.

When working with a carer in relation to emotional adjustment it may be important to share information within the team. However, it may be appropriate to share only on a 'need-to-know' basis to protect confidentiality. The danger of emotional involvement means team members will need to have recourse to supervision to help them deal with issues that arise (UKCC, 1987).

If specialist resources are not available within the team, referral to outside agencies may be necessary. Established contacts within organizations such as

Relate can facilitate easy referral, although it is important that confidentiality is maintained. A referral letter on rehabilitation centre notepaper, read and agreed by the client and carer, will signal to counsellors that brain injury is a factor, without any further information being disclosed. Counsellors will need an awareness of possible consequences of brain injury so that appropriate techniques are adopted. Memory issues, for example, may limit opportunities for people to take on home assignments as part of the counselling process.

Specialist bereavement intervention or counselling for specific problems may be necessary. Again, local specialist services will need to be accessed. This often incurs a cost and the NHS can be reluctant to fund such intervention.

As well as formal referral there are less structured ways in which options can be presented – leaflets, booklets and contact numbers, as long as they are up to date, may be a more acceptable introduction to counselling for some people.

Outcomes

Head injury affects an entire family, not just the injured person (Frosh et al., 1997). Throughout this volume authors have indicated that carers and families are essential to the rehabilitation process. Working with carers can be satisfying, but the outcome of intervention by the therapist or team is often judged subjectively. The feedback given is often verbal and, even when questionnaires or feedback forms are used, it is almost impossible to be objective. In research by Hawley et al. (2000) it was stated that 'measurement of outcomes after rehabilitation was problematic as no outcome measures existed which were able to capture improvements in community-based outcome following rehabilitation, and also take account of the patient's and carer's own viewpoints'. There are some materials that may have value in monitoring change and evaluating outcome of intervention, including the Aylesbury Family Roles Questionnaire (Tyerman, Young and Booth, 1994) and the Personal Assessment of Intimacy in Relationships (Schaefer and Olson, 1981). Family outcome research has progressed substantially during the last decade, but it is an area that demands more attention in order to justify necessary funding and ensure that valuable work with carers can continue.

Conclusions

It is widely recognized that traumatic brain injury represents a major long-term burden for health and social services (Hawley et al., 2000). Rehabilitation teams should explore creative ways to involve carers in the rehabilitation process, whilst remembering that carers are not therapists. They are a valuable resource and their contribution to providing care probably exceeds the combined efforts of statutory and voluntary agencies. Warner and Wexler (1998) highlight the enormous financial burden that statutory services would have to meet if people were not prepared to take on the role of caring for their relatives or friends. They should therefore command recognition and respect from the team, and be given the information and practical help they need to enable them to make a choice as to their level of involvement. Once that decision is made, the team must accept it and work within its parameters to produce the best quality of rehabilitation for both client and carer.

Appendix: contact addresses

Carers National Association
20/25 Glasshouse Yard
London EC1A 4JT

Crossroads – Caring for Carers
10 Regent Place
Rugby CV21 2PN

Headway
National Head Injury Association
King Edward Court
King Edward Street
Nottingham NG1 1EW

National Association of Citizens Advice Bureaux
Myddleton House
115-123 Pentonville Road
London N1 9LZ

National Debt Line
0800 808 4000

Princess Royal Trust for Carers
142 Minories
London EC3N 1LB
Relate
National Marriage Guidance
Herbert Gray College
Little Church Street
Rugby
Warwickshire CV21 3AP

SPOD - The Association to aid the Sexual and Personal Relationships of
People with Disabilities
286 Camden Road
London N7 0BJ

References

Barnes M (1997) Organisation of neurological rehabilitation services. In Greenwood R,
    Barnes MP, McMillan TM, Ward CD (eds) Neurological Rehabilitation 3. Hove:
    Psychology Press, pp. 29–39.
Booth J (1998) Supporting families. Paper presented to the Head Injury Social Work Group,
    Derby, 22 April.
Brooks DN, McKinlay W (1983) Personality and behavioural change after severe blunt head
    injury. A relative's view. Journal of Neurology, Neurosurgery, and Psychiatry 46: 336–44.
Department of Health (2000) The National Health Service Plan – A Plan for Investment. A
    Plan for Reform. Norwich: The Stationery Office.
Edelstein EL (1989) Denial. New York: Penium.
Epstein NB, Baldwin LM, Bishop DS (1983) The McMaster Family Assessment Device.
    Journal of Marital and Family Therapy 9: 171–80.
Frosch S, Gruber A, Jones C, Myres S, Noel E, Westerlund A, Zavisin T (1997) The long term
    effects of traumatic brain injury on the roles of caregivers. Brain Injury 11(12): 891–906.
Geddes JML, Claydon AD, Chamberlain MA (1989) The Leeds Family Placement Scheme: an
    evaluation of its use as a rehabilitation resource. Clinical Rehabilitation 3: 189–97.
George C (2000) Welfare Benefits Handbook. London: Child Poverty Action Group.
Great Britain (2000) Supporting People. (Government consultation paper.) London: HMSO.
Harrison JJ (1986) The Young Disabled Adult. London: Royal College of Physicians.
Hawley C, Stilwell J, Davies C, Stilwell P (2000) Post-acute rehabilitation after traumatic
    brain injury. British Journal of Therapy and Rehabilitation 7(3): 116–21.
Heap K (1977) Group Theory For Social Workers. Oxford: Pergamon Press.
King's Fund (1999) Quality Standards for Local Carer Support Services Consultation Paper.
    London: Kings Fund.
Kinsella GJ, Duffy FD (1979) Psychosocial re-adjustment in the spouses of aphasic patients.
    Scandinavian Journal of Rehabilitation Medicine 11: 129–32.
Kübler-Ross E (1969) On Death and Dying. New York: Tavistock Publications.
Lezak MD (1978) Living with the characterologically altered brain injured patient. The
    Journal of Clinical Psychiatry 39: 592–8.
Martin J, White A (1998) The Financial Circumstances of Disabled Adults Living in Private
    Households. OPCS Surveys of Disability in Great Britain Report 2. London: HMSO.
McKinlay W, Brooks DN, Bond MR, Martinage DP, Marshall MM (1981) The short-term out-
    come of severe blunt head injury as reported by relatives of the injured persons. Journal
    of Neurology, Neurosurgery, and Psychiatry 44: 527–33.
Oddy M (1997) Psychosocial consequences of brain injury. In Greenwood R, Barnes MP,
    McMillan Tm, Ward CD (Eds) Neurological Rehabilitation. Hove: Psychology Press.
    423-33.
Oddy M, Humphrey M, Uttley D (1978) Stresses upon the relatives of head-injured patients.
    Brit J Psychiat 133: 507–13.

Oddy M, Coughlan T, Tyerman A, Jenkins D (1985) Social adjustment after closed head injury: a further follow-up seven years after injury. Journal of Neurology, Neurosurgery, and Psychiatry 48: 564–8.

Panting A, Merry PH (1972) The long term rehabilitation of severe head injuries with particular reference to the need for social and medical support for the patient's family. Rehabilitation 38: 33–7.

Preston-Shoot M (1987) Effective Groupwork. Basingstoke: Macmillan.

Romano MD (1974) Family response to traumatic head injury. Scand J Rehab Med 6: 1–4.

Rosenbaum M, Najenson T (1976) Changes in life patterns and symptoms of low mood as reported by wives of severely brain-injured soldiers. Journal of Consulting and Clinical Psychology 44: 881–8.

Rust J, Bennum I, Crowe M, Golombok S (1988) Golombok Rust Inventory of Marital State (GRIMS) Questionnaire. Windsor: NFER-Nelson.

Schaefer MT, Olsen DH (1981) Assessing intimacy – personal assessment of intimacy in relationship inventory. Journal of Marital and Family Therapy 7: 47–60.

Social Services Inspectorate Department of Health (1996) A Hidden Disability: a Report of the SSI Traumatic Brain Injury Rehabilitation Project. London: Department of Health.

Stewart W (1985) Counselling in Rehabilitation. London: Croom Helm.

Suffolk Carers Charter Group (1999) Charter For Carers in Suffolk (Leaflet).

Tate RL, Lulham JM, Broe GA, Strettles B, Pfaff A. (1989) Psychosocial outcome for the survivors of severe blunt head injury; the results from a consecutive series of 100 patients. Journal of Neurology, Neurosurgery and Psychiatry 52: 1128–34.

Thomsen IV (1984) Late outcome of very severe blunt head trauma. A 10–15 year second follow-up. Journal of Neurology, Neurosurgery and Psychiatry 47: 260–8.

Tyerman A (1997) Outcome Measures in a Community Head Injury Service. Neuropsychologial Rehabilitation 9 (3/4): 481–91.

Tyerman A, Young K, Booth J (1994) Aylesbury Family Roles Questionnaire II. Unpublished document. Aylesbury: Community Head Injury Service, Bedgrove Health Centre.

UKCC (United Kingdom Central Council for Nursing, Midwifery and Health Visiting) (1987) Confidentiality Advisory Paper. London: UKCC.

Urbach JR (1989) The impact of parental head trauma on families with children. Psychiatric Medicine 7: 17–36.

Walker AE (1972) Long term evaluation of the social and family adjustment to head injuries. Scandinvian Journal of Rehabilitation Medicine 4: 5–8.

Ward C, McIntosh S (1987) The rehabilitation process: a neurological perspective. Neurological Rehabilitation 2: 13–27.

Warner L, Wexler S, Institute of Actuaries (1998) Eight Hours A Day Taken For Granted. The Princess Royal Trust for Carers supported by Glaxo Wellcome. London: Princess Royal Trust for Carers.

CHAPTER 10

Legal issues and driving after head injury

OLIVER GRAVELL, SUSAN FREEBURN, WARREN COLLINS, ROSEMARY GRAVELL

Many issues arise in a rehabilitation setting that do not fall into the remit of a particular discipline. Some of these, such as sexual difficulties after head injury, have been discussed elsewhere in this volume but there are two areas that seem to crop up time and time again in clinical practice, which have not been specifically addressed in this volume. Those areas are legal matters and the question of returning to driving after head injury. This short chapter will offer a brief overview, with the aim of enabling clinicians to understand terms that arise and to direct clients to those who have the necessary specialist knowledge. It is intended therefore to offer third party, rather than comprehensive, cover.

Legal issues

In a community rehabilitation setting, the legal issues that arise seem to fall into three areas - compensation claims, relationship matters and criminal proceedings.

Compensation claims

Compensation claims are generally pursued by a solicitor on behalf of the client. It is recommended, if there has been some form of brain injury, that specialist solicitors are used who have experience with what are termed 'maximum severity' personal injury claims. In the UK, the Association of Personal Injury Lawyers will be able to provide details of local specialists. However, compensation is not paid just because an accident has happened and solicitors will need to consider the prospects of establishing legal fault or 'liability' - for example, if health and safety failings led to an injury at work, or if the driver of a car caused an accident that injured either a passenger in that car or another person. They will also consider the possibility of contributory negligence, which may reduce the amount of compensation, such as the failure to wear a seat belt.

There are a number of ways by which clients may fund a claim. Trade unions or other organizations may offer legal assistance. Legal aid, now known as Legal Service Commission Funding, is only available for compensation claims in very limited circumstances. Home or motor insurance may cover legal costs. 'No win-no fee', or conditional fee arrangements, are much misunderstood. Solicitors in the UK are not allowed to act on the basis of taking a percentage of damages in civil litigation cases. Solicitors may agree to waive fees if a claim fails, but the client may still be liable for the other side's costs, so it is a condition of such deals that insurance is taken out against this possibility. If the claim is successful, the solicitor's costs will include an extra 'success fee', which reflects the risk taken, but this cost will generally be met by the other side and will therefore not reduce the compensation amount.

Most claims are pursued through the civil courts, but there may be cases where the injury occurs as the result of a criminal act, such as an assault in the street, and claims may be made through the Criminal Injuries Compensation Authority. In civil courts the burden of proof is on the 'balance of probabilities', whereas in criminal cases the case must be proved 'beyond reasonable doubt'. This means that there may be a civil claim even if police decide not to prosecute, or if a prosecution fails. Generally people need to issue proceedings within three years of the date of an accident, but different rules apply to head-injured claimants if they are deemed to have insufficient mental capacity to instruct a solicitor. In this event the Court of Protection will be involved and a 'litigation friend' may be appointed, both of which terms are defined later in this chapter.

A full court trial is not always necessary and many claims are settled out of court. The claim will involve three types of damages. General damages cover those things that cannot be given a monetary value, such as loss of lifestyle, pain and suffering. Special damages are for the consequential financial loss suffered as a result of the injury, and establishing the amount of compensation will involve assessing rehabilitation needs, employment issues, housing and equipment needs, nursing care (including gratuitous care provided by family and friends), and long-term case management, as well as loss of future earnings and pension. This will also include an amount for losses incurred by carers. Members of the rehabilitation team may be asked for reports detailing the specific rehabilitation needs of clients. The third type of damages is future losses and this covers the ongoing costs of special damages, taking into account the likely prognosis. It may be possible to ask for provisional damages if there is a risk that a medical condition, such as epilepsy, will manifest itself in the future, which allows a return to court in the future should this happen.

The procedure for making a claim begins with a letter of claim sent to the defendant's insurers, who normally deal with issues of liability within three months. If liability is admitted, the value of the claim is then dealt with as a separate issue. Both sides will obtain witness statements and other documentary evidence, including reports from rehabilitation staff.

Until recently a major problem was the length of time needed to assess the full loss, which led to delays before the award of damages and obtaining payment. All too often the delay in payment led to delays in instigating appropriate rehabilitation until it was too late to make substantial differences. However, recently, lawyers and insurers drew up a Code of Best Practice that recommends interim payments to meet the immediate therapeutic and treatment needs of the client. The insurer pays for an assessment of needs and for the implementation of recommendations.

Payment of damages may be as a one-off lump sum or by structured settlements, when the insurance company sets up a fund to provide an annual income, designed to meet the ongoing needs of the client throughout his life.

The award of substantial compensation damages can lead to difficulties for clients and families unused to handling large amounts of money. This is, of course, complicated by the likelihood that the client will have cognitive impairments. Specialist solicitors can advise on such matters as enduring power of attorney, and on wills, tax and estate planning, Court of Protection receivership applications and trusts.

Some of the terms that have been used so far in this discussion, such as enduring power of attorney and Court of Protection, will be terms that rehabilitation clinicians may well encounter in the course of their work, and it is worth defining both.

Enduring power of attorney

When someone grants a power of attorney to another person, they are effectively granting them their authority to carry out all, or a specified but limited part, of their affairs. This authority only lasts if the donor retains his mental capacity to manage his affairs. To overcome this problem, it is now possible to grant an enduring power of attorney. Then, at the time when the donor loses capacity, the enduring power of attorney is suspended until it has been registered at the Court of Protection. Thereafter it remains in force until either the donor recovers, or the attorney ceases to act because of retirement or death, or he asks the Court of Protection to release him.

In broad terms the test for whether someone has the mental capacity to manage his affairs is that he knows the nature and extent of his assets and has the ability to process the information.

Court of Protection

Unfortunately, most people do not sign an enduring power of attorney and it is obviously too late to do so after a brain injury has been sustained. In these cases, an application must be made to the Court of Protection. The Court of Protection is an office of the Supreme Court and under the Mental Health Act 1983 it has the authority to make Orders and give directions in relation to the estate of persons (known as patients) who, by reason of mental disorder, are incapable of managing their affairs and property. When that happens, it is necessary to apply to the Court for an Order appointing someone, known as a Receiver, to deal with the patient's affairs.

There is no satisfactory definition of mental disorder other than 'mental illness, arrested or incomplete development of mind, psychopathic disorder and any other disorder or disability of the mind.' This may well include those with cognitive impairments as a result of a head injury. If the Court concludes, on considering medical evidence provided to it in a standard form, that the patient is incapable of managing his affairs (and if his property totals more than £5,000) it will sanction the appointment of a Receiver to manage the estate in accordance with strict rules that it sets down.

To involve the Court, there must be an application to it, which is normally made by the nearest relative of the patient, who is also usually the proposed Receiver. If the nearest relative is unable or unwilling to apply, another relative or friend or a professional, such as a solicitor, can apply, provided that notice is given to all closer relatives who have been 'overlooked'. The application must include a detailed certificate (which can be obtained direct from the Court) setting out the patient's immediate family and his property. If the proposed Receiver is of advanced age or resident outside England and Wales the Court will tend not to appoint him or her and generally joint Receivers are not appointed.

On receipt of the papers the Court will normally set a date, about four weeks later, on which the appointment will be considered. When approval is given, the Court issues an Order and any supplementary directions as to the management of the patient's estate. If the patient recovers the ability to manage his affairs the Receiver can stand down, following an application to the Court.

The Receiver is entitled to expenses incurred in the exercise of his duties, but not to remuneration, unless the Court directs otherwise. Annual accounts are submitted to the Court and unusual items of expenditure have to be cleared in advance. The Receiver has to give security to the Court to guard himself against claims of any fraud or negligence, usually by a 'fidelity guarantee bond', which is an insurance policy based on the value of the estate. Necessary amounts to 'maintain' the patient (that is, pay for his upkeep) will be agreed by the Court. The Court of Protection can allow legal costs to be met from the patient's estate and levies an annual fee based on the patient's income.

Relationship issues

Unfortunately, severe brain injury of any type can place a great strain on the client's relationship. It is important to note that the law in England and Wales does not treat married and unmarried couples equally at the time that a relationship breaks down, even if children are involved. The label 'common-law spouse', whilst appearing regularly in the media, in fact has had no meaning in English law since the 18th Century.

Where a marriage has broken down, the spouse who files for divorce (the petitioner) only needs to establish that the relationship has irretrievably broken down, even if the other person does not want a divorce. To get a divorce without waiting for up to five years the petitioner must assert that the other person has behaved unreasonably. It is largely a subjective test and therefore the behaviour alleged can be as a result of a change in personality caused by a head injury.

As part of the divorce, the Court has the power to intervene and resolve any outstanding financial issues, dealing with the question of whether maintenance should be paid by one spouse to the other (and how much) and also with the appropriate division of the family home and other assets. In doing this the Court will take into account all the relevant circumstances, including the impact of the brain injury. If clients have received, or are likely to receive, significant compensation, it is essential that specialist legal advice be taken from a matrimonial lawyer with experience of handling clients who suffer from a disability and who have large assets, to ensure that their ongoing needs are not prejudiced through any divorce settlement. The solicitors' Family Law Association should be able to provide a list of local specialists.

There is no similar jurisdiction for unmarried couples, and there is no duty to pay maintenance to a former partner, even after a long-standing relationship and even if the non-brain injured party has a high income and could afford to support the injured person. Additionally, where there has been no marriage, the Court has no power to alter the ownership of a property so that, if one partner has made no financial contribution to the purchase of the family home, and the property is registered in only one name, there is no entitlement to any equity built up during the relationship. The only exception is if the 'non-owner' can prove, under complex trust law, that there was an agreement to share the equity, reached at the time the property was bought.

Maintenance may have to be considered when there are children, and depends on the non-resident parent's income. If agreement cannot be reached the Child Support Agency will need to be involved. If there is a question over where the child should live (residence) or whether the child should see someone (contact) the guiding principle is 'what is right for this particular child', taking into account all the circumstances of the case, including the medical/psychological state of the parents. Whether a brain injury suffered by a parent will be a significant factor will, naturally, depend on the extent and, more importantly, the impact it has had on the parent's behaviour and abilities. There is a presumption, however, that it is always better for a child to know and have a relationship with both parents, unless it can be shown not to be in that child's best interests.

If there are Court proceedings because of a financial issue with filing of the divorce petition, or, indeed if there is a compensation claim, the Court will ensure that, if the brain-injured person does not have the necessary mental capacity to represent himself (that is, he is not able to manage his own affairs), a 'litigation friend' is appointed to represent him. This litigation friend must confirm to the Court that the person has a disability and that there is no legal conflict that might prevent him acting as friend. The friend may be a relative, a professional person or the Official Solicitor (who acts through his staff).

The Official Solicitor is appointed by the Lord Chancellor to look after the interests of those involved in some form of litigation who cannot, for whatever reason, look after their own affairs. If rehabilitation staff are working with someone whom they believe to be involved in litigation, but who is unable to cope with it because of their injury, they can approach the Official Solicitor, whose office will investigate and take appropriate steps. This referral does not have to be through a solicitor.

Criminal proceedings

Most rehabilitation centres specializing in head injury will have clients involved with criminal proceedings at some time. Individuals who have a head injury may be detained on suspicion of committing a crime. If they have committed an offence it may be related to their injury - for example, an assault may be due to disinhibition and lack of anger control - or unrelated to any effects of the head injury. There may also be clients who were injured at the time of the criminal offence - either as an innocent victim or who may themselves be subject to criminal proceedings. Whatever the nature of the suspected crime or possible contributory factors, in the first instance individuals need to be aware of their rights following arrest.

Any person, regardless of means, is entitled to free legal advice whilst at a police station - whether arrested or attending voluntarily. The duty solicitor can be requested if the individual does not know a named solicitor, and it is the solicitor's role to advance and protect the rights of the detained person. If a custody officer is told or suspects that a person is not able to understand questions put to him, for any reason, including head injury, extra rights and protections come into effect. Most importantly, the custody officer should contact an appropriate adult.

An appropriate adult can be a relative, guardian, person experienced with dealing with people deemed to be mentally incapable (such as cognitively impaired people), or a social worker. He or she assists and advises the individual and can exercise the right to legal advice, even if the head-injured person has refused it. The police must repeat the detained person's rights in the presence of this adult, and consent for any processes (such as a search or samples) is only valid if given in that adult's presence. However, there is no duty of confidentiality as is the case with a solicitor, so an admission of guilt made, for example, to a social worker in this role may be passed on to the police.

The solicitor will advise on the best approach to take in interviews and monitor behaviour, requesting breaks or further consultations when appropriate. He or she may request a full psychiatric, neurological or other appropriate examination if there are concerns regarding the person's fitness to be detained. Rehabilitation staff may be able to tell the solicitor which of these would be most appropriate. If the brain injury is very severe and the client lacks any insight, it is unlikely that he would be charged.

If the individual is charged with an offence, he should contact a solicitor as soon as possible. This does not need to be the same solicitor who represented him at interview. The solicitor can apply for legal aid, but if the accused person will be dealt with in a Magistrate's Court there is no guarantee that such aid will be granted – it has to be seen to be 'in the interests of justice' and the decision will take into account considerations such as whether the person is able to understand what is happening in court, among others. In a Crown Court the accused person may have to make a contribution towards costs, depending on their financial circumstances.

The solicitor will advise on any defences and can also put forward mitigating factors that might influence sentencing. This may include the effects of any head injury.

Fitness to plead is an important issue to consider when head-injured clients are charged. If this is a possible factor the solicitor should instruct a psychiatrist or other expert to assess whether the individual can follow the evidence, give evidence or give instructions. If deemed unable to plead, it will affect the way in which the Court deals with the person.

Driving after a head injury

An issue that is often of great concern to clients is their ability to drive after a head injury. It is increasingly rare for adults not to be able to drive and many people depend on the car to maintain their lifestyle – for example, many people do jobs that require driving skills or would be unable to reach work unless they had access to a car. Despite government attempts to encourage use of public transport, it is a fact at present that the public services are not efficient and frequent enough to meet people's needs. This is especially true in rural areas. Undoubtedly the ability to drive will be a factor in rehabilitation as it will enable some clients to access facilities and services in the wider community. Those who cannot drive will be more restricted. However, the overriding concern, of course, is that only those who can drive safely should be allowed to drive.

Whether an individual can drive after having had a head injury is a common question put to all members of the rehabilitation team. In some cases it becomes apparent that clients are asking many different people the same question, in order to try to find a professional who will 'allow' them to resume driving.

It seems obvious that the cognitive, behavioural and other issues that can arise after head injury could affect the ability of individuals to return to driving. Problems with decision making, attention and in other respects have been identified amongst people who had returned to driving after brain injury (Lundqvist and Ronnberg, 2001). Hawley (2001) wrote that 'poor judgement and impulsivity must be major sources of risk, with physical problems playing only a minor role'. In Hawley's paper, he looked at samples of people who had and had not returned to driving after head injury. Those who had were as a group more independent (measured by FIM/FAM scores) and had less severe injury (although 56.2% were still deemed to have had severe injury). However *both* groups, and their families, reported problems with anger, aggression, irritability, memory, concentration and vision.

Only 10.8% of those driving before the injury had actually been banned by the DVLA and most of these cases were due to epilepsy. Another 5.3% were advised by a clinician not to drive. However, the large majority had had no advice regarding return to driving, particularly if they had made a good physical recovery.

Occasionally it is obvious whether a client is or is not safe to drive, but in the majority of cases there will be some doubt. It is important that correct advice is offered to clients and that members of the team include the ability to drive in their discussions, to ensure that a consistent approach is taken. This chapter offers a brief summary of the guidelines suggested by the Driver and Vehicle Licensing Agency (DVLA), but readers should refer to the fuller reference (DVLA, 2001) for more detail. It is worth noting that in many countries patients with brain injury are required to have a medical examination before a driver's licence can be renewed (Van Zomeren, Brouwer and Minderhoud, 1987).

Fitness to drive

In the UK, the Secretary of State for Transport has the responsibility, via his or her medical advisors, to ensure that all licence holders are fit to drive. In relation to fitness to drive there are three categories of disability.

Prescribed disability is a legal bar to holding a licence unless certain specified conditions are met. An example of this would be epilepsy, where there are strict conditions in relation to length of time since a fit. The conditions are clearly set out in the DVLA guide for medical practitioners.

The second category is 'relevant disability' which covers any medical condition likely to render the person a source of danger whilst driving, such as a visual field defect.

Finally there is prospective disability, which relates to medical conditions that are intermittent or progressive and therefore may cause the driver at some time to have a prescribed or relevant disability. Licences in this group of people are held subject to medical review at agreed intervals – an example would be diabetes.

The DVLA guidelines list medical conditions and recommendations in relation to fitness to drive. In the case of serious head injury, for instance, the recommendation is that the client takes six to 12 months off driving if consciousness was lost but there were no complications such as intracranial haematoma. The client may then resume driving without notifying the DVLA. However, persistent behaviour disorder due to head injury (or another cause) means the DVLA must be informed and medical reports will determine fitness to drive. Similarly, impairment of cognitive function may mean reports and assessment are necessary. Epilepsy, visual field defects and other possible sequelae of head injury will all be factors. There is no single marker after head injury that can categorically lead to a decision about fitness to drive, and all cases will need to be considered individually.

Responsibilities

It is the legal obligation of the licence holder to notify the DVLA of any medical condition either at the time of application or at any time subsequently if a condition develops. This is stated on the driving licence. Obviously there will be some people who, after head injury, are unable personally to inform the DVLA, but there may also be those who do not want to inform them because they are frightened that they will not be able to regain their licence. Some will believe themselves able to drive, even when advised against it by rehabilitation staff, whereas others may realize they cannot drive yet but expect to achieve sufficient recovery to drive in the future.

The DVLA guidelines for medical practitioners state that the client must be advised and given an explanation for why he should inform the DVLA, and if the client is unable to understand the practitioner should immediately inform the DVLA herself.

If the client does not accept the medical opinion then a second opinion should be offered, but the client should be advised not to drive until that is obtained.

It is common to find that clients have continued to drive despite not being considered fit to do so. In such cases, the medical practitioner is advised to make every reasonable effort to persuade them to stop – which may include telling their next of kin. It can help, to convince someone not to drive, to point out that insurance cover may be invalid if they have not complied with DVLA rules. If all else fails a doctor may choose to disclose relevant medical information in confidence to the medical advisor at the DVLA. Before giving the information, however, the practitioner must inform the client and subsequently write to confirm a disclosure has been made.

On receipt of all the relevant information, the DVLA medical advisor decides whether to issue, revoke or refuse a licence. The client must then contact the drivers' medical unit at the DVLA if he wants to discuss or challenge the decision.

Assessment of driving ability

Guidelines about the assessment of skills necessary for driving, together with suggestions about retraining driving skills, are provided by Brouwer and Withaar (1997).

In addition to medical and neuropsychological information it is usually best to 'test' the individual's ability to drive. There are centres across the country which offer driving assessments to disabled people and it may well be valuable to suggest this to clients if there is some doubt over their ability. However, this involves a cost to the client and there are some who feel the expense is too great. In addition, Van Zomeren et al. (1988) question whether these assessments do adequately assess the higher cognitive levels required in driving. The difficulties of identifying measures of cognitive function which can reliably predict fitness to drive are discussed by Christie et al. (2001).

Drivers whose licences have been revoked on health grounds are unable to regain their right to drive until they are no longer considered to have a relevant disability. In some cases this cannot be done purely on the basis of medical information. Until recently the assessment centres were only able to evaluate abilities, such as reaction time in off-the-road situations as no one is allowed to drive on-road without a valid licence. It is much more useful, however, to be able to see how an individual copes with 'real' (that is, on-road) situations.

To circumvent this problem, new regulations, which came into force on 1 January 2001, allow for a 'disability assessment licence', which covers the driver for such an assessment. The decision whether to allocate such a licence lies with the DVLA's medical advisor. The person conducting the assessment must be an examiner who has been appointed by the Secretary of State for that purpose. This new licence allows for a period of retraining if deemed necessary and is valid for 12 months, but ceases to be valid once the assessment has taken place. Entitlement to drive can be reinstated if a further period of practice and assessment is thought appropriate. The assessment result will lead to reinstatement of a full licence or refusal of a licence.

If no formal assessment is required and there are any concerns about a client who has been given permission to drive again, then it is sensible to encourage him to do a few sessions with a driving instructor to re-establish his confidence and check he can cope. Many driving schools are familiar with requests of this sort and will provide an appropriate service.

Long-term support

Hawley (2001) recommends that all clients be informed by the rehabilitation team of their entitlement to drive after a head injury. To ensure this it would seem sensible to agree within the team whose responsibility this will be, and to establish a policy and procedures appropriately.

Many clients become quite agitated about returning to driving and can be very persistent in their demands for an answer from therapists or other team members. It is therefore often helpful to emphasize to the client that this is a DVLA decision.

If clients are told that they can no longer drive it may be very distressing. It is likely that it will affect their ability to resume various activities that they enjoyed before and it will affect their independence. There may be enforced role changes within relationships as a result and these may cause friction. Consideration of the ability to drive is not traditionally part of any particular discipline's brief, but the team does need to recognize the possible ramifications of the loss of this activity. As well as considering the practical difficulties, team members must respond sensitively to the emotional response of the client.

Many clients have their driving licence reinstated, perhaps after a good report from one of the driving assessment centres. Nevertheless it is not uncommon for therapists to have some concern about the client's safety, because of evident cognitive problems or sometimes because worries are expressed by family members. Driving is an 'overlearned' skill and therefore many people with cognitive impairments can nevertheless drive competently. An element of risk arises when they have to react quickly to unexpected or complex situations, which inevitably arise from time to time when driving. Many clients report changes in their driving habits and the key precautions that are likely to enhance safety after brain injury are: not to drive too fast; to avoid fatigue by not driving long distances or for long periods of time without a break; to avoid driving at night as this seems to place greater demands on concentration.

References

Brouwer WH, Withaar FK (1997) Fitness to drive after traumatic brain injury. Neuropsychological Rehabilitation 7: 177–93.

Christie N, Savill T, Buttress S, Newby G, Tyerman A (2001) Assessing fitness to drive after head injury: a survey of clinical psychologists. Neuropsychological Rehabilitation 11: 45–55.

DVLA (2001) At a Glance Guide to the Current Medical Standards of Fitness to Drive. Swansea: DVLA.

Hawley CA (2001) Return to driving after head injury. Journal of Neurology, Neurosurgery and Psychiatry 70: 761–6.

Lundqvist A, Ronnberg J (2001) Driving problems and adaptive driving behaviour after brain injury: a qualitative assessment. Neuropsychological Rehabilitation 11: 171–85.

Van Zomeren AH, Brouwer WH, Minderhoud JM (1987) Acquired brain damage and driving: a review. Arch Phys Med Rehab 68: 697–705.

Van Zomeren AH, Brouwer WH, Rothengatter JA, Snoek JW (1988) Fitness to drive a car after recovery after severe head injury. Arch Phys Med Rehab 69: 90–6.

CHAPTER 11

Conclusions and future trends

ROGER JOHNSON

Brain injury rehabilitation is a neglected service. It might be hoped that this will change in the near future. The House of Commons Select Committee Report (Great Britain, 2001) highlighted the urgent need for improvement in rehabilitation services for head-injured people. They advocate that acute hospitals should be responsible for setting up managers to coordinate brain injury services, and that they should identify care pathways that ensure that the needs of people with head injury are met after discharge. They suggest there should be managers with responsibility for rehabilitation services and they recommend a case management system. They state that 'it may also be necessary to increase capacity of specialised staff.' The latter suggestion may be the more important. Greenwood et al. (1994) concluded that case management was no substitute for developing skilled and specialist rehabilitation services. The House of Commons Select Committee Report also recommended extra resources should be made available where necessary to set up specialist, post acute, inpatient rehabilitation facilities. They identified a lack of community support and continued rehabilitation after discharge as the greatest problem area. They recommended that Health Authorities be 'required to provide rehabilitation in the community'.

Given the limited rehabilitation services that already exist it would clearly involve considerable investment to bring services up to standards in line withthese recommendations. Additional funding is likely to remain a problem. The National Service Framework for neurological conditions, to which proposals for head injury rehabilitation are to be linked, is not due for implementation until 2004 (Frontline, 2001).

Nor does history give grounds for optimism. The lack of resources and shortage of people with expertise and experience in brain injury rehabilitation has been stated many times in the past (Lewin, 1959, 1970; Lancet, 1982; Gloag, 1985). In 1988 a Medical Disability Society report said: 'The rehabilitation of people with brain injury is very unsatisfactory in most British hospitals.' Ten years later an updated report from the society (now called the British Society for Rehabilitation Medicine) stated that rehabilitation needed to be given greater priority and observed that some health authorities had failed to establish any specialist rehabilitation in their district (British Society of Rehabilitation Medicine, 1998).

The Royal College of Surgeons (1999) stated that all those attending hospital with head injury should be followed up. At present, this does not happen. This is no doubt in part because of the very large number of patients who attend an accident and emergency department with a minor head injury but are not admitted. A majority will quickly recover and the difficulty is to identify those who may not do so well. However, some of those who are admitted to hospital and have a severe head injury have little or no follow-up too. Paradoxically this is at a time when the technology and neurosurgical skills available to ensure their survival are at an unprecedented level of development. Once the acute and immediate post-acute care are completed patients may be discharged home with little or no follow-up and no further therapy (McMillan et al., 1988). In some areas this is because there is no service available but, more worryingly, it is common, even where there is a brain injury rehabilitation service, for patients not to be referred to it. These days this can be because of the pressure of hospital waiting lists so that patients are discharged from acute care very early and without time to organize adequate follow-up plans. Alternatively, it may be because they have made a good physical recovery and there are no resources or time to identify the less evident but perhaps serious neuropsychological or behavioural consequences of the injury. There may be undue optimism that patients are well on their way to a full recovery.

This problem is not new – attention was drawn to the need for better screening and assessment facilities for those with head injury, and the importance of routine and expert follow-up, by the Medical Disability Society report in 1988. This recommended that outpatient clinics should have a core team of medical staff, psychologist and social worker, which must work in co-operation with others such as nurses, therapists and teachers. What is surprising is that in many areas there has been no progress in developments of this kind and, at least in some areas, the opportunities for rehabilitation may have declined despite apparent increases in therapy posts (Nocon and Baldwin, 1998). The Royal College of Surgeons report (1999) drew attention to the fact that in many hospitals general or orthopaedic surgeons are responsible for head-injured patients but few have had recent or specific training in their management. Many patients are lost to follow-up.

Rehabilitation services are familiar with the client who is referred for the first time one or even two years or more after injury. Typically, their history is of discharge home following acute care and being left to make their own plans about return to work. They lose their jobs and fail in subsequent attempts to work, their family and social life fall apart and the symptoms due to head injury become entangled with problems of depression, anxiety and loss of confidence. Clients such as this may have had one or two follow-up appointments early on. They have usually made a good physical recovery, and perhaps their own report is of good recovery in other respects – not least due to their lack of insight. Perhaps it is therefore not surprising that they are encouraged to return to work and are discharged. The Medical Disability Society Report of 1988 advised that a checklist system should be used 'to avoid problems being missed by junior level medical staff rotating through the department'. This was reiterated in their subsequent report (British Society of Rehabilitation Medicine, 1998). There is clearly a need for rehabilitation specialists to take a lead in developing criteria by which acute care staff can identify those clients who need to be referred on to a rehabilitation service, and in establishing the best possible links with those responsible for medical follow-up.

Probably one of the most useful criteria for predicting longer term neuropsychological problems, and hence those with a need for rehabilitation intervention, is duration of post-traumatic amnesia (PTA). There is some controversy about it (McMillan, Robertson and Wilson, 1996; Ahmed et al., 2000) and clinically it has rather fallen into disuse in many areas, or it is widely misunderstood. Although it is not always easy to identify exactly, the research literature, starting with Cairns in 1942, gives useful predictions. Anyone with a PTA of a few days or more should be properly assessed, at least from a neuropsychological point of view. Once the duration of PTA is of one to two weeks, long-term problems are likely (Tate, 1987) and will affect (but not necessarily preclude) return to work. These people have an essential need for assessment by the rehabilitation team and should be provided with advice and, where necessary, therapy or other intervention. If PTA has lasted for more than two weeks then persisting cognitive and behavioural disability will follow (Brooks et al., 1987), and rehabilitation and support will be needed in the longer term. These and other criteria need to be developed by rehabilitation teams and communicated to those responsible for medical follow-up, and in other areas of head-injury management. This might reduce the number of head-injured clients who are either never referred to rehabilitation services or else only after they have run into significant practical problems.

Better links between rehabilitation and primary care also need to be developed, particularly in the context of a community rehabilitation service. Once the patient is discharged from hospital the general practitioner often finds himself in the key role of advising the patient and judging the need to refer back to medical or rehabilitation specialists (Royal College of Surgeons,

1999). The difficulty for GPs is that, in a working life, on average, each will see only about two people severely disabled by head injury (British Society for Rehabilitation Medicine, 1998) and most therefore have rather little experience of managing their complex problems. The need for better education opportunities about head injuries for GPs was highlighted by the Government Select Committee (Great Britain, 2001).

The majority of people with severe head injury make rapid progress from the point of view of their medical problems and the physical injuries they may have. Their principal problems, and those that will prove most persistent, will be neuropsychological and behavioural. Within a few weeks a majority are fit enough to be at home. Most of them will not only prefer to be at home but often, with appropriate management and advice, they can benefit from an early return, as far as possible, to their normal environment and circumstances. The danger for them is that the problems they still have as a result of their head injury have the potential to disrupt their social, leisure and domestic activities and can have a profound impact on their ability to work. Moreover, both they and their families will often have a poor understanding of the effects of their injury and many clients will have defective insight as a direct consequence of brain injury. If left to their own devices, they will be vulnerable to taking on too much too soon and to other misjudgements.

The chapters of this book have described the difficulties these people face and the many different facets of head-injury rehabilitation. Head-injured people have complex and diverse needs and a multidisciplinary approach is essential, together with good networks with other agencies and resources. Rehabilitation over an extended period of time is also essential because of the slow and protracted recovery after head injury and because some problems, such as employment and social difficulties, or expression of behaviour problems, may only emerge late on in the course of recovery. The expertise needed within the multidisciplinary team cannot be overestimated. Too often services are set up with inadequate funding and economies are made in the level of experience and training of the staff. Head injury rehabilitation is too complex for this to be a sensible strategy. Rehabilitation professionals working in the field of head injury must be adequately trained (Royal College of Surgeons, 1999). Most rehabilitationists have a general training in their professional area and encounter few opportunities for specialist teaching about the rehabilitation of head injury. It is to be hoped that the respective professional bodies, or the special interest groups who already promote training courses, will give priority to improving this situation in the future.

It is my view that a community service is the key to successful rehabilitation for the majority of people after head injury. It is a relatively new model of service delivery but one that should become more widely available.

Community rehabilitation may be particularly relevant for rural areas, such as Suffolk, where the head-injured population is widely dispersed, but many of the advantages of community rehabilitation programmes are equally relevant in urban areas. In particular the scope for *in vivo* training is important as it provides the best learning environment for those with brain injury, and the best approach to circumventing the problems with insight that commonly follow head injury. Community rehabilitation is also able to provide continuity of support for a long period and modify that support according to the client's changing needs over the two years or more during which recovery and the gradual process of adaptation may take place. Head-injured people do not pursue their rehabilitation in isolation and community rehabilitation is well placed to involve families, work colleagues and employers, and to meet their needs too. Moreover, compared to inpatient rehabilitation, it is a low-cost service in which resources can be focused on therapy staff without also having to provide for the accommodation and care of the clients.

Research should be supported or pursued by a head-injury rehabilitation team. This book demonstrates the large body of knowledge about the nature of head injury disability and rehabilitation that has been built up – particularly over the past 20 to 30 years. Nevertheless, major gaps are evident. The greatest of these is the very poor knowledge we have of the nature of recovery after brain injury and exactly what factors and therapies might aid this process. There remains a great need for more effective outcome measures and ways of demonstrating more clearly the elements of therapy that are beneficial. At present, there are perhaps only two certainties about recovery from head injury. First, it is largely a natural process, due to gradual resolution of oedema, for example, or possibly due to some development or reorganization of connections between brain cells. A good deal of progress will occur with or without therapy. Secondly, where the brain has been damaged, this is probably permanent and therefore full recovery is not possible. It may be that future developments will lead to a better understanding of how to promote natural brain plasticity and regeneration of neurones. This may be possible under optimum conditions but at present there is little evidence that it occurs in adult humans (McMillan, Robertson and Wilson, 1999). Future progress is also likely to come from the research into 'brain repair' technologies that involve the transplant of neuronal tissue into an area of damaged brain (Barker and Dunnett, 1999). It is unlikely this will lead to the demise of rehabilitation – the initial work of this kind with animals has indicated that far from reducing the need for rehabilitation these techniques are only successful where they are accompanied by intensive programmes of retraining.

Despite the present limitations to recovery once the brain has been damaged, there is plenty of evidence that clients are able to achieve a great deal through rehabilitation that would not have been possible without specialist therapy and expert help and advice. It has been stated that there is no proof that brain injury rehabilitation is effective and methodological difficulties make it unlikely that any 'proof' will be forthcoming (Cope, 1995). However, in evaluating the benefits of rehabilitation there can be a confusion between measures of recovery – in the sense of restoration of abilities (which is largely a natural process) and measures of adaptation and functional improvement (which is largely a product of good rehabilitation). The Warwick Study (National Traumatic Brain Injury Study, 1998) suggested the benefits of rehabilitation were more clearly associated with input aimed at organizing or advising on levels of occupation and support whereas no link was found between duration of therapy interventions and outcome. Good outcome was as likely from a short, well-directed and specific intervention as from a lengthy therapy. Thus, good outcome may depend on the level of experience and skill of the therapist, who can tailor her therapy to the needs of the individual, rather than on intensive application of a prescriptive intervention.

Rehabilitation programmes may aim to improve communication or memory skills, for example, but it is notoriously difficult to discriminate between the possibility that a cognitive treatment is the cause of the progress that is observed or whether it is due to natural recovery. The important and clearer benefits of rehabilitation may be to train the client in the use of a communication aid, or to use particular compensatory strategies for memory such as a mnemonic. Moreover, advice and management plans geared to individual circumstances may avoid a disastrously early return to work, whereas a successful one may be possible later once the client's ability to handle his problems with communication or memory has progressed.

This book illustrates the skills and knowledge employed by the various disciplines but also that there is a need for specialists to develop new rehabilitation methods and to advance their knowledge of the techniques that are effective. Evaluation of therapy is essential in order to improve the service for the clients and it is evident that there are many areas in which improvements might be achieved. Trying to demonstrate the efficacy of cognitive treatments (Cicerone et al., 2000) may, in a clinical context, be tackling the wrong question. The important benefits of rehabilitation are to channel progress so that the client can capitalize on natural recovery. Avoiding the development of 'bad habits' is important, and particularly so in some areas such as where there are behaviour problems (Eames et al., 1996), in certain aspects of physical recovery – preventing the development of contractures for example – or minimizing the development of secondary symptoms of anxiety, depression or loss of confidence. Once symptoms of these kinds have become established they can be very hard to reverse.

The rehabilitation process must also help the client to understand the nature of their disabilities, the likely limitations to recovery, and the time scales involved. This ensures the development of the right aims and expectations. It has been shown that accurate expectation can be important to good outcome in other fields of recovery (for example, Rutter, 1979), but relatively little attention has been paid to it in work with head-injured people. These factors can help the client achieve as successful a level of adaptation as possible and avoid the all-too-common establishment of hopes of full recovery or unrealistic plans that ignore the implications of their disabilities. If these matters are not dealt with early on in the rehabilitation process, for clients and their families, then they become increasingly difficult to tackle successfully. It is likely that further development and research into the part that education can play in rehabilitation following head injury will lead to considerable outcome benefits. These aspects of rehabilitation are not easy to deal with and it is one of the reasons why expertise in the field of head-injury rehabilitation is so important. Unless the therapists have the experience and knowledge to make good judgements about these issues then it is, of course, impossible for them to help the client to make them. Probably one of the commonest failures in head-injury rehabilitation is misjudgement about when and how to return to work. Many people lose their jobs as a result and then fail to settle back into work at all, although there is evidence this often could have been achieved if advice or a wiser approach had been available to them to begin with.

Measures of functional outcome and level of handicap show benefits from programmes of rehabilitation that cannot be easily disputed. Yet the history of the evaluation of outcome in rehabilitation has all too often been biased by the 'medical model' of a prescribed period of treatment and efforts to demonstrate reduced impairment as a result. The difficulty in obtaining good evidence of this sort sometimes results in the benefits of investment in rehabilitation being underestimated – not least by those who hold budgets in the health services and other statutory bodies.

Measurement of outcome and the benefits of intervention are perhaps particularly difficult to establish in the context of community rehabilitation because individually tailored programmes, and the range of problems and contexts in which the client may be seen, do not lend themselves to conventionally designed studies. Ironically, the fact that services can be so poor in some areas and relatively well-developed in others provides an opportunity for comparative studies that could be exploited along the lines suggested by High, Boake and Lehmkuhl (1995).

Clearly comparison of 'good' and 'bad' areas in terms of return-to-work rates, levels of stress amongst relatives, or number of visits by clients to their GPs, for example, could provide useful insights into service benefits. There is a responsibility on the part of therapists and others working in the field of rehabilitation to evaluate the interventions they devise and seek to improve understanding of the rehabilitation process. Advances in this respect are needed, not least in order to be able to argue more powerfully for the much-needed investment in the development of rehabilitation services for people with head injury.

References

Ahmed S, Bierley R, Sheikh JI, Date ES (2000) Post-traumatic amnesia after closed head injury: a review of the literature and some suggestions for further research. Brain Injury 14: 765–80.

Barker RA, Dunnett SB (1999) Neural repair, transplantation and rehabilitation. Psychology Press: Hove.

British Society of Rehabilitation Medicine (1998) Working Party Report: Rehabilitation after Traumatic Brain injury. London: BSRM.

Brooks N, McKinley W, Symington C, Beattie A, Campsie L (1987) Return to work within the first seven years of severe head injury. Brain Injury 1: 5–19.

Cairns H (1942) Discussion on rehabilitation after injuries to the central nervous system. Proceedings of the Royal Society of Medicine 35: 299–302.

Cicerone KD, Dahlberg C, Kalmar K, Langenbahn DM, Malec JF, Berquist TF, Felicitti T, Giacino JT, Harley JP, Harrington DE, Herzog J, Kneipp S, Laatsch L, Morse PA (2000) Evidence-based cognitive rehabilitation: recommendations for clinical practice. Archives of Physical Medicine and Rehabilitation 81: 1596–615.

Cope DN (1995) The effectiveness of traumatic brain injury rehabilitation: a review. Brain Injury 9: 649–70.

Eames P, Cotterill G, Kneale TA, Storrar AL, Yeomans P (1996) Outcome of intensive rehabilitation after severe brain injury: a long term follow up study. Brain Injury 10: 631–50.

Frontline (2001) Head injury rehabilitation reforms are delayed. Frontline (August 1): .9.

Gloag D (1985) Rehabilitation after head injury: 2. Behaviour and emotional problems, long term needs, and the requirements for services. British Medical Journal 290: 913–16.

Great Britain (2001) House of Commons Select Committee Report. Third Report. Health Committee. Head Injury: Rehabilitation. London: HMSO.

Greenwood RJ, McMillan TM, Brooks DN, Dunn G, Brock D, Dinsdale S, Murphy LD, Price JR (1994) Effects of case management after severe brain injury. British Medical Journal 308: 1199–205.

High WM, Boake C, Lehmkuhl LD (1995) Critical analysis of studies evaluating the effectiveness of rehabilitation after traumatic brain injury. Journal of Head Trauma Rehabilitation 10: 14–26.

Lancet (1982) Rehabilitation. Research aspects of rehabilitation after acute brain damage in adults. Report of a co-ordinating group. The Lancet ii, 1034–1036.

Lewin W (1959) Planning for head injuries. British Medical Journal 1: 131–4.

Lewin W (1970) Rehabilitation needs of the brain injured patient. Proceedings of the Royal Society of Medicine 63: 28–32.

McMillan TM, Greenwood RJ, Morris JR, Brooks N, Murphy L, Dunn G (1988) An introduction to the concept of case management with respect to the need for service proviosion. Clinical Rehabilitation 2: 319–22.

McMillan TM. Jongen TL. Greenwood RJ. (1996). Assessment of post-traumatic amnesia after severe closed head injury: retrospective or prospective? Journal of Neurology, Neurosurgery and Psychiatry 60: 422–7.

McMillan TM, Robertson IH, Wilson BA (1999) Neurogenesis after brain injury: implications for neurorehabilitation. Neuropsychological Rehabilitation 9: 129–33.

Medical Disability Society (1988) Report of the working party on the management of traumatic brain injury. London: The Development Trust for the Young Disabled on behalf of the Medical Disability Society.

National Traumatic Brain Injury Study (1998) Report of the National Brain Injury Study. Coventry: University of Warwick.

Nocon A, Baldwin S (1998) Trends in rehabilitation policy: a review of the literature. London: Kings Fund, Audit Commission.

Royal College of Surgeons of England (1999) Report of the Working Party on the Management of Patients with Head Injuries. London: Royal College of Surgeons.

Rutter BM (1979) The prognostic significance of psychological factors in the management of chronic bronchitis. Psychological Medicine 9: 63–70.

Tate RL (1987) Issues in the management of behaviour disturbance as a consequence of severe head injury. Scandanavian Journal of Rehabilitation Medicine 19: 13–18.

Index

acute management 50-3
adjustment to disability 18-9, 270, 273, 281, 328
akinesia 167
aggression 161-3, 166, 175, 178
agnosia 141, 143-4
alcohol *see* substance abuse
anger management 182-5, 196
anosognosia 90,143
anxiety 164, 166-7, 230, 278-81
apathy 43, 102, 161, 163, 167-8, 278, 280
aphasia *see* dysphasia
apraxia *see* dyspraxia
articulatory dyspraxia 218
assessment 28, 114-9
   behaviour problems 173-8, 198-9
   cognitive problems 90-1, 118-21, 136, 140, 145, 221-3
   driving 319-20
   employment 249-51
   language problems 218-26
   physical problems 76, 84, 89, 94-8, 106
   psychosocial problems 281-3, 296-7, 306
   rating scales 77, 97-8, 146, 177-81, 224-5, 237, 282-3
   self-rating scales 116, 146, 147-8, 282, 297, 306
   swallowing 103
asteriognosis 89, 141, 155
ataxia 74-6, 217
attention disorders 113, 177-8, 125-8, 148-9, 213-4, 220, 229, 245, 255
axonal injury 45

behavioural disorders 43, 159
   behaviour modification 187-93
   definition 163
   environmental factors 185-6
   return to work 248
   self control strategies 193-7
   special units 180, 187-9, 201
   treatment 181-97
body-scheme disorders *see* somatosog-nosia
brain repair 326
brain swelling 47

cardiovascular fitness 87-8, 94
carers 6, 10, 24-5, 27, 66, 104-5, 115-6, 128, 173, 177, 181, 194, 226, 234-6, 282, 291
case management 21-2, 322
cerebellar ataxia *see* ataxia
cognitive communication disorder 210-2, 213-5
cognitive impairment 112, 164, 245-6, 247-8, 249, 294-5
cognitive rehabilitation 123-5, 127-8, 131-5, 137-9, 144, 229-30, 327
community rehabilitation 14, 27-32, 189, 325-6
compensation claims 9, 21, 310-4
compensatory strategies 18, 27, 29, 100
   cognitive 124, 128, 133-5, 138-9, 144, 148-55, 232
   communication 231-2
   physical 75-6
confidentiality 24, 305

331